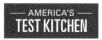

ALSO BY THE EDITORS AT AMERICA'S TEST KITCHEN

100 Recipes: The Absolute Best Ways to Make the True Essentials

The New Family Cookbook

Kitchen Hacks

The Complete Vegetarian Cookbook

The Complete Cooking for Two Cookbook

The Cook's Illustrated Meat Book

The Cook's Illustrated Baking Book

The Cook's Illustrated Cookbook

The Science of Good Cooking

Pressure Cooker Perfection

The America's Test Kitchen Cooking School Cookbook

The America's Test Kitchen Menu Cookbook

The America's Test Kitchen Quick Family Cookbook

The America's Test Kitchen Healthy Family Cookbook

The America's Test Kitchen Family Baking Book

THE AMERICA'S TEST KITCHEN LIBRARY SERIES

The Best Mexican Recipes

The Make-Ahead Cook

The How Can It Be Gluten-Free Cookbook: Volume 2

The How Can It Be Gluten-Free Cookbook

Healthy Slow Cooker Revolution

Slow Cooker Revolution Volume 2: The Easy-Prep Edition

Slow Cooker Revolution

The Six-Ingredient Solution

Comfort Food Makeovers

The America's Test Kitchen D.I.Y. Cookbook

Pasta Revolution

Simple Weeknight Favorites

The Best Simple Recipes

THE TV COMPANION SERIES

The Complete Cook's Country TV Show Cookbook

The Complete America's Test Kitchen TV Show Cookbook 2001–2016

America's Test Kitchen: The TV Companion Cookbook (2009 and 2011–2015 Editions)

Behind the Scenes with America's Test Kitchen

Test Kitchen Favorites

Cooking at Home with America's Test Kitchen

America's Test Kitchen Live!

Inside America's Test Kitchen

Here in America's Test Kitchen

The America's Test Kitchen Cookbook

AMERICA'S TEST KITCHEN ANNUALS

The Best of America's Test Kitchen (2007–2016 Editions)

Cooking for Two (2010–2013 Editions)

Light & Healthy (2010–2012 Editions)

THE COOK'S COUNTRY SERIES

Cook's Country Eats Local

From Our Grandmothers' Kitchens

Cook's Country Blue Ribbon Desserts

Cook's Country Best Potluck Recipes

Cook's Country Best Lost Suppers

Cook's Country Best Grilling Recipes

The Cook's Country Cookbook

America's Best Lost Recipes

THE BEST RECIPE SERIES

The New Best Recipe

More Best Recipes

The Best One-Dish Suppers

Soups, Stews & Chilis

The Best Skillet Recipes

The Best Slow & Easy Recipes

The Best Chicken Recipes

The Best International Recipe

The Best 30-Minute Recipe

The Best Light Recipe

The Cook's Illustrated Guide to Grilling and Barbecue

Best American Side Dishes

Cover & Bake

Italian Classics

American Classics

FOR A FULL LISTING OF ALL OUR BOOKS

CooksIllustrated.com

AmericasTestKitchen.com

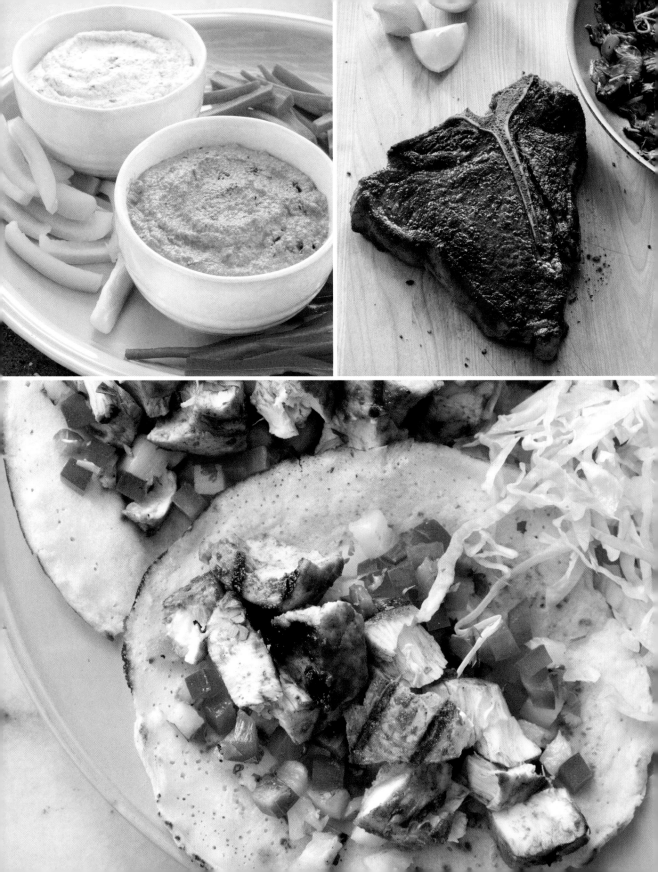

PALEO
PERFECTED

A REVOLUTION IN EATING WELL
WITH 150 KITCHEN-TESTED RECIPES

BY THE EDITORS AT
America's Test Kitchen

AMERICA'S TEST KITCHEN
17 Station Street, Brookline, MA 02445

Library of Congress Cataloging-in-Publication Data

Paleo perfected : a revolution in eating well with 150 kitchen-tested recipes / by the editors at America's Test Kitchen.

pages cm

Includes index.

ISBN 978-1-940352-42-8

1. Cooking (Natural foods) 2. High-protein diet--Recipes. 3. Prehistoric peoples--Nutrition. I. America's Test Kitchen (Firm)

TX741.P35 2016

641.3'02--dc23

2015029865

Manufactured in the United States of America

10 9 8 7 6 5 4 3 2 1

Paperback: US $26.95 / $29.95 CAN

Distributed by:

Penguin Random House Publisher Services

tel: 800-733-3000

EDITORIAL DIRECTOR: Jack Bishop

EDITORIAL DIRECTOR, BOOKS: Elizabeth Carduff

EXECUTIVE FOOD EDITOR: Julia Collin Davison

SENIOR EDITOR: Dan Zuccarello

ASSOCIATE EDITORS: Danielle DeSiato, Melissa Herrick, Sebastian Nava, and Russell Selander

EDITORIAL ASSISTANT: Samantha Ronan

TEST COOKS: Leah Collins, Lawman Johnson, and Nicole Konstantinakos

DESIGN DIRECTOR: Greg Galvan

ART DIRECTOR: Carole Goodman

DEPUTY ART DIRECTOR: Taylor Argenzio

DESIGNER: Jen Kanavos Hoffman

PHOTOGRAPHY DIRECTOR: Julie Cote

ASSOCIATE ART DIRECTOR, PHOTOGRAPHY: Steve Klise

STAFF PHOTOGRAPHER: Daniel J. van Ackere

ADDITIONAL PHOTOGRAPHY: Keller + Keller and Carl Tremblay

FOOD STYLING: Catrine Kelty, Marie Piraino, and Maeve Sheriden

PHOTO SHOOT KITCHEN TEAM:

   ASSOCIATE EDITOR: Chris O'Connor

   TEST COOK: Dan Cellucci

   ASSISTANT TEST COOKS: Allison Berkey and Matthew Fairman

PRODUCTION DIRECTOR: Guy Rochford

SENIOR PRODUCTION MANAGER: Jessica Quirk

PRODUCTION MANAGER: Christine Walsh

IMAGING MANAGER: Lauren Robbins

PRODUCTION AND IMAGING SPECIALISTS: Heather Dube, Sean MacDonald, Dennis Noble, and Jessica Voas

PROJECT MANAGER: Britt Dresser

COPY EDITOR: Cheryl Redmond

PROOFREADER: Christine Corcoran Cox

INDEXER: Elizabeth Parson

PICTURED ON FRONT COVER: Zucchini "Spaghetti" and Meatballs (page 165)

PICTURED OPPOSITE TITLE PAGE: Whipped Cashew Nut Dip with Roasted Red Peppers and Olives and Whipped Cashew Nut Dip with Chipotle and Lime (page 31), Tuscan-Style Steaks with Garlicky Spinach (page 157), and Grilled Fish Tacos with Pineapple Salsa (page 234)

PICTURED ON OPPOSITE PAGE: Grilled Vegetable Kebabs (page 259) and Greek Lamb Meatballs with Cauliflower Rice (page 195)

PICTURED ON BACK COVER: Tomato and Zucchini Tart (page 263), Gingery Stir-Fried Chicken with Asparagus and Bell Pepper (page 121), Almond Yogurt Parfaits (page 85), Shredded Beef Tacos with Cabbage Slaw (page 162), Ultimate Burgers (page 146), and Blueberry Pancakes (page 78)

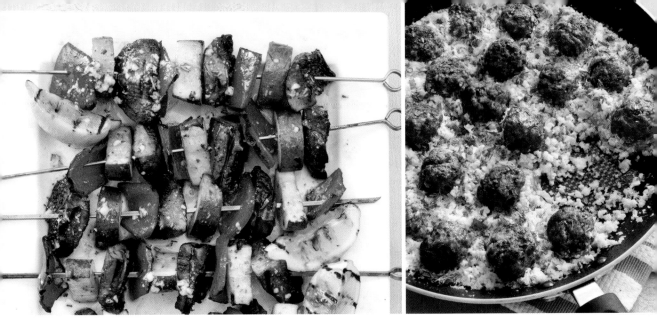

CONTENTS

This book has been tested, written, and edited by the folks at America's Test Kitchen, a very real 2,500-square-foot kitchen located just outside of Boston. It is the home of *Cook's Illustrated* magazine and *Cook's Country* magazine and is the Monday-through-Friday destination for more than four dozen test cooks, editors, food scientists, tasters, and cookware specialists. Our mission is to test recipes over and over again until we understand how and why they work and until we arrive at the "best" version.

We start the process of testing a recipe with a complete lack of conviction, which means that we accept no claim, no theory, no technique, and no recipe at face value. We simply assemble as many variations as possible, test a half-dozen of the most promising, and taste the results blind. We then construct our own hybrid recipe and continue to test it, varying ingredients, techniques, and cooking times until we reach a consensus. The result, we hope, is the best version of a particular recipe, but we realize that only you can be the final judge of our success (or failure). As we like to say in the test kitchen, "We make the mistakes, so you don't have to."

All of this would not be possible without a belief that good cooking, much like good music, is indeed based on a foundation of objective technique. Some people like spicy foods and others don't, but there is a right way to sauté, there is a best way to cook a pot roast, and there are measurable scientific principles involved in producing perfectly beaten, stable egg whites. This is our ultimate goal: to investigate the fundamental principles of cooking so that you become a better cook. It is as simple as that.

If you're curious to see what goes on behind the scenes at America's Test Kitchen, check out our daily blog, AmericasTestKitchenFeed.com, which features kitchen snapshots, exclusive recipes, video tips, and much more. You can watch us work (in our actual test kitchen) by tuning in to *America's Test Kitchen* (AmericasTestKitchen.com) or *Cook's Country from*

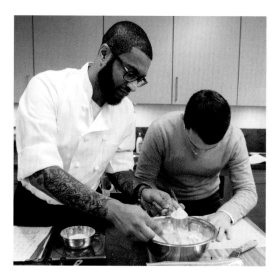

America's Test Kitchen (CooksCountryTV.com) on public television. Tune in to America's Test Kitchen Radio (AmericasTestKitchen.com) on public radio to listen to insights, tips, and techniques that illuminate the truth about real home cooking. And find information about subscribing to *Cook's Illustrated* magazine at CooksIllustrated.com or *Cook's Country* magazine at CooksCountry.com. Both magazines are published every other month. However you choose to visit us, we welcome you into our kitchen, where you can stand by our side as we test our way to the best recipes in America.

FACEBOOK.COM/AMERICASTESTKITCHEN

TWITTER.COM/TESTKITCHEN

YOUTUBE.COM/AMERICASTESTKITCHEN

INSTAGRAM.COM/TESTKITCHEN

PINTEREST.COM/TESTKITCHEN

AMERICASTESTKITCHEN.TUMBLR.COM

GOOGLE.COM/+AMERICASTESTKITCHEN

PREFACE

I once interviewed Dr. David Katz of Yale University about the paleo diet. He pointed out that hunters in the Paleolithic era often came back empty-handed or with just one or two small animals. So there goes the notion of paleo as a meat-centric approach to meal planning. Even today, scientists have visited remote tribes in the Amazon and found much the same thing about meat consumption—it is a luxury, not a staple.

Instead, the central concept of paleo is returning to an unprocessed, non-agricultural diet, one that depends less on the pantry staples we take for granted—flour, pasta, soy sauce, cornstarch, wine, vegetable oil, rice, potatoes, and commercial broths to name a few—and more on less-processed foods that are free from sugars, stabilizers, and other unwanted additives.

One might then ask, "Why America's Test Kitchen?" Well, try to make spaghetti and meatballs, fried chicken, blueberry muffins, beef stew, or granola bars without the usual ingredients. This requires heavy-duty kitchen testing to sort out what to use in place of the spaghetti (spiralized zucchini does the trick), the batter for the chicken (arrowroot and almond flours mixed with seltzer), the basic flour mixture for the muffins (almond flour, coconut flour, and arrowroot flour, with a resting time for proper hydration), the store-bought broth in the beef stew (beef bones provide meaty depth), and the oats in the granola bars (nuts and seeds work well, plus maple syrup and processed dates for both texture and sweetness).

After more than a year of kitchen work, we discovered how to use pureed vegetables as a thickener; how to make a great pan sauce without wine or butter; how to replace flour with different non-wheat flours and starches in different combinations depending on the recipe; how to make a stir-fry without most of the usual suspects, including soy sauce, sugar, and Chinese wine; and how to replace milk and cream and still get a creamy final result.

Plus we came up with recipes for a true "paleo pantry," including chicken and beef broths, mayonnaise, ketchup, barbecue sauce, mustard, and tomato sauce. You also get building block recipes for pie pastry, almond yogurt, sandwich rolls, wraps, "cheese," and almond milk. And we also found creative ways to use the slow cooker to solve many paleo recipe problems.

Look, I'm not a fad diet person but I do care deeply about what and how I eat. In fact, I often do consume a diet that is mostly paleo—I like fresh, minimally processed foods as a starting point. So the recipes in this book are, for the most part, just common-sense healthy—the type of foods that sensible healthy folks would want to cook for their family and friends.

There is an old Vermont story that reminds me of trying a newfangled diet. Fred Wilcox used to come down from the mountains into town about twice a year. One autumn, he was sideswiped by a tourist driving a car. The visitor, shaken and anxious to help, jumped out and asked if the old-timer was hurt. Fred stood up slowly, looked him in the eye, and said, "Well, it ain't done me any good!"

Unlike old Fred, we think that this natural approach to food and cooking will do you a lot of good. But, perhaps even better, the food will taste good—very good—along the way. The most important thing is to enjoy the cooking and the food. That's the best way I know to stay happy and healthy.

CHRISTOPHER KIMBALL
Founder and Editor,
Cook's Illustrated and *Cook's Country*
Host, *America's Test Kitchen* and
Cook's Country from America's Test Kitchen

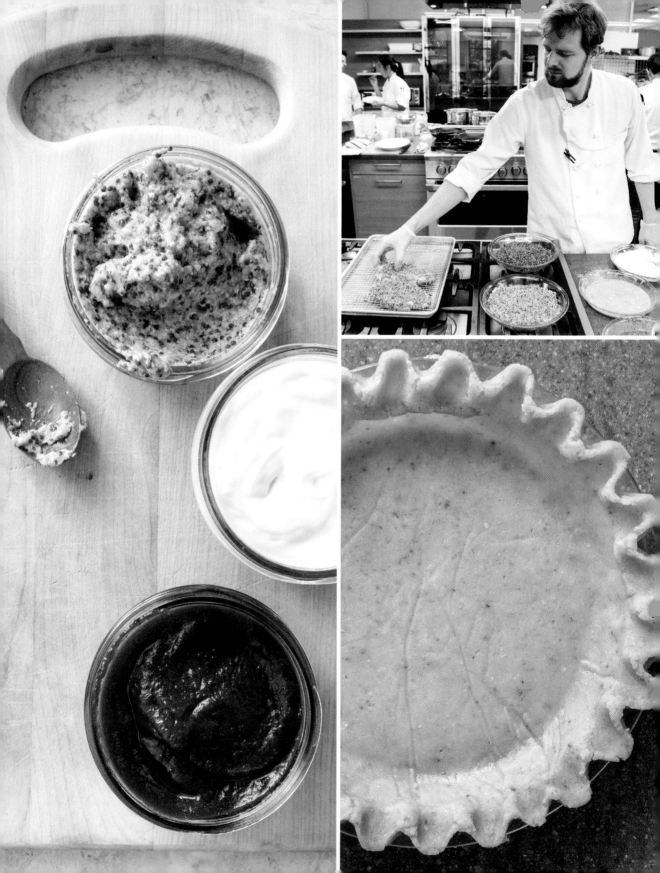

THE PALEO KITCHEN: GETTING STARTED

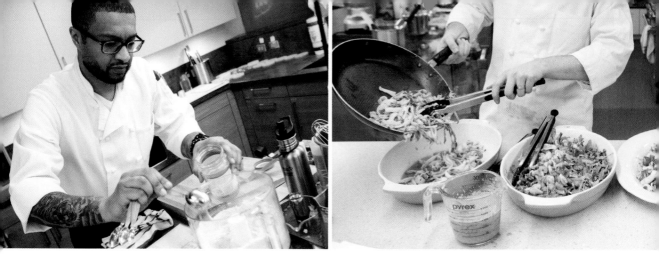

Introduction

Here in the test kitchen, we're always looking for new challenges: recipes and techniques that will test our skills and make us better, more knowledgeable cooks. And although we don't usually concern ourselves with "diets" in the traditional sense of the word, there was something about the paleo diet that intrigued us—the focus on whole foods, the emphasis on cutting out processed junk foods, and the importance of cooking at home. The widespread popularity of paleo made us think that this was more than just a trend. And as with many diet-oriented books, there seemed to be room for the test kitchen to contribute and add value.

We quickly realized that a lot of the staple ingredients that we rely on every day were off the table. Things like cornstarch, vegetable oil, soy sauce—even table salt—were out. Half the challenge of making successful paleo dishes was in coming up with replacements for these items. We still wanted pan sauces, stir-fries, and creamy dips, so to get these things right, we tested every method we could come up with.

Meat is an important part of the typical paleo diet, so we knew we would need to move beyond the standard beef, pork, and chicken. Proteins like lamb shoulder chops, duck breasts, and even venison steaks made their way onto our table of contents. (The venison recipe even inspired us to develop a rich, beautifully creamy paleo béarnaise sauce.)

But the most challenging thing we tackled in this book was paleo baking. We discovered a whole new world of flours: almond, arrowroot, coconut, and tapioca. We developed recipes for muffins, pancakes, crackers, and pie dough, each of which required dozens of rounds of testing and retesting. Sometimes, a mere teaspoon of coconut flour or ghee was the difference between good and great. Our tasters doggedly ate their way to the final version of every recipe (though it wasn't always easy), and we're confident that the results are the best they can be.

A surprising obstacle we came up against was the fluid definition of what paleo means. Our solution was to build our recipes around strict paleo guidelines. We used limited natural sweeteners, moderate amounts of nuts and seeds, and no dairy. We relied on grass-fed or pasture-raised meats, paleo-friendly tomato paste and bacon, and homemade stocks. But we also know that not everyone reading this book is going to want to follow the paleo diet to the letter. Not everyone has time to stock their pantry with homemade chicken broth and mayonnaise every week. So we made sure our recipes would also work with store-bought versions of these ingredients, and provided plenty of shopping tips.

We were constantly surprised by the challenges we faced: Recipes that we thought would be merely a matter of switching out a couple of ingredients (like stuffed mushrooms, chicken stir-fry, and crab cakes) ended up being some of the most interesting and eye-opening of all. We hope you're just as pleasantly surprised as we were.

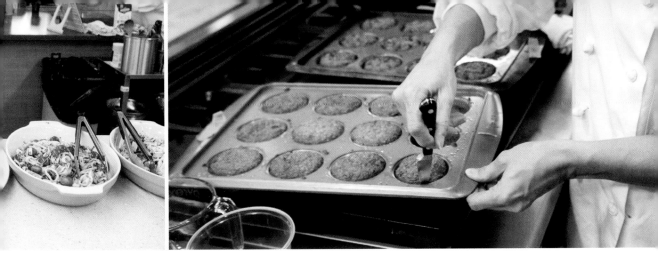

Eating the Paleo Way

At the center of the paleo diet is the philosophy that eating minimally processed, whole foods is the key to good health. Taking inspiration from our Paleolithic-era, hunter-gatherer ancestors, the modern paleo template centers around eating plenty of meat and vegetables while avoiding dairy, grains, refined sugar, alcohol, and more—processed foods that, as a result of organized agriculture, were introduced to human diets after the Paleolithic period. The chart below summarizes the essence of the paleo diet.

YES	NO	IN MODERATION
Meat (pasture-raised/ grass-fed/wild)	Processed foods	Fruit (organic)
Seafood (wild-caught/ sustainable)	Sugar, artificial or processed sweeteners (including agave and stevia)	Nuts (like cashews, almonds, walnuts, pecans, macadamia nuts, and pine nuts)
Eggs (from pasture-raised birds)	Grains and cereals (like wheat, corn, rice, and oats)	Seeds (like sesame seeds, poppy seeds, and sunflower seeds)
Vegetables (organic)	Legumes (including peanuts)	
Fermented foods	Highly processed fats and oils (like vegetable oil, canola oil, safflower oil, and corn oil)	Starches (like arrowroot or tapioca, which come from nutrient-dense plants)
Spices		
Healthy fats (like animal fats, olive oil, coconut oil, nut oils, avocados and avocado oil)	Alcohol	Natural sweeteners (like honey, coconut sugar, maple syrup, and maple sugar)
	Dairy	

The Paleo Swap at a Glance:
Ten Crucial Ingredients You Need to Rethink

Given the restrictions this diet presents, people serious about following it need to rethink not only how they shop and stock their pantry but also how they cook. Many fundamental ingredients that we depend on when cooking are off-limits, and you must make homemade versions of other key ingredients since the commercial versions are highly processed or contain stabilizers and gums (think mayonnaise, broths, and canned tomatoes). Before you even get started, take a look at the chart below, which we developed to make paleo cooking less intimidating to those who may not be familiar with it yet. We've provided some of the test kitchen's favorite alternatives for some nonpaleo ingredients that are normally crucial to most recipes. Although these substitutes won't work in every recipe—nor are they simply one-for-one swaps—this chart will help you start to understand how to approach paleo cooking.

INSTEAD OF THIS	USE THIS	WHY?
Vegetable oil	Coconut oil or extra-virgin olive oil	Instead of reaching for highly processed vegetable oil, we often use coconut oil or ghee, both of which perform well at high temperatures. The coconut flavor in our preferred coconut oil is too faint to detect in most dishes. Extra-virgin olive oil also works well for cooking, but save the expensive, high-end versions for raw applications.
Butter	Ghee	Because ghee, which is made by straining the milk solids from melted butter, is dairy-free, it's widely considered to be paleo-friendly. Although ghee won't work in all recipes, it is fairly high-heat-stable, so it performs well in applications like sautéing or pan-frying.
Milk, cream, and yogurt	Whipped cashews, coconut or almond yogurt	Soaked and pureed cashews make a surprisingly good substitute for dairy in creamy fillings and panades (paste made from bread and milk used to keep ground meat tender and moist). Nut-based yogurts also make a great stand-in for dairy-based yogurt in parfaits and creamy sauces.
All-purpose flour	Nut flours	Since no single nut-based flour can perform the same functions as all-purpose flour, we use a combination of almond flour and coconut flour, along with arrowroot flour (see page 5 for more information), to give baked goods structure.

INSTEAD OF THIS	USE THIS	WHY?
Cornstarch	Arrowroot flour or tapioca flour	We found that arrowroot flour works well to thicken sauces and gravies and helps to lighten the texture of baked goods. Tapioca flour works well in coatings, such as velveting chicken for stir-fries.
Sugar	Honey, maple syrup, coconut sugar, maple sugar, dried or fresh fruit	Sugar—even raw sugar—is a highly processed food. Instead, we use natural sweeteners, like honey, maple syrup, maple sugar, coconut sugar, and fruit. Each of these sweeteners has different characteristics (like flavor and moisture content); we chose which one to use based on the specific recipe.
Store-bought broths	Homemade broths or water	Most store-bought broths contain additives, preservatives, and sugar—and those that don't can be hard to find. Homemade broths (see the recipes on pages 16-18) have a depth and intensity that store-bought broths lack, and even a small amount can provide a boost of savory flavor to many recipes. When possible, we make a broth within the body of a recipe to help keep things streamlined. That means using bone-in cuts or adding marrow-rich bones to recipes like beef stew. In recipes that already have a lot of flavor but need a small amount of liquid, water does the trick.
Canned tomatoes	Fresh tomatoes and/or tomato paste	Most brands of canned tomatoes contain preservatives and some even contain added sugar. We use fresh tomatoes wherever possible, processing them to approximate canned diced tomatoes. When appropriate, we also boost tomato flavor with tomato paste, which is simply tomato puree that is cooked to remove moisture.
Rice and potatoes	Cauliflower or celery root	We use cauliflower to make "rice" by processing the raw florets into rice-size pieces. Hardy root vegetables like celery root, rutabaga, or parsnips, which hold their shape nicely when cooked, work well in place of potatoes.
Soy sauce	Coconut aminos and fish sauce	To replace soy sauce, we use two ingredients to create a similarly salty, savory flavor profile: coconut aminos, which looks like soy sauce but has a slightly sweeter, less intense flavor (see page 11 for more information), and fish sauce, which helps deepen savory flavor but doesn't taste fishy when used in small quantities.

Buying Produce, Meat, and Seafood

Paleo meals should be nutrient-dense, satisfying, and, most of all, delicious. Meat and vegetables are the building blocks of paleo cooking, and what you buy will make a difference in how your dishes turn out. Although shopping for paleo-friendly ingredients like pasture-raised pork or wild-caught salmon might take some extra effort, the resulting dishes will be well worth the time spent.

Produce

The paleo diet encourages you to eat organic, non-GMO fruits and vegetables whenever possible, since these are not grown using pesticides and so will not contain any trace chemicals. If you can't buy all organic produce, try buying organic for the items known as the "Dirty Dozen" (below, left). This list is published annually by the Environmental Working Group (EWG), and you can find the latest updates at ewg.org/foodnews. The food with the highest pesticide residue is at the top.

On the other hand, the EWG also publishes the "Clean 15" (below, right), which lists the items with the least amount of pesticide. These are considered safer to buy conventionally grown. This list starts with the food with the lowest pesticide residue.

DIRTY DOZEN	CLEAN 15
Apples	Avocados
Peaches	Sweet Corn (not paleo)
Nectarines	Pineapples
Strawberries	Cabbage
Grapes	Sweet Peas (frozen) (not paleo)
Celery	
Spinach	Onions
Sweet Bell Peppers	Asparagus
Cucumbers	Mangos
Cherry Tomatoes	Papayas
Snap Peas (imported)	Kiwi
Potatoes	Eggplant
	Grapefruit
	Cantaloupe
	Cauliflower
	Sweet Potatoes

Meat

Most beef sold in supermarkets today is grain-fed, meaning that after the animals are 6 months old, they are fed a diet of corn and other grains. These grains are cheap and fatten the animals quickly, lowering production costs for large-scale farms and increasing the marbling in the meat. But since cows' bodies are not designed to digest corn, this type of diet makes them sick, often requiring antibiotics. Grass-fed animals, on the other hand, eat grass and hay, are not fed antibiotics or growth hormones, and are not confined. Grass-fed meat is generally leaner than grain-fed, but after some testing, we discovered that the differences are minimal. Note that because it has less fat, grass-fed beef is less forgiving when it comes to overcooking, so be sure to check the temperature of the meat at the beginning of the time range. The best way to source grass-fed beef, lamb, and bison is to seek out a high-end grocery store or a local butcher shop.

Unlike cows, pigs and chickens are naturally omnivorous and have no trouble digesting grain. But conventionally raised pigs and chickens are often confined to tiny cages in unhygienic conditions with no room to roam. So when shopping for pork, poultry, and eggs, try to purchase pasture-raised. Note that the term "pasture-raised" is not government regulated, so you'll have to look for third-party certifications, like Certified Humane, Animal Welfare Approved, or American Humane Certified. ("Free-range" means that animals must have access to the outdoors, but the amount, duration, and quality of access are not defined.) If you can't find pasture-raised chickens, go for organic: Certified organic producers must follow stricter guidelines than conventional producers. Birds must be fed organic (and therefore non-GMO) feed, be raised without antibiotics, and have access to the outdoors (though how much is not regulated).

In addition, be sure to avoid pork or chicken that has been "enhanced," meaning it has been injected with flavorings. It's not paleo, and it compromises the flavor and texture of the meat. We also recommend that you avoid water-chilled chicken, which is chilled after slaughter in a water bath that may contain chemicals like chlorine. Instead, look for labels that say "air-chilled." Besides not containing added chemicals, air-chilled birds don't absorb extra water (which you would pay for at the market).

Seafood

When purchasing fish and other seafood, your best bet is to find a reliable high-end grocery store or local seafood purveyor, and look for fish that is wild-caught and sustainable. For the most up-to-date recommendations on sustainable seafood choices, look for the Marine Stewardship Council logo at the store, or check the Monterey Bay Aquarium Seafood Watch website (montereybayaquarium.org).

When buying shrimp, there are a few things to keep in mind. Just because shrimp is raw doesn't mean it's fresh. Since only 10 percent of the shrimp sold in this country comes from U.S. sources, chances are the shrimp has been previously frozen.

Unless you live near a coastal area, "fresh" shrimp likely means defrosted shrimp. We recommend skipping the seafood counter and going straight for the freezer section. There, you'll find wild shrimp that have been individually quick-frozen (IQF). IQF shrimp are frozen at sea, locking in quality and freshness. Make sure to read the ingredient list carefully; "shrimp" should be the only ingredient listed on the bag or box. (In an effort to prevent darkening or water loss during thawing, some manufacturers add salt or sodium tripolyphosphate [STPP]. Not only are these additives not paleo-friendly, our tasters found an unpleasant texture and taste in salt-treated and STPP-enhanced shrimp.) Finally, look for shrimp with the shells still on; they have more flavor and better texture.

Shellfish like lobsters and crab are all wild-caught and are well suited for a paleo diet as long as they are not processed. For example, canned crab meat often contains additives that are not paleo-friendly. Look for fresh, in-season crab if you can find it. Some other shellfish, such as clams and mussels, are mostly farmed, but are still good options. When shopping for scallops, make sure that your scallops are "dry," not "wet." Wet scallops have been treated with a chemical solution to extend their shelf life, which compromises their quality and isn't paleo-friendly. Dry scallops will look ivory or pinkish; wet scallops are bright white.

PROTEIN	CHOOSE	AVOID
Beef, Bison, Lamb	Grass-fed	Conventional/grain-fed
Pork	Pasture-raised (via third-party certifications), organic	Enhanced (read label and avoid anything with extraneous ingredients)
Chicken	Pasture-raised (via third-party certifications), organic, air-chilled	Enhanced (read label and avoid anything with extraneous ingredients)
Fish	Wild-caught and sustainable	Farm-raised, frozen
Shrimp	IQF, shell-on	STPP- or salt-injected
Scallops	Dry (ask at counter)	Wet

Restocking Your Pantry: What's In, What's Off-Limits, and Why

Getting started on a paleo diet can be intimidating, but familiarizing yourself with paleo ingredients and having a well-stocked pantry ensures that cooking paleo is easy and approachable. Below are a few essentials that we rely on throughout the book. Be sure to read all labels carefully when shopping, as some surprising items can contain nonpaleo ingredients like preservatives, stabilizers, or sugar.

Oils and Fats

Vegetable oil and other common cooking oils like canola, sunflower, or corn oil are generally made from genetically modified organisms (GMOs) and are often chemically refined. Although all oils are processed to some degree, these oils are more highly processed than other oils. In this book, we use minimally processed oils and fats.

GHEE: Ghee is made from butter that has had all of the milk solids removed. It is solid at room temperature and can be stored in the pantry—it does not need to be refrigerated. It is fairly high-heat stable, which means that it can be used as a cooking medium. Although you can buy ghee at many grocery stores, it is easy to make yourself (see the recipe on page 16).

COCONUT OIL: Made by extracting oil from the meat of coconuts, coconut oil comes in "refined" and "unrefined" versions. We generally prefer to use refined coconut oil, since its coconut flavor is less pronounced. Some refined coconut oil undergoes chemical processing, so check labels carefully and look for oils that are expeller pressed. Coconut oil is solid at room temperature—we don't recommend keeping it in the fridge, since it gets very hard.

EXTRA-VIRGIN OLIVE OIL: Real extra-virgin olive oil is pressed without using heat or chemicals. It has a lower smoke point than ghee or coconut oil but can still be used for cooking in most cases. It also works well in raw applications like dressings. Our favorite high-end olive oil, which is best enjoyed in raw applications, is **Columela**. For cooking, we like **California Olive Ranch Arbequina** or **Lucini Italia Premium Select**.

MACADAMIA NUT OIL: This nut-based oil has a light, pleasant flavor that makes it well suited for homemade mayonnaise. Macadamia oil has a high smoke point, which means you can use it for cooking, but we recommend saving this relatively pricey oil for raw applications like mayo and salad dressing.

AVOCADO OIL: Avocado oil is extracted from the soft flesh of avocados, not the seeds as many other oils are. We prefer the neutral flavor of refined avocado oil to unrefined, which has a strong and distinct flavor. Like macadamia oil, we recommend saving this pricey oil for raw applications, although it does have a high smoke point and can be used for cooking.

TOASTED SESAME OIL: This flavorful, nutty-tasting oil is made from toasted sesame seeds. We use it largely in raw applications, though it also provides flavor to some of our stir-fry recipes. Purchase sesame oil in a glass bottle and refrigerate it to extend its shelf life.

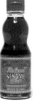

RENDERED BACON FAT: Bacon is a great way to enhance the meaty depth of a dish, and it makes a savory addition to a variety of recipes. If we're already using bacon in a recipe, we sometimes use the bacon fat as a cooking medium or as an ingredient. If you're serving bacon but not using the fat right away, you can reserve the rendered fat to use later. Keep rendered bacon fat in the fridge for up to one month.

Flours, Starches, and Other Baking Essentials

Many of the fundamental ingredients used in baking, such as wheat flour, sugar, and butter, aren't included in the paleo diet. And even many common "alternative" flours, like rice flour or chickpea flour, are grain- or legume-based. We had to completely rethink our baking pantry essentials. See page 13 for more information.

ALMOND FLOUR: We use high-protein almond flour as the bulk of the flour in most of our baking recipes—its mild, subtly sweet, nutty flavor works well in a variety of applications. Almond flour is usually made with blanched almonds, while almond meal can be made with blanched almonds or almonds with their skins on. We prefer flour (or meal) made from blanched almonds since the lighter color tends to be more versatile and appealing. You can make your own almond flour by grinding blanched almonds in the food processor. Store almond flour in the refrigerator or freezer to extend its shelf life.

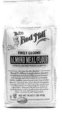

COCONUT FLOUR: Coconut flour is made from dried ground coconut meat. It has a noticeable coconut flavor when used on its own, but we tend to use it in small amounts to break up the denseness of almond flour, giving baked goods more structure and a better crumb. We also use it to help absorb the fat and liquid that almond flour can't. Store coconut flour in the refrigerator or freezer to extend its shelf life.

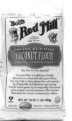

ARROWROOT FLOUR: Arrowroot flour is a pure starch. We use it for a range of purposes, including as an ingredient in baked goods, where it provides balance to protein-heavy almond and coconut flours. We also use arrowroot to make a batter for fried chicken: The starch crisps up nicely in the hot oil without becoming heavy or saturated. We find that to prevent a gritty texture in baked goods and batters, it is important to let the uncooked mixture rest to allow the arrowroot to fully hydrate. Arrowroot is also useful as a thickener; just a small amount gives pan sauce a better consistency. Arrowroot should be stored in the pantry.

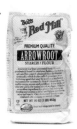

TAPIOCA FLOUR: Made from the starchy tuberous root of the cassava plant, this white powder, like arrowroot, is a pure starch. But different starches absorb water, swell, and gel at different temperatures and to different degrees; we found that tapioca and arrowroot are not interchangeable. Tapioca starch works best in coatings, such as when velveting meat for a stir-fry or dredging chicken for a bound "breading." It also makes a good thickener in our stir-fry sauces, where an ultrasmooth, satiny texture is desirable. In addition, we use tapioca in our Paleo Wraps (page 24), since it gives the finished wraps some elasticity and stretch. Tapioca flour is sometimes labeled tapioca starch. Either product can be used in our recipes. Tapioca should be stored in the pantry.

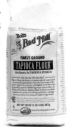

BAKING SODA: Containing just bicarbonate of soda, baking soda provides lift to baked goods. When baking soda, which is alkaline, encounters an acidic ingredient (such as lemon juice), carbon and oxygen combine to form carbon dioxide. The tiny bubbles of carbon dioxide then lift up the dough or batter. In addition to lift, baking soda improves browning in everything from pie dough to batter-fried chicken, and can help tenderize tough proteins like lamb shoulder chops or calamari.

CREAM OF TARTAR: This fine white powder is sold in small bottles in the spice aisle, but it's not actually a spice—it's a byproduct of the wine-making process. Since cream of tartar is naturally acidic, we use cream of tartar and baking soda to approximate the effects of baking powder. Baking powder contains both baking soda and an acidic ingredient and is traditionally used in recipes where there is no natural acidity. Since it generally contains cornstarch to keep the powder dry, baking powder is not paleo-friendly.

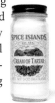

PSYLLIUM HUSK: We use psyllium husk powder in our Paleo Sandwich Rolls (page 25) to help create an open crumb and good structure. Psyllium interacts with proteins to create a strong network capable of holding in lots of gas and steam during baking. It provides a strong enough structure to support the rolls even when they've cooled. It also adds a pleasant, wheaty flavor. We tested a number of widely available brands of powdered psyllium husk and found their performance varied. We had the best luck using **Now Foods Psyllium Husk Powder**, which is available online.

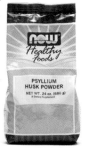

Natural Sweeteners

White sugar is highly processed; chemicals must be used to purify the cane syrup and turn it into refined sugar. Instead, the paleo diet relies on natural sweeteners, like the ones listed here. We choose which sweetener to use based on each individual recipe; because each option has a distinct flavor and interacts with other ingredients differently, it's helpful to have a variety of sweeteners on hand.

HONEY: The flavor of honey, which is made by bees from the nectar of flowers, varies depending on the source of the nectar and on the style of processing. Honey comes in two styles: traditional translucent honey and raw honey. All honey is heated and strained to remove impurities: Traditional honey is strained under high pressure to remove pollen, while raw honey is gently strained, just enough to rid it of wax or debris. We prefer the more nuanced flavor of raw honey— our favorite is **Nature Nate's 100% Pure Raw and Unfiltered Honey**. Since it has such a distinct flavor, it is best used in specific applications where the flavor is desirable or won't be noticed. Store honey in the pantry; it will keep indefinitely.

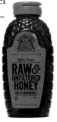

MAPLE SYRUP: Although maple syrup ranges in color and flavor, from mild-tasting light amber to boldly flavored, dark-colored syrups, all maple syrup is produced the same way—by boiling the sap of maple trees. Choose one that best suits your tastes, and make sure the ingredient label reads only "maple syrup."

MAPLE SUGAR: Maple sugar is made by boiling the liquid out of maple syrup. Like cane sugar, it is granulated and can be used in a wide variety of applications. We like to use maple sugar in recipes where a maple flavor is desirable, but extra moisture (as would be found in maple syrup) is not.

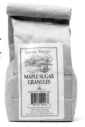

COCONUT SUGAR: Coconut sugar is made from coconut palm flower sap, from which the liquid is evaporated over moderate heat. Like maple sugar, it usually comes granulated. Its flavor is more mild than maple sugar's, but, like maple sugar, it doesn't add extra moisture to a recipe. We use coconut sugar in muffins to give them a neutral-flavored sweetness.

DRIED FRUIT: Dried fruits, like dates and raisins, can make great natural sweeteners. Since every fruit has its own distinct flavor profile, it's important to choose the fruit carefully based on the recipe. Sometimes we puree dried fruit (as in our All-Morning Energy Bars [page 82]) to create uniform sweetness or flavor, but we also use small pieces of dried fruit to provide bursts of sweetness in a dish.

Seasonings and Flavorings

While most herbs and spices are paleo-friendly, some other ingredients that we use to boost flavor are not—like soy sauce, Parmesan cheese, and wine, to name a few. But without these ingredients, some dishes can taste flat. Keeping your pantry stocked with the ingredients below can help ensure that your food tastes great.

KOSHER SALT: Table salt often contains anti-caking agents and other additives that are not part of the paleo diet. All of the salt called for in this book is kosher salt. The larger crystals in kosher salt mean that it weighs less than table salt, so you must use more of it to achieve the same flavor. Do not use table salt in the recipes in this book, as it will make dishes taste overly salty. We use **Diamond Crystal Kosher Salt** in the test kitchen (note that Morton's Kosher Salt, another common brand, contains anticaking agents and should be avoided). You can substitute finely ground sea salt for the kosher salt; reduce the amount of salt by half if using sea salt.

VINEGAR: Vinegar isn't just for making vinaigrettes; we also use it to perk up sauces, stews, and braises. Much like lemon or lime juice, a drizzle of acidic vinegar before serving can brighten and balance a dish. Different types lend distinct flavors to dishes, and we rely on several varieties in this book to lend nuanced flavor to recipes. We recommend keeping a variety of vinegars on hand, such as sherry vinegar, balsamic vinegar, white and red wine vinegars, and cider vinegar. Check labels carefully to make sure the vinegar does not contain added sugars, artificial colors, or other additives.

COCONUT AMINOS: Coconut aminos is often used as a paleo replacement for soy sauce. It's made by aging coconut tree sap. The dark, almost black liquid looks similar to soy sauce, though we find the flavor of coconut aminos to be sweeter and less intense than that of soy sauce. Look for coconut aminos in the international aisle of well-stocked supermarkets, specialty stores, or online.

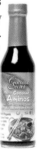

FISH SAUCE: At its most basic, fish sauce is made from just fermented anchovies and salt. The amber-colored liquid is used both as an ingredient and a condiment in Asian cuisines. We use small amounts of fish sauce to add well-rounded savory flavor to many dishes, including stir-fries. But many brands of fish sauce contain additives or preservatives; make sure to read labels carefully and buy one with only anchovies and salt on the ingredient list. We use **Red Boat 40° N Fish Sauce** in our recipes.

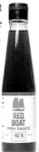

DRIED MUSHROOMS: Mushrooms are particularly high in savory umami flavor, and are especially useful when cooking paleo dishes that use water instead of broth. Dried mushrooms have highly concentrated flavor, giving recipes a major dose of meatiness; dried porcini or shiitake are good options. When buying dried mushrooms, always inspect them closely. Avoid those with small holes, which indicate the mushrooms may have been subjected to pinworms. The mushrooms should also be free of dust and grit.

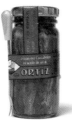

ANCHOVIES: These small fish are salt-cured and then packed in either salt or olive oil. Like fish sauce, they can add savory depth to everything from stews to braises. Anchovy paste provides a similar flavor; you can substitute ¼ teaspoon of paste for one anchovy fillet. (However, when a recipe calls for more than a couple of anchovies, skip the paste and use jarred fillets; the intensity of the paste can be overwhelming in larger quantities.) Be sure to read labels carefully to ensure that your anchovies (or anchovy paste) are paleo-friendly. Our favorite brand of anchovies is **Ortiz.**

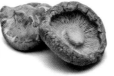

THAI RED CURRY PASTE: Thai red curry paste combines a number of hard-to-find, authentic Thai aromatics—including galangal (Thai ginger), bird's eye chiles, lemon grass, and kaffir lime leaves—in one easy-to-find ingredient. It is usually sold in small jars with the Thai ingredients at the supermarket. Be sure to check the label to make sure the ingredients are paleo-friendly.

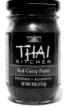

Miscellaneous Essentials

Just as in nonpaleo cooking, it's important to keep your pantry stocked with a few key ingredients that you'll use often. Here are some that we think are important to know about.

TOMATO PASTE: Most canned tomatoes contain sugar and chemical additives, so they're not considered paleo. The exception: tomato paste (but be sure to check labels). Tomato paste is tomato puree that has been cooked to remove almost all moisture. It can provide long-simmered tomato flavor in dishes that would normally rely on canned tomatoes. We also use tomato paste to add savory flavor to recipes. Because it's so concentrated, it's naturally full of glutamates, which provide the meaty flavor known as umami.

MUSTARD: Mustard is useful for more than just topping burgers; it also lends bright, tangy flavor to many dishes and dressings. Not all mustards are paleo-friendly; many contain added sugar or preservatives, so check the labels carefully. We like to have Dijon and whole-grain mustards on hand. If you'd like to make your own, see our recipes on pages 20-21.

NUT MILK YOGURTS: Like regular cow's milk yogurt, nut-based yogurts are made by culturing nut milks. But because nut milks don't naturally thicken the way that cow's milk does when cultured, they usually require some type of thickening agent—and often, store-bought nut yogurts utilize multiple thickening agents, stabilizers, and gums to achieve the right consistency. To avoid these, we make our own almond yogurt (see the recipe on page 23), which is great for breakfast parfaits or making creamy yogurt sauces.

Baking with Alternative Flours

All-purpose flour is milled from wheat berries, which contain starches, proteins, and fats. When flour comes in contact with water, gluten forms, which gives finished baked goods their structure and chew. When developing recipes like Blueberry Muffins and Paleo Single-Crust Pie Dough, we were charged with the task of figuring out how to create structure without using wheat flour. And since nut-based flours do not contain the proteins that create gluten, nor does any single nut flour work exactly like all-purpose flour, we had to use a combination of paleo-friendly almond flour, coconut flour, and arrowroot flour to give baked goods just the right structure, texture, and flavor.

FLOUR	WHY WE USE IT
Almond	Almond flour is perfect for creating volume—its mild, pleasant flavor makes a great base for a wide variety of recipes. But since it's made from nuts, it has a much higher fat and protein content than regular all-purpose flour (all-purpose flour contains 10 to 12 percent protein, while almond flour contains a whopping 21 percent). While you might think that all that protein would provide a lot of structural integrity, the opposite is in fact true: The high fat content disrupts the protein network, so baked goods made from almond flour alone have little structure and turn out dense. Almond flour is also low in starch, which means it can't absorb liquid. Combine the lack of absorption power with the fact that the fat from the nuts tends to leach out when baked, and you've got heavy, greasy baked goods. To counteract these problems, we decrease the amount of fat in our recipes (relative to traditional versions), and, more importantly, we supplement with coconut and arrowroot flours.
Coconut	Coconut flour works very differently than almond flour. For one thing, it is much higher in starch than almond flour, which means that it can easily absorb and trap liquid during mixing and baking. Plus, coconut flour is defatted and dehydrated during production, so its ability to absorb liquids is increased even further. Because of this, it can turn baked goods too dry when used in large amounts, but when used judiciously, it can help give baked goods structure, improve their texture, and create a more open crumb.
Arrowroot	Arrowroot flour is a pure starch, which means it contains no protein at all. Because it is a starch, it absorbs liquids easily and helps to lighten the texture of baked goods without making them overly dry. We found that when using arrowroot in doughs or batters, a resting period is often necessary to allow the starch granules to fully hydrate and not taste gritty or starchy. (Tapioca flour, like arrowroot flour, is a pure starch, but tasters found that it gave baked goods an off-flavor and a pasty texture. We like tapioca better as a coating for meat in stir-fries and when creating a bound breading.)

Spiralizing 101

Vegetables are an integral part of the paleo diet, so it's important to have creative ways to incorporate them into your meals. Spiralized vegetables can work as a main meal, a side dish, or a colorful and healthy addition to soups and stews—almost anywhere that traditional recipes might call for pasta.

The Best Veggies to Use

During our testing, we found that vegetables with solid cores were a must for spiralizing—hollow vegetables like acorn squash or very soft vegetables like tomatoes do not spiralize well. We chose noodles that paired well with the other flavors and textures in each recipe; overall, we favored summer squash, zucchini, butternut squash, and carrots. Summer squash and zucchini have delicate, neutral flavor profiles that meld seamlessly with flavorful sauces. They have a pasta-like texture with pleasant chew, and hold their shape nicely once cooked. They are quite easy to spiralize, and they work as short noodles or longer, spaghetti-like strands. Carrots, with their sturdy texture, spiralize beautifully, and make a great base for a side dish where their distinct flavor can shine.

Tasters also loved the flavor of butternut squash noodles; their subtle sweetness works well with bold sauces. However, butternut squash is more difficult to spiralize than zucchini and summer squashes, since it is a harder vegetable. We cut off the seed-filled bulbs and reserve them for other uses, spiralizing only the solid necks. Cooked, butternut squash noodles are considerably more delicate than zucchini and summer squash, making it more difficult to get long strands.

Although the flavors of zucchini, summer squash, carrots, and butternut squash work best with the recipes in this book, vegetables like beets, celery root, cucumbers, parsnips, rutabaga, and sweet potatoes can also be successfully spiralized.

Cooking Spiralized Noodles

In addition to finding the best types of noodles, we had to test a number of different cooking techniques to find the best way to prepare them. Zucchini noodles tasted great raw in some applications, but most recipes worked best with cooked noodles. Boiling the noodles in salted water didn't work, since the water later leached out of the noodles and into the sauce. We also tried sautéing, but fitting a full batch of noodles in a skillet was challenging, and even with constant stirring, the noodles cooked unevenly. We liked roasting best: It was easy to spread all of the noodles out on a baking sheet, and the noodles softened evenly while maintaining some texture and chew. Roasting also eliminated excess moisture, preventing the finished dishes from becoming watery.

When roasting tender vegetable noodles like summer squash and zucchini, we roast them uncovered for the entire cooking time. This allows moisture to evaporate and results in tender, flexible noodles. We find that draining the noodles after cooking helps to further ensure that we don't end up with unwanted moisture in the finished dish.

When roasting firmer vegetable noodles, like butternut squash, beets, celery root, or sweet potatoes, we recommend cooking them covered with foil for part of the cooking time so that they will steam slightly and become tender. Removing the foil partway through allows the surface moisture to evaporate. Don't drain these noodles; because they contain less moisture to begin with, they are less pliable once cooked, and transferring them to and from a colander results in unnecessary breakage.

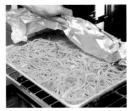

Buying a Spiralizer

If you plan on making spiralized vegetables often, it's worth purchasing a spiral slicer, or spiralizer. Spiralizers are relatively inexpensive and will save you time in the kitchen—if you buy the right one. There is a wide array of styles available, and we tested several models and found that not all of them work equally well. Our favorite model is the **Paderno World Cuisine Tri-Blade Plastic Spiral Vegetable Slicer**, which rapidly and effortlessly produces mounds of long, thick or thin strands and wide, curling ribbons. It works by holding food on prongs against a cutting blade while you turn a crank; our testers found it easy and intuitive. Its rectangular, 12-inch-long chamber can hold vegetables up to 10 inches long or 7 inches thick. It comes with three blades that store in the base of the unit and sets up in seconds.

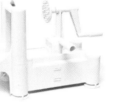

What If You Don't Have a Spiralizer?

If you don't own a spiralizer, you can also use a mandoline or a V-slicer fitted with an ⅛-inch julienne attachment. Make sure to position the vegetable on the mandoline vertically so that your noodles are as long as possible. Our favorite mandoline is the **Swissmar Börner Original V-Slicer Plus Mandoline**, which cuts effortlessly and produces stunningly precise results.

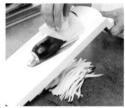

Although it's a little bit less efficient, you can also use a julienne peeler to create decent vegetable noodles. We do not recommend cutting vegetable noodles by hand.

How to Spiralize

Depending on your spiralizer, the amount of trimming required will vary. Be sure to check the recipe for specific instructions on peeling the vegetables and cutting the noodles.

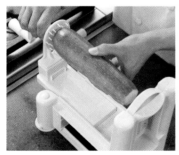

1. Trim vegetable so it will fit on prongs. Secure vegetable between prongs and blade surface.

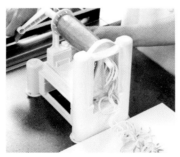

2. Spiralize by turning crank.

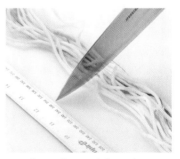

3. Pull noodles straight and cut into correct lengths as directed by recipe.

Paleo Basics

Since many of the store-bought items we rely on every day are not paleo-friendly (and versions that are can be difficult—if not impossible—to find), we created homemade versions that not only adhere to paleo standards, but also taste far better than anything we could buy.

Ghee

MAKES ABOUT 1½ CUPS

✔ **WHY THIS RECIPE WORKS** Traditional ghee is made by slowly simmering butter until the liquid has evaporated and the milk solids have started to brown. The solids are then strained out so that all that's left is pure butterfat. Because the milk solids have been removed, ghee no longer contains dairy, making it paleo-friendly. It's an invaluable ingredient in the paleo pantry, since it is well suited for most high-heat cooking methods, and provides a rich, buttery flavor to many a dish. Making ghee at home is very simple and more economical than buying it. We first tried making ghee on the stovetop, but the direct heat increased the risk of burning the milk solids and ruining the ghee. Instead, we turned to the gentle, even heat of a low oven, and put the butter in an uncovered Dutch oven to ensure that all of the water evaporated. To give the ghee its signature nutty flavor, it was important to let it cook until the milk solids were well toasted. Finally, we lined a fine-mesh strainer with cheesecloth to ensure that none of the solids would slip through, which would compromise the ghee's flavor and shelf life. Be sure to use unsalted butter here. This recipe can be doubled.

1 **pound (4 sticks) unsalted butter**

1. Adjust oven rack to middle position and heat oven to 250 degrees. Place butter in Dutch oven and bake uncovered until all water evaporates and solids are golden brown, 2½ to 3½ hours.

2. Line fine-mesh strainer with triple layer of cheesecloth that overhangs edges and set over large bowl. Let ghee cool slightly, then transfer to prepared strainer and let sit until all ghee is extracted; discard solids. (Cooled ghee can be stored at room temperature for up to 3 months or refrigerated for up to 1 year.)

Paleo Chicken Broth

MAKES ABOUT 8 CUPS

✔ **WHY THIS RECIPE WORKS** This rich and well-rounded chicken broth is perfect for use across a wide range of paleo recipes—as a base for soups, stews, and sauces; as a cooking medium; and even on its own. Many recipes for chicken stock call for simmering a whole chicken, but we found that cutting the chicken into pieces yielded more flavor by providing more surface area for browning. We tested a variety of vegetables to round out our broth and found that onion enhanced the chicken flavor while also imparting a gentle sweetness. Chopping and then sautéing the onion in the pot after browning the chicken helped concentrate the onion's flavor. We simmered pots of broth from 1 to 24 hours, and tasters agreed that at 4 hours, our broth had the best flavor— a deep, well-rounded chicken base with a slightly aromatic sweetness. After 8 hours, the broth began to taste slightly metallic, and further cooking gave way to bitter, harsh, and even burnt tones. If using a slow cooker, you will need one that holds 5½ to 7 quarts. You can reserve the separated chicken fat in step 4 and substitute it in savory recipes where olive oil, coconut oil, or ghee are called for.

1 **tablespoon extra-virgin olive oil**
3 **pounds whole chicken legs, backs, and/or wings, hacked into 2-inch pieces**
1 **onion, chopped**
8 **cups water**
3 **bay leaves**
 Kosher salt

1. Heat oil in Dutch oven over medium-high heat until just smoking. Pat chicken dry with paper towels. Brown half of chicken, about 5 minutes; transfer to large bowl. Repeat with remaining chicken; transfer to bowl.

2. Add onion to fat left in pot and cook over medium heat until softened, about 5 minutes. Stir in 2 cups water, bay leaves, and 1 teaspoon salt, scraping up any browned bits.

3A. FOR THE STOVETOP: Stir remaining 6 cups water into pot, then return browned chicken and any accumulated juices and bring to simmer. Reduce heat to low, cover, and simmer gently until broth is rich and flavorful, about 4 hours.

3B. FOR THE SLOW COOKER: Transfer browned chicken and any accumulated juices and onion mixture to slow cooker. Stir in remaining 6 cups water. Cover and cook until broth is rich and flavorful, about 4 hours on low.

4. Remove large bones from pot, then strain broth through fine-mesh strainer into large container; discard solids. Let broth settle for 5 to 10 minutes, then defat using wide, shallow spoon or fat separator. (Cooled broth can be refrigerated for up to 4 days or frozen for up to 1 month.)

Paleo Beef Broth
MAKES ABOUT 8 CUPS

☑ **WHY THIS RECIPE WORKS** We set out to create a deeply flavorful, nuanced beef broth that we could use in recipes or enjoy as a drinking broth. We started with the most important ingredient: the beef. Although many recipes call for roasting beef bones, we found that these broths didn't have much beefy flavor. Using meat alone produced thin broths that lacked body. Finally, we settled on oxtails—they were economical, widely available, and served as all-in-one bundles of flavor-packed meat, fat, collagen-rich connective tissue, and bone marrow. Plus, since they're sold precut, they didn't require any special preparation at home. Next, we needed to figure out how to extract the most flavor from the oxtails. We browned them first to create fond, then simmered broths for 4, 8, 12, 24, and 48 hours. The range of colors and flavors amazed tasters; at 4 hours, the broth resembled chicken broth and had

barely any beefy flavor, but by 48 hours, it had a burnt, metallic taste. Although the 12-hour broth had decent flavor, the 24-hour broth was the runaway winner: The beautiful mahogany color, rich beefy flavor, and luxurious, almost silky texture had tasters going back for seconds. An onion, a bit of tomato paste, and some bay leaves enhanced the broth's meaty flavor while adding a touch of aromatic sweetness, and white mushrooms played a crucial role in rounding out the overall flavor with their warm, savory tones. We found that the long, slow simmer could be accomplished in a 200-degree oven or in a slow cooker set on low, keeping our recipe streamlined and hands-off. Try to buy oxtails that are approximately 2 inches thick and 2 to 4 inches in diameter; they will yield more flavor for the broth. Oxtails can often be found in the freezer section of the grocery store; if using frozen oxtails, be sure to thaw them completely before using. If using a slow cooker, you will need one that holds 5½ to 7 quarts. You can reserve the separated beef fat in step 4 and substitute it in savory recipes where olive oil, coconut oil, or ghee are called for.

2	**tablespoons extra-virgin olive oil**
6	**pounds oxtails**
1	**large onion, chopped**
8	**ounces white mushrooms, trimmed and chopped**
2	**tablespoons tomato paste**
10	**cups water**
3	**bay leaves**
	Kosher salt and pepper

1. Heat 1 tablespoon oil in Dutch oven over medium-high heat until just smoking. Pat oxtails dry with paper towels. Brown half of oxtails, 7 to 10 minutes; transfer to large bowl. Repeat with remaining 1 tablespoon oil and remaining oxtails; transfer to bowl.

2. Add onion and mushrooms to fat left in pot and cook until softened and lightly browned, about 5 minutes. Stir in tomato paste and cook until fragrant, about 1 minute. Stir in 2 cups water, bay leaves,

1 teaspoon salt, and ¼ teaspoon pepper, scraping up any browned bits.

3A. FOR THE OVEN: Adjust oven rack to middle position and heat oven to 200 degrees. Stir remaining 8 cups water into pot, then return browned oxtails and any accumulated juices to pot and bring to simmer. Fit large piece of aluminum foil over pot, pressing to seal, then cover tightly with lid. Transfer pot to oven and cook until broth is rich and flavorful, about 24 hours.

3B. FOR THE SLOW COOKER: Transfer browned oxtails and any accumulated juices and vegetable mixture to slow cooker. Stir in remaining 8 cups water. Cover and cook until broth is rich and flavorful, about 24 hours on low.

4. Remove oxtails, then strain broth through fine-mesh strainer into large container; discard solids. Let broth settle for 5 to 10 minutes, then defat using wide, shallow spoon or fat separator. (Cooled broth can be refrigerated for up to 4 days or frozen for up to 1 month.)

Paleo Vegetable Broth

MAKES ABOUT 1¾ CUPS BASE; ENOUGH FOR 7 QUARTS BROTH

✅ **WHY THIS RECIPE WORKS** A good vegetable broth is an important ingredient to have on hand, but supermarket offerings don't taste like vegetables—and they often include preservatives or additives. For a simple, economical, and space-saving solution, we decided to grind a selection of fresh vegetables, salt, and savory ingredients into a paste that we could store in the freezer and reconstitute as needed. Leeks provided an aromatic backbone, and a small amount of freeze-dried onions rounded out the flavor of the leeks. Tomato paste and coconut aminos provided a savory boost. Adding 2 tablespoons of kosher salt to the broth base not only helped with seasoning, but also kept it from freezing solid, making it easy to remove 1 tablespoon at a time. To make 1 cup of broth, stir 1 tablespoon of fresh or frozen broth base into 1 cup of boiling water. If particle-free broth is desired, let the broth steep for 5 minutes and then strain it through a fine-mesh strainer. For more information on coconut aminos, see page 11.

1	pound leeks, white and light green parts only, chopped and washed thoroughly (2½ cups)
2	carrots, peeled and chopped (⅔ cup)
¾	cup chopped celery root
½	cup fresh parsley leaves and thin stems
3	tablespoons dried minced onions
2	tablespoons kosher salt
1½	tablespoons tomato paste
3	tablespoons coconut aminos

1. Process leeks, carrots, celery root, parsley, minced onions, and salt in food processor to fine paste, about 4 minutes, scraping down sides of bowl as needed. Add tomato paste and process for 1 minute, scraping down sides of bowl every 20 seconds. Add coconut aminos and process for 1 minute.

2. Transfer mixture to airtight container and tap firmly on counter to remove air bubbles. Press small piece of parchment paper flush against surface of mixture and cover. (Paste can be frozen for up to 6 months.)

Paleo Mayonnaise

MAKES ABOUT 1 CUP

✅ **WHY THIS RECIPE WORKS** Most store-bought mayonnaises have long ingredient lists that include preservatives, stabilizers, and unwanted additives, and even homemade mayo recipes often call for vegetable oil. We wanted to create a simple, paleo-friendly mayonnaise that could be used in many different applications. Most mayo recipes contain egg yolks, and for good reason: Egg yolks contain a natural emulsifier, which first helps bind the ingredients and then prevents them from separating, creating a uniformly creamy consistency. To make our mayo even more foolproof, we wanted to boost the emulsifying power of the egg yolks with another ingredient. We found that just a bit of Dijon mustard further emulsified the mixture and added a pleasant hint of acidity. Since vegetable oil was off the table, we replaced it with extra-virgin olive oil. We decided to use a food processor to mix our mayo since the mechanical agitation forms a much more stable emulsion than most cooks can achieve by hand. However, our mayonnaise ended up with an unpleasant bitter flavor. We were puzzled until we remembered a recent test kitchen discovery: Extra-virgin olive oil tends to become bitter when processed because it contains bitter-tasting compounds that break into small droplets at high processing speeds and become more prominent. We decided to cut the bitterness by supplementing with another oil. Our tests revealed that mild-flavored macadamia nut oil worked well; we could put it in the food processor without it becoming bitter. To balance out the flavor of the macadamia nut oil and create a more traditional-tasting mayo, we whisked in some olive oil by hand at the end. You can substitute refined avocado oil for the macadamia nut oil, if desired. This recipe can be doubled.

2	large egg yolks
1	tablespoon white wine vinegar
½	teaspoon Dijon mustard
	Kosher salt and pepper
¾	cup macadamia nut oil
¼	cup extra-virgin olive oil

Process egg yolks, vinegar, mustard, and ½ teaspoon salt in food processor until combined, about 10 seconds. With machine running, slowly drizzle in macadamia nut oil until completely incorporated. Transfer mixture to medium bowl and, whisking constantly, slowly drizzle olive oil into egg mixture. If pools of oil gather on surface as you whisk, stop addition of oil and whisk mixture until well combined, then resume whisking in oil in slow stream. Mayonnaise should be thick and glossy with no pools of oil on its surface. Adjust mayonnaise consistency with water as needed, 1 teaspoon at a time. Season with salt and pepper to taste. (Mayonnaise can be refrigerated for up to 3 days.)

Paleo Ketchup

MAKES ABOUT 1 CUP

✓ WHY THIS RECIPE WORKS At its most basic, ketchup is a simple combination of tomatoes, vinegar, salt, and spices, but most store-bought ketchup also contains high-fructose corn syrup—a red flag for paleo dieters. We wanted to create a recipe for classic ketchup without the added preservatives and refined sugars. We started out with deeply flavored tomato paste as our base, which gave us the thick texture and tomatoey backbone we wanted. Simple white vinegar provided brightness and tang. Ground mustard, onion powder, garlic powder, and just a pinch of ground allspice offered complexity, while coconut sugar gave the rich mixture some much-needed sweetness. To bring all the flavors together and achieve the perfect, spreadable consistency, we simmered the ketchup for about 10 minutes. When reducing the ketchup, make sure to occasionally scrape the bottom of the saucepan with a rubber spatula to prevent scorching. This recipe can be doubled or tripled.

1	(6-ounce) can tomato paste
½	cup distilled white vinegar
½	cup coconut sugar
¼	cup water
1	teaspoon kosher salt
¼	teaspoon dry mustard
¼	teaspoon onion powder
⅛	teaspoon garlic powder
	Pinch ground allspice

Whisk all ingredients together in medium saucepan. Bring to gentle simmer over medium-low heat and cook, stirring occasionally, until ketchup is thickened and measures about 1 cup, about 10 minutes. Let cool to room temperature. (Ketchup can be refrigerated for up to 1 week.)

Paleo Barbecue Sauce

MAKES ABOUT 2 CUPS

✓ **WHY THIS RECIPE WORKS** We wanted to come up with a versatile, paleo-friendly barbecue sauce that could be used to marinade, baste, or finish a range of grilled or roasted meats. Most recipes for home-made sauces include hefty amounts of refined sugar, much like their store-bought counterparts. Instead, we created a naturally sweet foundation for our sauce by gently coaxing out and caramelizing the sugars from an onion. We built up our sauce with tomato paste and cider vinegar, and we added a touch of woodsy sweetness with maple syrup. A combination of garlic, chili powder, cayenne pepper, and Dijon mustard gave the sauce its necessary kick, with a hint of smokiness from smoked paprika. We found that in order for the flavors to meld, a long, slow simmer was key. When reducing the barbecue sauce, make sure to occasionally scrape the bottom of the saucepan with a rubber spatula while stirring to prevent scorching. This recipe can be doubled or tripled.

2	tablespoons extra-virgin olive oil
1	onion, chopped fine
	Kosher salt and pepper
3	garlic cloves, minced
1	teaspoon chili powder
1	teaspoon smoked paprika
⅛	teaspoon cayenne pepper
1	cup tomato paste
1½	cups water
3	tablespoons maple syrup
3	tablespoons cider vinegar
2	tablespoons Dijon mustard

1. Heat oil in medium saucepan over medium-low heat until shimmering. Add onion and 1 teaspoon salt and cook until softened and golden brown, about 10 minutes. Stir in garlic, chili powder, paprika, and cayenne and cook until fragrant, about 30 seconds. Stir in tomato paste and cook until beginning to brown, about 2 minutes.

2. Whisk in water, maple syrup, vinegar, and mustard, scraping up any browned bits. Bring to gentle simmer and cook, stirring occasionally, until sauce is thickened and measures about 2 cups, about 30 minutes. Let cool to room temperature. Season with salt and pepper to taste. (Barbecue sauce can be refrigerated for up to 1 week.)

Paleo Dijon Mustard

MAKES ABOUT 1 CUP

✓ **WHY THIS RECIPE WORKS** Mustard is a must-have condiment: Not only does it make a great spread, but it also brightens up dressings and sauces. We wanted to make a flavorful Dijon mustard without any of the artificial flavors, preservatives, or addi-tives often found in store-bought mustards. We also wanted to ensure that our recipe stayed simple and straightforward. To that end, we started with a base of three simple ingredients: yellow mustard seeds, vinegar, and salt. Many recipes also called for wine for additional flavor; to keep our recipe paleo, we opted to use water and white wine vinegar instead. Happily, tasters didn't miss the flavor of the alcohol. We also incorporated mustard powder for some kick and garlic powder and cinnamon for additional aromatic flavor. A little turmeric helped to enhance the yellow color. Before processing the ingredients together, we let the seeds soak for at least 8 hours to soften. A quick simmer on the stovetop thickened the mus-tard slightly, while passing the finished mustard through a fine-mesh strainer ensured a smooth, velvety texture. Finally, we found that letting our mustard sit for five days before using helped it to develop a more balanced and complex flavor.

1½	cups water
6	tablespoons yellow mustard seeds
3	tablespoons white wine vinegar
2	tablespoons dry mustard
1	tablespoon onion powder
2	teaspoons kosher salt
½	teaspoon garlic powder
¼	teaspoon ground cinnamon
⅛	teaspoon ground turmeric

1. Combine all ingredients in bowl, cover, and let sit at room temperature for at least 8 hours or up to 12 hours.

2. Process soaked mustard mixture in blender until smooth, about 2 minutes, scraping down sides of bowl as needed. Transfer mixture to medium saucepan, bring to simmer over medium-low heat, and cook, stirring often, until thickened slightly, 3 to 5 minutes.

3. Strain mustard through fine-mesh strainer set over bowl, pressing on solids to extract as much mustard as possible. Let mustard cool to room temperature. Transfer mustard to jar with tight-fitting lid and refrigerate for at least 5 days before using. (Mustard can be refrigerated for up to 2 months.)

Paleo Whole-Grain Mustard
MAKES ABOUT 1 CUP

✔ **WHY THIS RECIPE WORKS** For a more rustic version of our Paleo Dijon Mustard (left), we skipped the mustard powder in favor of spicier and more pungent brown mustard seeds. Cider vinegar, which has a mild acidity and a rounder flavor than white wine vinegar, nicely balanced the intensity of the seeds. A small amount of honey also helped to temper the mustard's bite. Instead of processing the mixture in the blender until smooth, we turned to the food processor to attain mustard that was spreadable but still had the pleasant pop of seeds that tasters liked. As with our Dijon mustard, we let the seeds soak for at least 8 hours to soften before processing, then stored the mustard in the refrigerator for at least five days to allow the flavors to develop.

½   **cup cider vinegar**
¼   **cup yellow mustard seeds**
¼   **cup brown mustard seeds**
¼   **cup water**
1   **tablespoon honey**
1½ **teaspoons kosher salt**

Combine all ingredients in bowl, cover, and let sit at room temperature for at least 8 hours or up to 12 hours. Process soaked mixture in food processor

until coarsely ground and thickened, about 1 minute, scraping down sides of bowl as needed. Transfer mustard to jar with tight-fitting lid and refrigerate for at least 5 days before using. (Mustard can be refrigerated for up to 2 months.)

Paleo Tomato Sauce
MAKES ABOUT 8 CUPS

✔ **WHY THIS RECIPE WORKS** For many of us, jarred tomato sauce is a pantry staple. But along with traditional ingredients like tomatoes, basil, and garlic, many store-bought sauces contain calcium chloride, added sugars, and other nonpaleo ingredients. We wanted a fresh-tasting, paleo-friendly tomato sauce that took advantage of simple ingredients. We started with an ample quantity of fresh tomatoes. Although many rustic tomato sauces included the skins, we found them to be distracting in our finished sauce, so we peeled the tomatoes by scoring them on one end and blanching them in boiling water. After a quick dip in an ice bath, the skins loosened up nicely. We decided to puree the tomatoes before cooking to achieve maximum evaporation and more concentrated flavor. We processed the tomatoes in batches to ensure a consistent texture. Adding some tomato paste ensured a deep, rich tomato profile, and browning the paste in olive oil brought out its flavor even more. Although many recipes called for the basil to be added at the end of cooking, we found that its flavor was better distributed, subtler, and more well rounded when we added it at the beginning. Letting the sauce reduce for a couple of hours built deep, concentrated flavor. A splash of red wine vinegar added at the end of cooking provided welcome brightness.

7½ **pounds tomatoes**
3   **tablespoons extra-virgin olive oil**
¼   **cup tomato paste**
3   **garlic cloves, minced**
¼   **cup chopped fresh basil**
    Kosher salt and pepper
    Red wine vinegar

1. Bring 4 quarts water to boil in Dutch oven. Fill large bowl halfway with ice and water. Remove core from tomatoes and score small X in base. Working in batches, lower tomatoes into boiling water and cook until skins just begin to loosen, 15 to 45 seconds. Using slotted spoon, transfer tomatoes to ice bath to cool, about 2 minutes. Remove tomatoes from ice bath and remove loosened tomato skins; discard blanching water and skins.

2. Working in batches, process peeled tomatoes in food processor until almost smooth, 15 to 20 seconds; transfer to large bowl.

3. Heat oil in now-empty pot over medium heat until shimmering. Add tomato paste and garlic and cook until fragrant, about 1 minute. Stir in processed tomatoes, basil, and 1 tablespoon salt. Bring to simmer and cook, stirring occasionally, until sauce is thickened and measures about 8 cups, 1½ to 2 hours. Season with salt, pepper, and vinegar to taste. (Cooled sauce can be refrigerated for up to 1 week or frozen for up to 6 months.)

Paleo Coconut Milk
MAKES ABOUT 1¾ CUPS

✔ **WHY THIS RECIPE WORKS** Much of the coconut milk found in stores contains a great number of additives, preservatives, and stabilizers, and the one or two brands that don't are difficult to find. We felt that the best way to avoid all nonpaleo ingredients was to develop our own recipe. We tested blending shredded coconut with water of varying temperatures and determined that near-boiling water worked best; the heat softened the coconut and extracted the most flavor. We wanted our recipe to make the equivalent of one can of coconut milk; after some testing, we landed on using 1¾ cups each of water and unsweetened shredded coconut meat. We strained the processed coconut mixture through a fine-mesh strainer lined with cheesecloth so that our milk would turn out perfectly smooth. Since the milk tended to curdle when heated to a simmer, we added a touch of baking soda if we planned on cooking with it. This made the milk more alkaline and discouraged the

milk proteins from clumping. For an accurate measurement of water, bring a full pot of water to a near-boil and then measure out the desired amount. We do not recommend using coconut flakes here. This recipe can be doubled. For more information on processing the coconut mixture safely, see page 271.

1¾   **cups unsweetened shredded coconut**
1¾   **cups near-boiling water (200 degrees)**
¼   **teaspoon baking soda (optional)**

Line fine-mesh strainer with triple layer of cheesecloth that overhangs edges and set over medium bowl. Process coconut and water in blender until coconut is finely ground, about 2 minutes. Transfer mixture to prepared strainer and press to extract as much liquid as possible. Gather sides of cheesecloth around coconut pulp and gently squeeze remaining milk into bowl; discard spent pulp. Stir in baking soda, if using. (Coconut milk can be refrigerated for up to 2 weeks.)

Paleo Almond Milk
MAKES ABOUT 4 CUPS

✔ **WHY THIS RECIPE WORKS** Almond milk is a refreshing dairy-free alternative to milk. Unfortunately, much of the almond milk available in stores is loaded with thickeners, stabilizers, and gums. We wanted a simple recipe for almond milk that tasted great and would be welcome in a paleo kitchen. Before we could make the milk, we found it was essential to soak the nuts for at least 8 hours to soften them and ensure that our milk didn't turn out grainy. We tested several ratios of almonds to water to determine which produced both the best flavor and the best texture. We found that blending 1¼ cups of soaked almonds with 4 cups of water gave us the ideal flavor and consistency. We then poured the mixture through a cheesecloth-lined fine-mesh strainer to separate the almond milk from the pulp. Since the pulp still contained a great deal of milk, we squeezed the pulp in the cheesecloth until no liquid remained.

To round out the flavor of the almond milk, we added a small amount of salt and some honey. This recipe can be doubled.

1¼ cups whole blanched almonds
Water
¼ teaspoon kosher salt
2 teaspoons honey (optional)

1. Place almonds in bowl and add cold water to cover by 1 inch. Soak almonds at room temperature for at least 8 hours or up to 24 hours. Drain and rinse well.

2. Line fine-mesh strainer with triple layer of cheesecloth that overhangs edges and set over large bowl. Process soaked almonds and 4 cups water in blender until almonds are finely ground, about 2 minutes. Transfer mixture to prepared strainer and press to extract as much liquid as possible. Gather sides of cheesecloth around almond pulp and gently squeeze remaining milk into bowl; discard spent pulp. Stir in salt and honey, if using, until dissolved. (Almond milk can be refrigerated for up to 2 weeks.)

Paleo Almond Yogurt

MAKES ABOUT 3 CUPS

✓ **WHY THIS RECIPE WORKS** Following a paleo diet doesn't mean you have to sacrifice the creamy texture and tangy taste of yogurt. Although there are a number of nondairy and soy-free alternative yogurts sold in stores, many of them contain additives, preservatives, and various gums. Our challenge was to create a paleo-friendly recipe that would have all the appeal and versatility of traditional yogurt. We first needed to determine the best milk for the job. To ensure that our yogurt was paleo-friendly, we knew we wanted to use one of our homemade nut milks (see the recipes at left). Yogurts made with coconut milk turned out consistently grainy; the smooth-textured almond milk yogurts were the clear preference. To promote the fermentation required in making yogurt, we elected to use probiotic capsules,

since typical yogurt starters are often sourced from dairy products. But the probiotics alone weren't thickening the yogurt: Since almond milk contains less protein than dairy milk, we couldn't achieve the thick, creamy consistency we were after without introducing an additional thickening agent. We tested gelatin, tapioca, and agar-agar, a thickener made from algae. Tasters preferred the yogurt made with agar-agar for its smooth and creamy consistency. You can find agar-agar and probiotic capsules at your local natural foods store. The flavor of the yogurt may vary depending on the brand of probiotic used; we developed this recipe using Renew Life Ultimate Flora Critical Care 50 Billion probiotic capsules. Do not substitute agar-agar flakes for the agar-agar powder. You can substitute coconut milk for the almond milk; however, the yogurt will have a slightly grainy consistency.

1¾ teaspoons agar-agar powder
¼ cup water
3 cups Paleo Almond Milk (page 22)
1 50-billion probiotic capsule

1. Adjust oven rack to middle position. Sprinkle agar-agar over water in small bowl and let sit until softened, about 10 minutes.

2. Heat milk in large saucepan over medium-low heat until just simmering. Add softened agar-agar and cook, whisking constantly, until fully dissolved. Transfer mixture to bowl and let cool, stirring occasionally, until mixture registers 110 degrees, about 20 minutes.

3. Twist open probiotic capsule and whisk contents into cooled milk mixture; discard capsule's casing. Cover bowl tightly with plastic wrap, place in oven, and turn on oven light. Let yogurt sit undisturbed for at least 12 hours or up to 24 hours. (Yogurt will not thicken while sitting.)

4. Refrigerate yogurt until completely chilled and set, about 4 hours. Process yogurt in blender until smooth, about 30 seconds. (Yogurt can be refrigerated for up to 1 week.)

Paleo Cashew Nut Cheese

MAKES ABOUT 1 CUP

✓ **WHY THIS RECIPE WORKS** Made by soaking and pureeing cashews, versatile nut "cheese" is a staple in many paleo kitchens. We wanted to develop a simple, foolproof recipe that would taste great on its own and also work in a wide variety of applications. Our recipe started with trying to determine what type of nut to use. In a side-by-side comparison of cheeses made with macadamia nuts, almonds, and cashews, the cashew cheese was the crowd favorite— the cheese was creamy, smooth, and had a pleasant, neutral flavor. (The almond cheese, although it had a slightly coarser texture, was a close second.) Next, we moved on to fine-tuning our recipe. We found that soaking the cashews for at least 8 hours was crucial in obtaining a creamy texture. A small amount of extra-virgin olive oil also contributed to creaminess, while lemon juice gave the mixture a bit of tang. We were amazed at the versatility of the finished nut cheese: It could be enjoyed as is, used as the base for a dip or spread, or substituted into recipes that would normally call for a cheese filling. You can substitute an equal amount of slivered almonds for the cashews; however, the cheese will have a slightly coarser consistency. This recipe can be doubled.

- 1 **cup raw cashews**
  Water
- 2 **tablespoons extra-virgin olive oil**
- 2 **teaspoons lemon juice, plus extra for seasoning**
  Kosher salt and pepper

1. Place cashews in bowl and add water to cover by 1 inch. Soak cashews at room temperate for at least 8 hours or up to 24 hours. Drain and rinse well.

2. Process soaked cashews, ¼ cup water, oil, lemon juice, and ½ teaspoon salt in food processor until smooth, about 2 minutes, scraping down sides of bowl as needed. Adjust consistency with extra water as needed. Season with salt, pepper, and extra lemon juice to taste. (Cheese can be refrigerated for up to 1 week.)

Paleo Wraps

MAKES 12 (6-INCH) WRAPS

✓ **WHY THIS RECIPE WORKS** We wanted to create soft, pliable, and tasty paleo wraps that would work for sandwiches, tacos, and more. We started by creating a dough using almond flour for structure, mild-flavored tapioca flour to increase pliability, and olive oil and water for moisture. But this dough was too sticky to roll out, and adding more flour or reducing the liquid didn't increase the dough's workability. We decided instead to create a pourable batter that we could cook in a pan like a crêpe or pancake. We added three eggs for richness and coconut flour to help manage the moisture content of the finished wraps. For the sake of ease, we combined all the ingredients in a blender and then allowed the batter to rest so the flours could hydrate and the batter could thicken to the right consistency. Once the mixture was ready, we simply added some batter to the skillet and tilted gently to spread the batter over the bottom of the pan. But the resulting wraps were eggy-tasting and very delicate. To fix these problems, we reduced the number of eggs to two and increased the amount of tapioca flour, doing away with the dominant egg flavor and making the wraps sturdier. We also found that even though using the blender made combining the ingredients easier, the speed of the blender incorporated too much air into the batter, leaving tiny holes in the cooked wraps. By mixing the ingredients by hand, we were able to minimize the air bubbles and avoid leaky wraps. To allow for practice, the recipe yields extra batter. To make larger wraps, pour ⅓ cup of batter into a 10-inch skillet or ½ cup batter into a 12-inch skillet; cook as directed. To reheat wraps quickly we found it best to use the microwave. Simply stack the wraps on a plate, sprinkle them with a little water, cover them with a paper towel, and microwave until warm and soft, about 1 minute. Wraps can also be reheated one at a time in a skillet.

2 cups (6 ounces) almond flour
¾ cup (3 ounces) tapioca flour
¼ cup (1 ounce) coconut flour
2 teaspoons kosher salt
1¾ cups water
2 large eggs
3 tablespoons plus 1 teaspoon extra-virgin olive oil

1. Whisk almond flour, tapioca flour, coconut flour, and salt together in large bowl. In separate bowl, whisk water, eggs, and 3 tablespoons oil together until combined. Whisk water mixture into almond flour mixture until thoroughly combined. Let batter rest for 15 minutes.

2. Meanwhile, place remaining 1 teaspoon oil in 8-inch nonstick skillet and heat over low heat for at least 5 minutes. Using paper towel, wipe out skillet, leaving thin film of oil on bottom and sides of skillet. Increase heat to medium and let skillet heat for 1 minute. After 1 minute, test heat of skillet by placing 1 teaspoon batter in center and cooking for 20 seconds. If mini test wrap is golden brown on bottom, skillet is properly heated; if too light or too dark, adjust heat accordingly and retest.

3. Whisk batter to recombine. Pour ¼ cup batter into far side of skillet and tilt and shake gently until batter evenly covers bottom of skillet. Cook wrap without moving it until top surface is dry and wrap starts to brown at edges, loosening wrap from side of skillet with rubber spatula, 1 to 3 minutes. Gently slide spatula underneath edge of wrap, grasp edge with your fingertips, and flip wrap. Cook until second side is lightly spotted, 1 to 3 minutes. Transfer cooked wrap to wire rack, inverting so spotted side is facing up.

4. Return skillet to medium heat for 10 seconds before repeating with remaining batter, whisking batter often to recombine. As wraps are done, stack on rack. Serve immediately or let cool to room temperature. (Cooled wraps can be wrapped tightly in plastic wrap and refrigerated for up to 1 week.)

Paleo Sandwich Rolls
MAKES 8 ROLLS

✓ **WHY THIS RECIPE WORKS** Too often, paleo-friendly sandwich breads turn out dry, crumbly, and dense or spongy, webby, and almost custard-like; plus, they usually lack the structure needed to stand up to a substantial filling. We wanted a hearty, sturdy sandwich roll that would taste great. To create good structure, we needed to use multiple flours and starches. For the base of our rolls we decided to use almond flour for its neutral flavor. Arrowroot flour was also essential, since the pure starch lightened the texture of the rolls and helped absorb moisture. Since we were after a bready flavor and texture, we used yeast as our leavener and added enough water to make a dough. But these ingredients alone didn't give our rolls much structure—nor did they taste very good. A couple of eggs provided better structure and offered some subtle richness. Psyllium husk powder, a common ingredient in gluten-free breads, gave the rolls a more open crumb by creating a sturdier protein network. It also contributed a pleasant, wheaty flavor. Some cider vinegar gave the rolls a sourdough-like tang, while honey, olive oil, and salt rounded out the flavor nicely. But the rolls were still turning out rather wet and dense. We tried reducing the amount of water, but since we were counting on the water to create steam and help the rolls rise in the oven, we couldn't reduce the amount enough to get rid of the wetness. Instead, we added some coconut flour to the dough, which easily absorbed the excess liquid without making the rolls crumbly. Finally, since the dough was fairly soft and tended to spread in the oven, we made foil collars to hold the dough in place during proofing and some of the baking time. Halfway through baking, we removed the collars to ensure even browning. A sprinkling of sesame seeds before baking was a welcome final touch.

1 cup plus 2 tablespoons warm water (110 degrees)
3 tablespoons honey
2 teaspoons instant or rapid-rise yeast

2 large eggs
3 tablespoons extra-virgin olive oil
1 tablespoon cider vinegar
3 cups (9 ounces) almond flour
1 cup (4 ounces) arrowroot flour
3 tablespoons coconut flour
5 teaspoons powdered psyllium husk
1 tablespoon kosher salt
1 teaspoon sesame seeds (optional)

1. Adjust oven rack to middle position and heat oven to 200 degrees. As soon as oven reaches 200 degrees, turn it off. (This will be warm proofing box for dough. Do not begin step 2 until oven has been turned off.) Line rimmed baking sheet with greased parchment paper. Using double layer of aluminum foil, create eight 13½ by 2-inch strips, then shape each into 4-inch circle and secure with staples. Grease inside of collars and place on prepared sheet.

2. Combine warm water, honey, and yeast in medium bowl and let sit until bubbly, about 5 minutes. Whisk in eggs, oil, and vinegar. Using stand mixer fitted with paddle, mix almond flour, arrowroot flour, coconut flour, psyllium husk, and salt together on low speed until combined, about 1 minute. Slowly add yeast mixture and let dough come together, scraping down sides of bowl as needed,

about 1 minute. Increase speed to medium and beat until sticky and uniform, about 6 minutes. (Dough will resemble loose cookie dough.)

3. Moisten your hands and divide dough into 8 equal pieces (3½ ounces). Working with 1 piece of dough at a time, roll into rough round and place in foil collar. Cover loosely with plastic wrap, place sheet in warmed oven, and let rise for 10 minutes; do not let plastic touch oven rack.

4. Remove sheet from oven and let sit on counter until dough has doubled in size, about 20 minutes. Meanwhile, heat oven to 400 degrees.

5. Reduce oven temperature to 350 degrees. Remove plastic and adjust foil collars as needed to be flush with sheet. Spray rolls with water and sprinkle with sesame seeds, if using. Set sheet with rolls inside second rimmed baking sheet and bake until rolls are golden brown and firm, 30 to 35 minutes, rotating sheet and removing foil collars halfway through baking.

6. Transfer rolls to wire rack and let cool completely before serving, about 1 hour. (Split rolls can be wrapped in double layer of plastic wrap and stored at room temperature for up to 2 days or frozen for up to 1 month. If frozen, microwave at 50 percent power for 1 minute then toast until golden.)

TEST KITCHEN TIP USING FOIL COLLARS

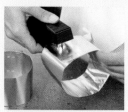

1. Using double layer of aluminum foil, create eight 13½ by 2-inch strips. Shape strips into 4-inch circles and secure with staples.

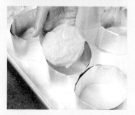

2. Grease inside of collars and place on greased parchment-lined baking sheet. Place shaped dough rounds in foil collars.

Paleo Single-Crust Pie Dough

MAKES ENOUGH FOR ONE 9-INCH PIE

✓ **WHY THIS RECIPE WORKS** Making a successful pie crust is difficult enough when you have the entire pantry at your disposal. Add the challenge of omitting conventional flours and fats and you have a tall order in front of you. We weren't deterred, however, and sought a single-crust pie dough that was just as light and flaky as a traditional one. We also wanted to make sure our pie crust was neutral-flavored enough to work in either sweet or savory applications. We began with almond flour, which provided an ideal base, but when used alone it cooked up dense and greasy. Adding some highly absorbent coconut flour made the shell more crisp and less oily, but it gave the dough a pliable texture that tasters didn't like.

A half-cup of arrowroot flour solved this problem, lightening the texture of the dough and helping it to crisp beautifully in the oven. A small amount of baking soda further lightened the shell and encouraged good browning. Our next challenge was to determine the fat and liquid components of the dough. Using an egg white instead of a whole egg provided structural support without making the dough taste eggy. Two tablespoons of water comprised the remainder of the liquid, while a generous amount of coconut oil gave the dough richness without adding unwanted flavor. Some lemon juice rounded out the dough's flavor with subtle, fresh notes. The dough was too fragile to roll out on the counter; luckily, we found we could easily roll it between two sheets of parchment and then use the parchment to help transfer the dough to the pie plate. As with many traditional recipes, our paleo pie crust needed to be parbaked to make sure it didn't turn gummy or soggy once we added fillings. Pie dough should be used immediately; do not store in refrigerator before rolling and baking.

- 2 **cups (6 ounces) almond flour**
- ½ **cup (2 ounces) arrowroot flour**
- 2 **tablespoons coconut flour**
- 1 **tablespoon coconut sugar**
- ½ **teaspoon baking soda**
- ½ **teaspoon kosher salt**
- ¼ **cup plus 1 teaspoon coconut oil, melted**
- 1 **large egg white**
- 2 **tablespoons water**
- 1 **tablespoon lemon juice**

1. Adjust oven rack to middle position and heat oven to 350 degrees. Grease 9-inch pie plate.

2. Whisk almond flour, arrowroot flour, coconut flour, coconut sugar, baking soda, and salt together in large bowl. In separate bowl, whisk ¼ cup melted coconut oil, egg white, water, and lemon juice together until thoroughly combined. Stir oil mixture into flour mixture with rubber spatula until dough comes together.

3. Turn dough onto sheet of parchment paper and flatten into 4-inch disk. Cover dough with second sheet of parchment paper and roll into 12-inch circle. Remove top parchment sheet, gently invert dough over prepared pie plate, and ease dough into plate. Remove remaining parchment and trim overhanging dough to ½ inch beyond lip of plate. Tuck overhang under itself; folded edge should be flush with edge of plate. (Dough rim may crack slightly, but will come back together once crimped). Using index finger of 1 hand and thumb and index finger of other hand, crimp edge of dough to make attractive fluted rim. Use excess dough to patch any holes. Gently brush dough with remaining 1 teaspoon melted coconut oil.

4A. FOR A PARTIALLY BAKED CRUST: Place pie plate on rimmed baking sheet and bake until crust looks dry and is lightly browned, 30 to 35 minutes. Transfer plate to wire rack. Following particular pie recipe, use crust while it is still warm or let it cool completely.

4B. FOR A FULLY BAKED CRUST: Place pie plate on rimmed baking sheet and bake until crust looks dry and is golden brown, 40 to 45 minutes. Transfer plate to wire rack. Following particular pie recipe, use crust while it is still warm or let it cool completely.

TEST KITCHEN TIP
SHAPING A SINGLE-CRUST PIE SHELL

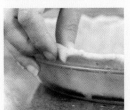

1. After trimming dough to ½ inch beyond lip of pie plate, tuck overhanging dough under itself to be flush with edge of plate.

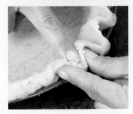

2. Using index finger of 1 hand and thumb and index finger of other hand, crimp edge of dough to make attractive fluted rim.

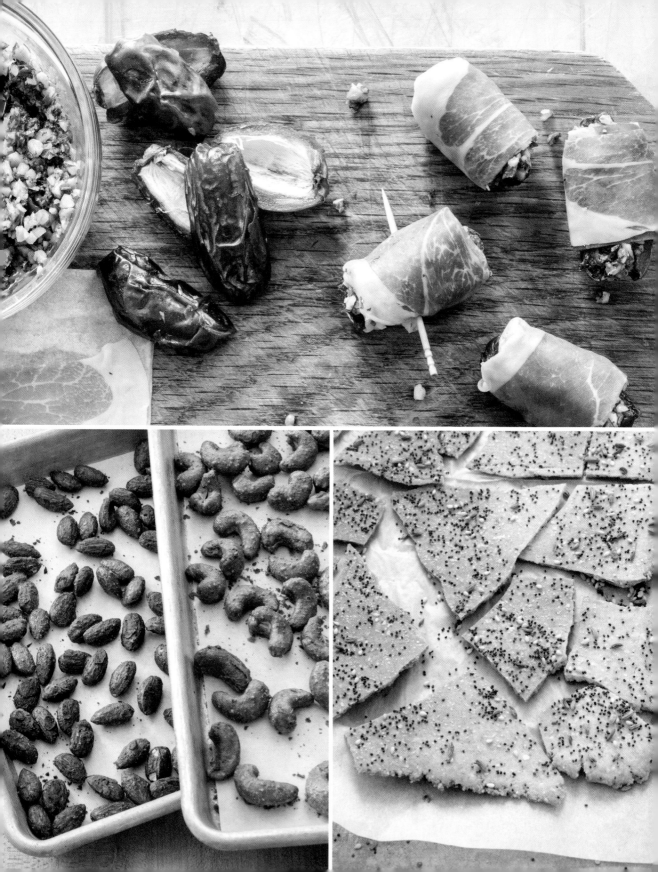

APPETIZERS AND SNACKS
CHAPTER 1

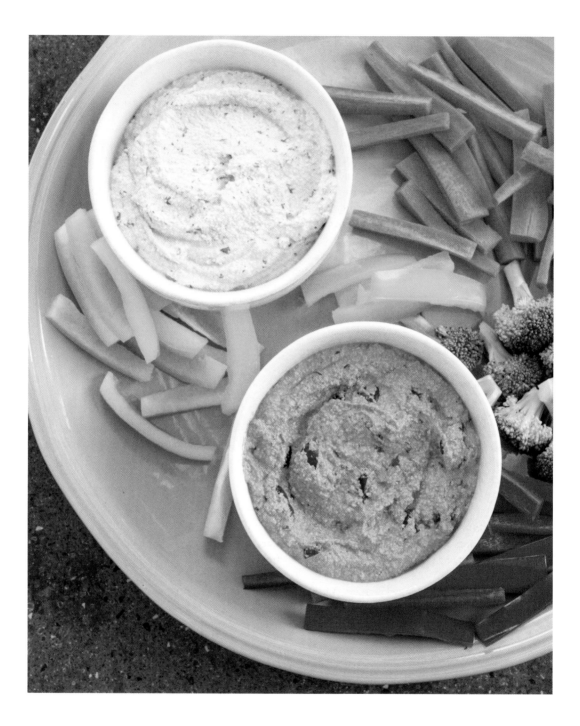

Whipped Cashew Nut Dip with Roasted Red Peppers and Olives

Serves 6 to 8

✓ **WHY THIS RECIPE WORKS** Creating a creamy, flavorful appetizer dip that's as good as any dairy-based one can be a challenge on a paleo diet, so we set out to create a foolproof, crowd-pleasing recipe. Cashews were an ideal starting point: When soaked and pureed, the nuts took on a creamy texture that made a perfect neutral-flavored base for our dip. We found that we needed to soak the raw cashews for at least 12 hours; any less, and the dip turned out grainy. Next, we turned to a variety of simple paleo-friendly ingredients to amp up the flavor of the dip. For our first combination, tasters liked the mildly smoky flavor of roasted red peppers with the briny, salty depth of chopped kalamata olives. A bit of olive oil and lemon juice boosted the flavor further and thinned the dip to a perfect spreadable consistency. Some parsley, stirred in with the olives after processing, provided welcome freshness. Since our dip had come together so quickly and easily, we decided to create two more flavorful variations, one using smoky chipotle, tangy lime juice, and fresh cilantro, and another with sweet sun-dried tomatoes and earthy rosemary. You can substitute an equal amount of slivered almonds for the cashews; however, the dip will have a slightly coarser consistency. Serve with Seeded Crackers (page 39), vegetable chips, or crudités.

1½ **cups raw cashews**
　　Water
½ **cup jarred roasted red peppers, rinsed, patted dry, and chopped**
3 **tablespoons extra-virgin olive oil**
3 **tablespoons lemon juice**
　　Kosher salt and pepper
1 **garlic clove, minced**
½ **cup minced fresh parsley**
½ **cup pitted kalamata olives, chopped**

1. Place cashews in bowl and add cold water to cover by 1 inch. Soak cashews at room temperature for at least 12 hours or up to 24 hours. Drain and rinse well.

2. Process soaked cashews, red peppers, 3 tablespoons water, oil, lemon juice, 1½ teaspoons salt, ½ teaspoon pepper, and garlic in food processor until smooth, about 2 minutes, scraping down sides of bowl as needed.

3. Transfer cashew mixture to serving bowl and stir in parsley and olives. Season with salt and pepper to taste. Cover with plastic wrap and let sit at room temperature until flavors meld, about 30 minutes. Serve. (Dip can be refrigerated for up to 5 days; if necessary, stir in 1 tablespoon warm water to loosen dip consistency before serving.)

VARIATIONS

Whipped Cashew Nut Dip with Chipotle and Lime

Omit red peppers and olives. Add ½ teaspoon chipotle chile powder and ½ teaspoon ground cumin to processor with soaked cashews and increase water to 6 tablespoons in step 2. Substitute ¼ cup lime juice (2 limes) for lemon juice and ⅓ cup minced fresh cilantro for parsley.

Whipped Cashew Nut Dip with Sun-Dried Tomatoes and Rosemary

Omit red peppers and parsley. Add 2 teaspoons minced fresh rosemary to processor with soaked cashews and increase water to 6 tablespoons in step 2. Substitute ½ cup finely chopped oil-packed sun-dried tomatoes for olives.

Baba Ghanoush

Serves 6 to 8

✓ **WHY THIS RECIPE WORKS** For baba ghanoush that boasted great eggplant flavor, we kept the flavorings simple: just tahini, lemon juice, garlic, and parsley. We found that it was critical to start with fresh eggplants and cook them until the flesh was very soft; undercooked eggplant tasted spongy and raw in the finished dish. Since the biggest hurdle when cooking eggplants is eliminating excess moisture, we pricked the skins with a fork before cooking to allow moisture to escape. To further avoid a watery texture in the finished baba ghanoush, we scooped out the softened, cooked pulp and let it drain for a few minutes before processing it. Look for eggplants with shiny, taut, and unbruised skins and an even shape (eggplants with a bulbous shape won't cook evenly). Serve with Seeded Crackers (page 39), tomato wedges, or cucumber slices.

- 2 **pounds eggplant**
- 2 **tablespoons tahini**
- 2 **tablespoons extra-virgin olive oil, plus extra for drizzling**
- 4 **teaspoons lemon juice, plus extra for seasoning**
  Kosher salt and pepper
- 1 **small garlic clove, minced**
- 2 **teaspoons chopped fresh parsley**

1. Adjust oven rack to middle position and heat oven to 500 degrees. Prick eggplants several times with fork, place on aluminum foil–lined rimmed baking sheet, and roast, turning eggplants every 15 minutes, until uniformly soft when pressed with tongs, 40 minutes to 1 hour. Let eggplants cool for 5 minutes on sheet.

2. Set colander over bowl. Trim top and bottom off each eggplant. Slice eggplants in half lengthwise and use spoon to scoop flesh from skins. Place flesh in colander (you should have about 2 cups); discard skins. Let eggplant drain for 3 minutes.

3. Transfer eggplant to food processor. Add tahini, oil, lemon juice, 1½ teaspoons salt, ¼ teaspoon pepper, and garlic. Pulse mixture into coarse paste, about 8 pulses, scraping down sides of bowl as needed. Season with salt and pepper to taste.

4. Transfer dip to serving bowl, cover with plastic wrap flush with surface of dip, and refrigerate until lightly chilled, about 1 hour. (Dip can be refrigerated for up to 1 day; let sit at room temperature for 30 minutes and season with extra lemon juice and salt before serving.) Drizzle with extra oil and sprinkle with parsley. Serve.

TEST KITCHEN TIP MAKING BABA GHANOUSH

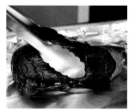

1. Roast eggplants until skins darken and wrinkle and eggplants are uniformly soft when pressed with tongs, 40 minutes to 1 hour.

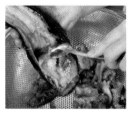

2. Trim top and bottom off each eggplant. Slice eggplants lengthwise and use spoon to scoop pulp from skins.

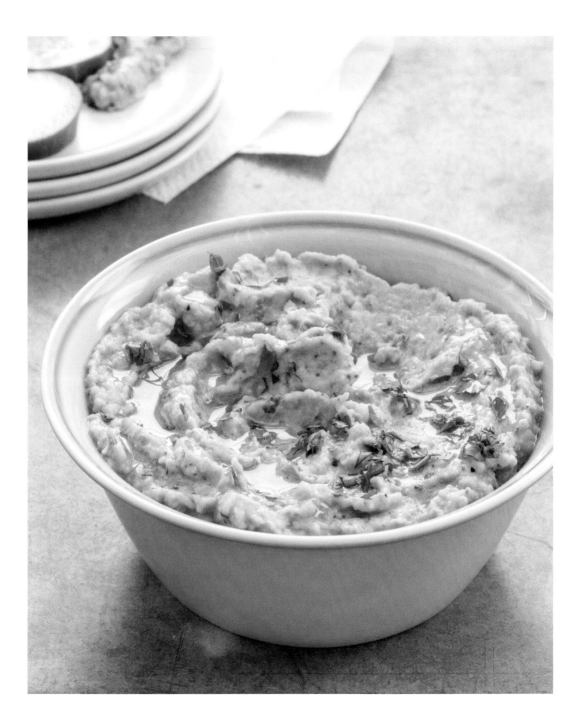

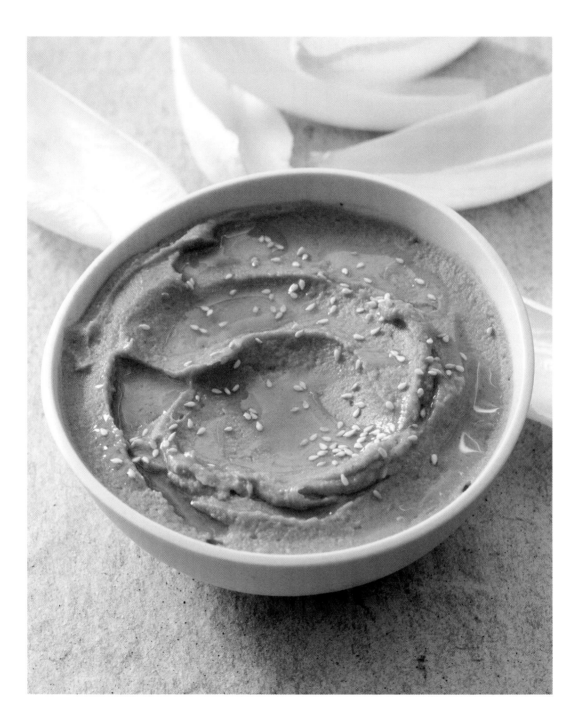

Sweet Potato Hummus

Serves 6 to 8

✓ **WHY THIS RECIPE WORKS** For a paleo version of hummus, we said goodbye to the chickpeas and hello to earthy, vibrant sweet potatoes. We aimed to bring out the sweet potatoes' subtle flavor by figuring out the best cooking method as well as the ideal balance of complementary ingredients. To keep things simple, we opted to microwave the sweet potatoes, which resulted in flavor that was nearly as intense as when we roasted them. Just ¼ cup of tahini was enough to stand up to the sweet potatoes without overwhelming the hummus. To round out the flavor of the hummus, we added some warm spices: paprika, coriander, and cumin. The addition of chipotle and a single clove of garlic curbed the sweetness and accented the spices well, while a couple tablespoons of lemon juice brought all the flavors into focus. Serve with Seeded Crackers (page 39), vegetable chips, or crudités.

1	**pound sweet potatoes, unpeeled**
¾	**cup water**
¼	**cup tahini**
3	**tablespoons extra-virgin olive oil, plus extra for drizzling**
2	**tablespoons lemon juice**
	Kosher salt and pepper
1	**garlic clove, minced**
1	**teaspoon paprika**
½	**teaspoon ground coriander**
¼	**teaspoon ground cumin**
¼	**teaspoon chipotle chile powder**
1	**tablespoon sesame seeds, toasted (optional)**

1. Prick sweet potatoes several times with fork, place on plate, and microwave until very soft, about 12 minutes, flipping potatoes halfway through microwaving. Let potatoes cool for 5 minutes on plate.

2. Slice potatoes in half lengthwise and use spoon to scoop flesh from skins; discard skins. Process sweet potato, water, tahini, oil, lemon juice, 1½ teaspoons salt, garlic, paprika, coriander, cumin, and chile powder in food processor until completely smooth, about 1 minute, scraping down sides of bowl as needed. Season with salt and pepper to taste.

3. Transfer hummus to serving bowl, cover with plastic wrap, and let sit at room temperature until flavors meld, about 30 minutes. Drizzle with extra oil and sprinkle with sesame seeds, if using. Serve. (Hummus can be refrigerated for up to 5 days; if necessary, stir in 1 tablespoon warm water to loosen dip consistency before serving.)

VARIATION

Parsnip Hummus

Look for tender, thin parsnips; large parsnips can taste bitter.

Substitute 1 pound parsnips, peeled and cut into 1-inch lengths, for sweet potatoes. Microwave parsnips in covered bowl until tender, about 10 minutes. Transfer parsnips to food processor and proceed with recipe.

Chicken Liver Pâté

Serves 6 to 8

WHY THIS RECIPE WORKS Rich and decadent, pâté is simple to put together and makes an occasion-worthy appetizer. Since classic pâté recipes include alcohol and cream, our challenge was to create a satisfying and flavorful version without using these ingredients. First, we needed to figure out how to cook the livers. Since our traditional recipe calls for simmering the livers in vermouth, we decided to try to build savory flavor by sautéing them in ghee. This produced well-browned livers, but the finished pâté was lackluster, so we turned our attention to re-creating the multidimensional flavor of classic pâté. Our first change was to add raisins and cider vinegar to the skillet. The raisins added a mild sweetness that offset the liver nicely and, combined with the vinegar, replicated the complex dried fruit flavor profile of the brandy used in traditional recipes. Adding extra ghee to the mixture made up for the lack of cream and helped create a smooth, luxurious texture. Although this pâté was greatly improved, tasters still wanted more depth of flavor. After several tests, we decided on an unorthodox method: We sautéed some chopped bacon, adding the bacon bits to the food processor with the other ingredients and using the rendered fat to cook the livers. This elevated the savory notes nicely without overpowering the other flavors in the pâté. As a final touch, we decided to pass the processed mixture through a fine-mesh strainer to ensure that the pâté was beautifully smooth, soft, and spreadable. Serve with Seeded Crackers (page 39), vegetable chips, or crudités.

2   slices bacon, chopped
12   ounces chicken livers, rinsed, patted dry, and trimmed of fat and connective tissue
    Kosher salt and pepper
3   shallots, sliced thin
7   tablespoons ghee
2   tablespoons raisins
2   teaspoons minced fresh thyme or ½ teaspoon dried
5   tablespoons water
1   tablespoon cider vinegar

1. Cook bacon in 12-inch skillet over medium heat until crisp, 5 to 7 minutes. Using slotted spoon, transfer bacon to food processor.

2. Season chicken livers with salt and pepper. Heat fat left in skillet over medium-high heat until shimmering. Add livers and cook, without moving, until lightly browned on first side, about 2 minutes. Flip livers and continue to cook until lightly browned on second side (livers should still have rosy interiors), about 2 minutes; transfer to processor.

3. Add shallots, 1 tablespoon ghee, raisins, and 1 teaspoon salt to now-empty skillet and cook until shallots are softened and lightly browned, about 3 minutes. Stir in thyme and cook until fragrant, about 30 seconds. Stir in 2 tablespoons water and vinegar, scraping up any browned bits. Cook until liquid is almost completely evaporated, about 1 minute.

4. Add shallot mixture, remaining 6 tablespoons ghee, and remaining 3 tablespoons water to processor and process until mixture is smooth, about 2 minutes, scraping down sides of bowl as needed. Transfer mixture to fine-mesh strainer set over bowl. Using back of ladle or rubber spatula, press liver mixture through strainer; discard solids. Season with salt and pepper to taste.

5. Transfer pâté to serving bowl and smooth top. Press plastic wrap flush to surface of pâté and refrigerate until firm, about 6 hours. (Pâté can be refrigerated for up to 3 days.) Before serving, let pâté sit at room temperature for 30 minutes and scrape off any discolored pâté from top.

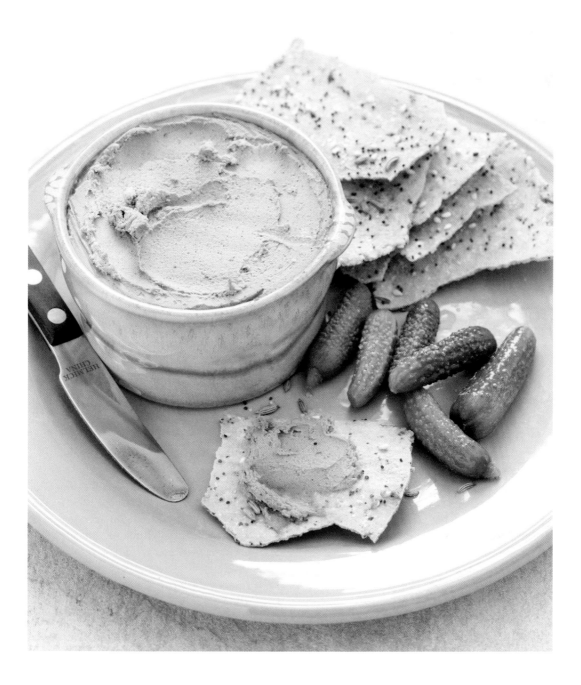

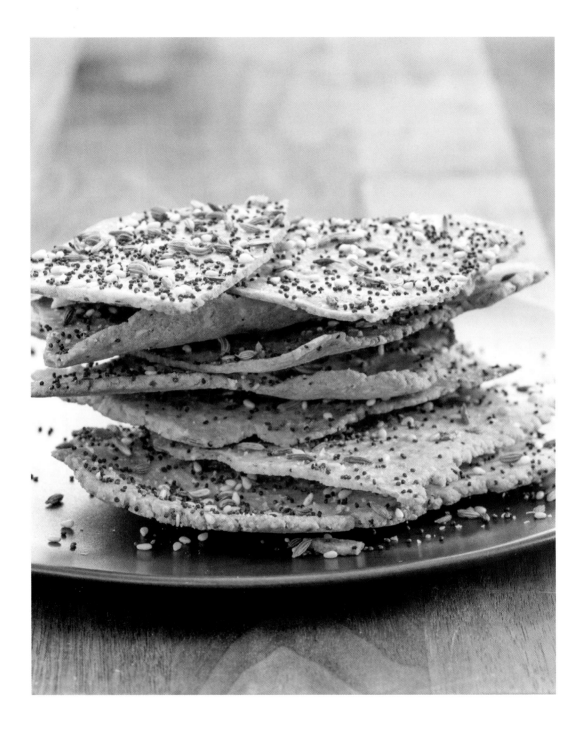

Seeded Crackers

Serves 6 to 8

✔ **WHY THIS RECIPE WORKS** We wanted to create a paleo cracker that was easy to make and that could accompany a number of paleo dips and spreads. Hoping to keep the recipe streamlined by using just one type of flour, we started with neutral-flavored almond flour. Unfortunately, these crackers turned out dense and greasy. It was clear that we would need a mix of flours for the right texture and flavor. Swapping in some highly absorbent coconut flour created crackers that were less greasy but unappealingly pliable and stale-tasting. We finally achieved the ideal texture by adding a small amount of arrowroot flour to our almond-coconut mixture; these crackers were crisper and lighter with great snap. With our flour mix settled, our next challenge was to find the right amounts of eggs, oil, and water. In a side-by-side test of crackers made with whole eggs, yolks, and egg whites, tasters preferred those made with just egg whites; the whites gave the crackers good crunch without adding any eggy flavor. A generous amount of olive oil provided a bit of richness. Next, we turned to flavorings: A combination of onion powder and sesame, poppy, and fennel seeds gave our crackers a well-rounded flavor profile. To make the dough easy to work with, we divided it in half before rolling it out. Rolling the dough between two sheets of parchment kept it from sticking to the rolling pin. We poked the dough with a fork to prevent it from puffing during baking. For extra crunch and flavor, we sprinkled more seeds on top of the crackers; a simple egg wash helped them adhere. Finally, we found that we could avoid the tedious task of cutting the dough into squares by simply breaking apart the sheets of baked dough into pleasantly rustic crackers.

1½ cups (4½ ounces) almond flour
¼ cup (1 ounce) coconut flour
¼ cup (1 ounce) arrowroot flour
1 tablespoon sesame seeds, toasted
1 tablespoon fennel seeds, toasted
1 tablespoon poppy seeds
 Kosher salt and pepper
¼ teaspoon onion powder
5 tablespoons extra-virgin olive oil
3 large egg whites (1 lightly beaten)
2 tablespoons water

1. Adjust oven racks to upper-middle and lower-middle positions and heat oven to 375 degrees. Whisk almond flour, coconut flour, arrowroot flour, 2 teaspoons sesame seeds, 2 teaspoons fennel seeds, 2 teaspoons poppy seeds, ½ teaspoon salt, ¼ teaspoon pepper, and onion powder together in large bowl. In separate bowl, whisk oil, 2 egg whites, and water together until thoroughly combined. Stir egg mixture into flour mixture with rubber spatula until dough comes together.

2. Divide dough in half. Working with 1 piece of dough at a time (keep remaining piece covered with plastic wrap), roll dough out between 2 pieces of parchment into ¹⁄₁₆-inch-thick rectangle (about 12 by 10 inches). Remove top piece of parchment and poke dough at 2-inch intervals using fork.

3. Slide rolled-out dough, still on parchment, onto separate baking sheets. Combine ½ teaspoon salt, remaining 1 teaspoon sesame seeds, remaining 1 teaspoon fennel seeds, and remaining 1 teaspoon poppy seeds in bowl. Brush dough lightly with beaten egg white and sprinkle evenly with seed mixture. Bake crackers until golden brown and edges are firm, 15 to 20 minutes, switching and rotating sheets halfway through baking. Slide crackers, still on parchment, onto wire racks and let cool completely, about 30 minutes.

4. Break cooled crackers into large pieces. (Crackers can be stored at room temperature in airtight container for up to 1 week.)

Kale Chips

Serves 4

✅ **WHY THIS RECIPE WORKS** Kale chips should boast a crisp texture and great earthy flavor, but often they just don't stay crispy. We found there were three key steps to getting kale chips with the perfect crisp texture. First, we used a very low oven to ensure that the kale would dry out but not burn, and we baked the chips for an hour or more to ensure that all of the moisture evaporated. We baked the leaves on a wire rack to allow the oven air to circulate above and beneath the kale. Finally, we made sure that we started with completely dry leaves—we spun them dry using a salad spinner and then blotted them between two dish towels to make sure no water was left clinging. Tossed with olive oil and seasoned lightly with crunchy kosher salt, these ultracrisp kale chips were a supersatisfying snack. We prefer to use Lacinato (Tuscan) kale in this recipe, but curly-leaf kale can be substituted; chips made with curly-leaf kale will taste a bit chewy at the edges and won't hold as well.

- 12 ounces Lacinato kale, stemmed and torn into 3-inch pieces
- 1 tablespoon extra-virgin olive oil
- 1 teaspoon kosher salt

1. Adjust oven racks to upper-middle and lower-middle positions and heat oven to 200 degrees. Set wire racks in 2 rimmed baking sheets. Dry kale thoroughly between clean dish towels, transfer to large bowl, and toss with oil.

2. Arrange kale evenly on prepared racks, making sure leaves overlap as little as possible. Sprinkle kale with salt and bake until very crisp, 1 to 1¼ hours, switching and rotating sheets halfway through baking.

3. Let chips cool completely on racks, about 10 minutes. Serve. (Kale chips can be stored in paper towel–lined airtight container for up to 1 day.)

VARIATIONS

Ranch-Style Kale Chips

Combine 2 teaspoons dried dill, 1 teaspoon garlic powder, and 1 teaspoon onion powder with salt before sprinkling over kale.

Spicy Sesame-Ginger Kale Chips

Substitute 1 tablespoon sesame oil for olive oil. Combine 2 teaspoons toasted sesame seeds, 1 teaspoon ground ginger, and ¼ teaspoon cayenne pepper with salt before sprinkling over kale.

TEST KITCHEN TIP MAKING KALE CHIPS

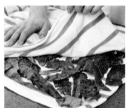

1. Stem kale, then tear leaves into rough 3-inch pieces. Wash and thoroughly dry kale between dish towels.

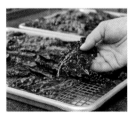

2. Arrange kale evenly on prepared racks, making sure leaves overlap as little as possible.

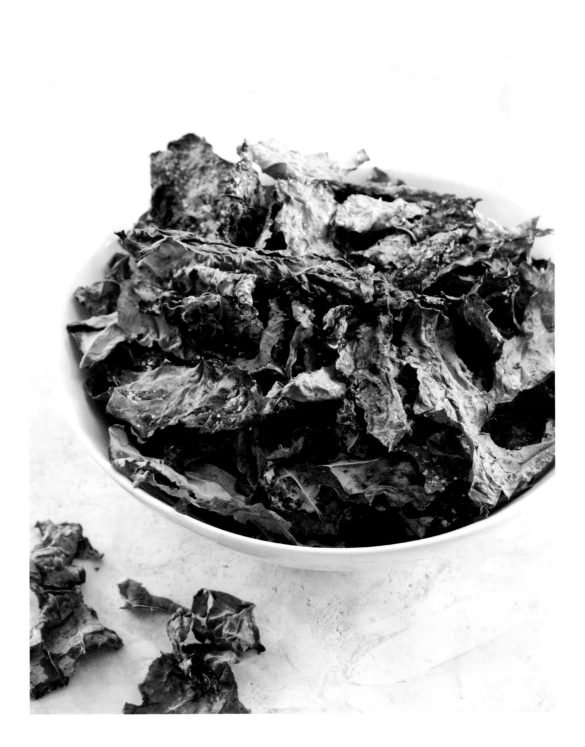

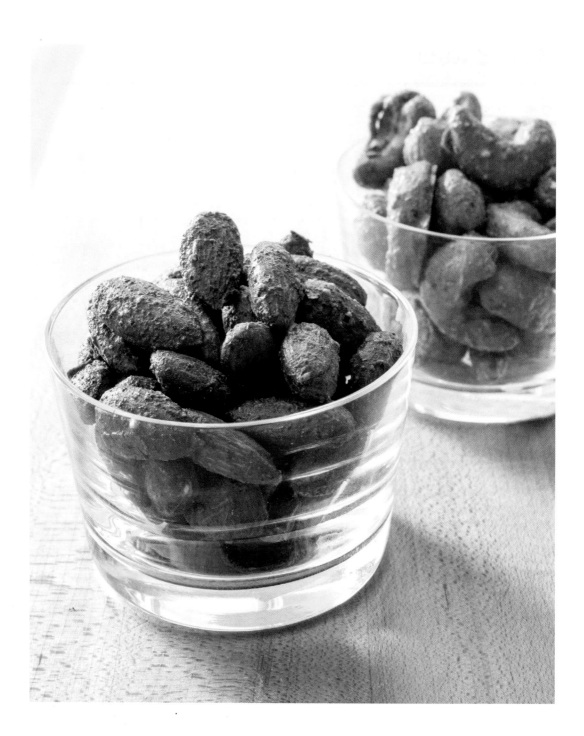

Spiced Nuts

Serves 8 to 10

✓ **WHY THIS RECIPE WORKS** Crunchy, aromatic, addictive spiced nuts make a perfect paleo-friendly snack. We wanted to create a recipe that would be simple to make and that would allow the flavor of the nuts to shine through. We decided to go with a simple spice combination of cinnamon, cloves, and cayenne, using just enough to complement the flavor of the nuts without overpowering it. To add a bit of background sweetness, we tested a variety of paleo-friendly sweeteners. Tasters preferred just ¼ cup of maple sugar, a natural sweetener made from maple syrup. To make sure the spices adhered to the nuts, we also needed a liquid component. Although some spiced nut recipes call for using butter or syrup, many call for a beaten egg white. Tasters preferred the nuts made with the egg white; the white created a crunchy shell around each nut without leaving the nuts tacky. Although tasters were happy with the finished nuts, some wanted a more savory option, so we decided to create a few variations. We chose bold spices but, as in our first recipe, used them in small amounts to create balanced flavors. A curried variation made use of a couple of flavorful spice blends, curry powder and garam masala; a second, slightly spicy, variation relied on chipotle chile powder, cumin, and garlic for a smoky, savory flavor; and a third variation combined orange zest and fennel for multidimensional, citrusy nuts. You can use any combination of nuts here; just be sure to have 1 pound of nuts in total. For more information on maple sugar, see page 10.

1	large egg white
¼	cup maple sugar
2	teaspoons ground cinnamon
2	teaspoons kosher salt
¾	teaspoon ground cloves
⅛	teaspoon cayenne pepper
1	pound cashews, pecans, walnuts, and/or whole almonds

1. Adjust oven racks to upper-middle and lower-middle positions and heat oven to 275 degrees. Line 2 rimmed baking sheet with parchment paper. Whisk egg white, sugar, cinnamon, salt, cloves, and cayenne together in bowl. Add nuts and toss to coat.

2. Spread nuts evenly over prepared sheets. Bake, stirring occasionally, until nuts are dry and crisp, 45 to 50 minutes, switching sheets halfway through baking.

3. Let nuts cool completely on sheets, about 30 minutes. Break nuts apart and serve. (Nuts can be stored at room temperature for up to 1 week.)

VARIATIONS

Curry-Spiced Nuts
Substitute 2 teaspoons curry powder, ½ teaspoon ground ginger, and ½ teaspoon garam masala for cinnamon, cloves, and cayenne.

Chipotle-Spiced Nuts
Substitute 2 teaspoons chipotle chile powder, 1 teaspoon ground cumin, and ¼ teaspoon garlic powder for cinnamon, cloves, and cayenne.

Orange and Fennel-Spiced Nuts
Substitute 4 teaspoons grated orange zest and 1 tablespoon ground fennel for cinnamon and cloves.

Prosciutto-Wrapped Stuffed Dates

Serves 6 to 8

✓ **WHY THIS RECIPE WORKS** These boldly flavored, sweet-salty stuffed dates are impressive enough for company, yet require only a few ingredients and minimal time. When developing this recipe, we knew we wanted to pair the sweet dates with some salty, savory ingredients, so prosciutto was a natural choice. To streamline the recipe as much as possible, we first tried combining the prosciutto with walnuts and parsley in a food processor. We quickly learned that this method wouldn't work; our pricey prosciutto was all but unrecognizable, and the walnuts were too small to lend any real texture. We decided instead to wrap the prosciutto around the stuffed dates. This put the prosciutto in the spotlight while still allowing the sweetness of the dates to come through. As for the stuffing, we found that chopping the walnuts and parsley by hand gave us more control over the final texture of the filling and yielded the best consistency. Some orange zest brightened the flavor of the stuffing nicely, and just a bit of olive oil helped the mixture bind together. The stuffing served as a nutty, crunchy counterpoint to the soft, sweet dates and, as an added benefit, came together in just minutes. High-quality dates and prosciutto are essential to the success of this recipe. Look for dates that are fresh, plump, and juicy; skip over any that look withered or dry. We prefer Medjool dates for this recipe, as they are particularly sweet with a dense texture.

⅔ cup walnuts, toasted and chopped fine
½ cup minced fresh parsley
2 tablespoons extra-virgin olive oil
½ teaspoon grated orange zest
  Kosher salt and pepper
12 large pitted dates, halved lengthwise
12 thin slices prosciutto, halved lengthwise

Combine walnuts, parsley, oil, and orange zest in bowl and season with salt and pepper to taste. Mound 1 generous teaspoon of filling into center each date half. Wrap prosciutto securely around dates. Serve. (Dates can be refrigerated for up to 8 hours; bring to room temperature before serving.)

VARIATION

Prosciutto-Wrapped Dates with Pistachios and Balsamic Vinegar

Omit orange zest. Substitute ⅔ cup shelled pistachios for walnuts and ¼ cup basil for parsley. Reduce olive oil to 1 tablespoon and add 1 tablespoon balsamic vinegar to nut mixture.

TEST KITCHEN TIP
MAKING PROSCIUTTO-WRAPPED DATES

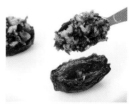

1. Mound 1 generous teaspoon of filling into center of each date half.

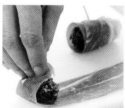

2. Wrap prosciutto securely around dates, leaving date ends uncovered.

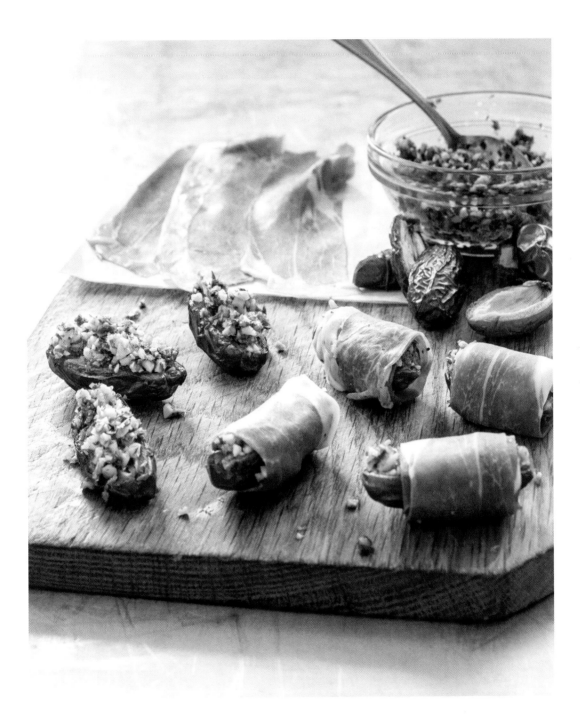

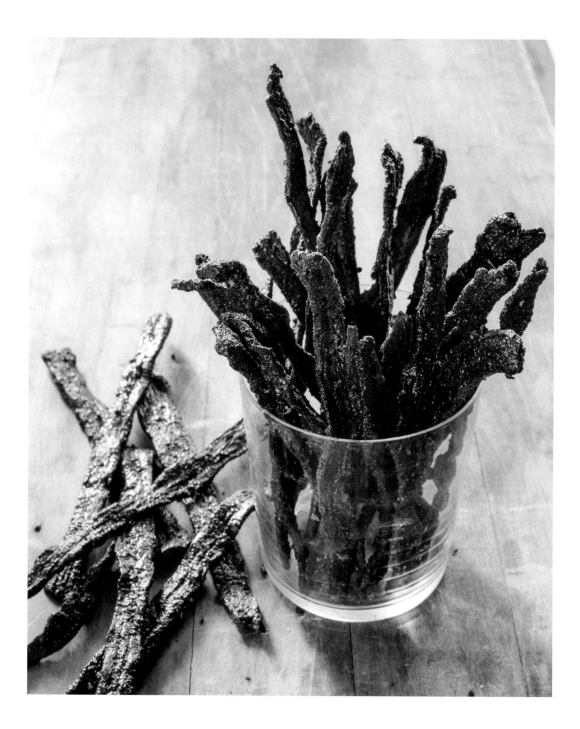

Beef Jerky

Serves 8 to 10

✔ **WHY THIS RECIPE WORKS** There are few things better suited to the paleo pantry than homemade beef jerky: Just a few seasonings and a low oven transform flank steak into an addictive, protein-packed snack. With this in mind, we set out to create a foolproof, flavorful recipe. Before being dried, the meat is almost always rubbed with salt and sometimes spices, which aid in preservation as well as flavoring. In modern jerky-making practices, this step is often achieved by soaking the meat in a salty liquid called a "wet-cure," which is essentially a marinade. Although nearly every homemade jerky recipe we found opted for this approach, we decided to go with a dry-rub method. There were two reasons for this decision: First, the wet-cure had a tendency to dilute the meat's flavor and break down its texture. We wanted jerky that was well seasoned but still had the texture and taste of beef. Second, there was the time consideration. Why add moisture to something you ultimately intend to dry? For our rub, we used salt and pepper along with paprika, fennel, and coriander to elevate the natural flavor of beefy flank steak. We also added a small amount of maple sugar to the rub, since its subtle sweetness would complement the earthy spices. We found that cutting the steak thin—into ⅛-inch-thick strips—and placing the strips on a wire rack during oven-drying greatly shortened the cooking time. For jerky that was more tender, we sliced the meat against the grain, while slicing with the grain yielded a chewier jerky. For spicier jerky, use the larger amount of pepper. To make slicing the flank steak easier, freeze it for 15 minutes. For more information on maple sugar, see page 10.

1–2   **tablespoons coarsely ground pepper**
2   **tablespoons maple sugar**
1½   **tablespoons kosher salt**
4   **teaspoons paprika**
1   **teaspoon ground fennel**
1   **teaspoon ground coriander**
1   **(1-pound) flank steak, trimmed**

1. Set wire racks in 2 rimmed baking sheets. Combine pepper, sugar, salt, paprika, fennel, and coriander in large bowl.

2. Pat steak dry with paper towels and slice into ⅛-inch-thick strips with grain (for chewy jerky) or against grain (for tender jerky). Add steak to spice mixture and toss until evenly coated. Arrange steak strips on prepared racks, spaced about ¼ inch apart, and refrigerate, uncovered, for at least 12 hours or up to 24 hours. Remove steak from refrigerator about 30 minutes before baking.

3. Adjust oven racks to upper-middle and lower-middle positions and heat oven to 225 degrees. Pat steak dry with paper towels. Bake until steak is dark, somewhat dry, and firm to touch but still pliable, 2 to 2½ hours, flipping steak strips and switching and rotating sheets halfway through baking.

4. Pat jerky with paper towels to remove any rendered fat and let cool completely, about 30 minutes. (Beef jerky can be refrigerated for up to 1 month.)

TEST KITCHEN TIP **SLICING FLANK STEAK**

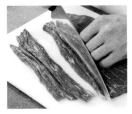

To easily slice flank steak, freeze for 15 minutes. Slice into ⅛-inch-thick strips with grain (for chewy jerky, as seen here) or against grain (for tender jerky).

Spinach and Bacon–Stuffed Mushrooms

Serves 6 to 8

✓ **WHY THIS RECIPE WORKS** Stuffed mushrooms are a popular appetizer, but the usual bread- or cheese-based stuffings mean that they're not paleo. We wanted to create a paleo-friendly filling with all the flavorful appeal of traditional ones. We decided that boiled and pureed cashews would provide a perfect base for our stuffing, since they make a creamy, neutral-flavored paste when processed. Next, we needed to figure out some flavorful additions that would complement the earthy mushrooms. We started with a classic stuffed mushroom ingredient: spinach. To maintain its vibrant green color and vegetal flavor, we cooked it only briefly. To build savory depth in our stuffing, we decided to sauté some chopped bacon and use the rendered fat to cook our aromatics and spinach. Finally, we turned to the mushrooms. To ensure that they were perfectly cooked and not soggy, we microwaved them before stuffing them to allow them to soften and release excess liquid. But once filled and baked, the mushrooms had a uniformly soft texture that tasters disliked. Some toasted cashews and the reserved crisped bacon bits, sprinkled over the tops of the mushrooms, served as a welcome crunchy element. Be sure to buy mushrooms with caps that measure at least 2 inches in diameter, as they shrink substantially when cooked. You can substitute an equal amount of slivered almonds for the cashews; however, the filling will have a slightly coarser consistency.

1   cup raw cashews, plus 3 tablespoons chopped fine and toasted
24   (2-inch-wide) white mushrooms, stemmed
¼   cup extra-virgin olive oil
     Kosher salt and pepper
3   slices bacon, chopped fine
1   onion, chopped fine
2   garlic cloves, minced
1   teaspoon minced fresh thyme or ¼ teaspoon dried
⅛   teaspoon red pepper flakes
6   ounces (6 cups) baby spinach

1. Bring 4 cups water to boil in medium saucepan over medium-high heat. Add cashews and cook until softened, about 15 minutes. Drain and rinse well.

2. Adjust oven rack to lower-middle position and heat oven to 450 degrees. Toss mushroom caps with 2 tablespoons oil and season with salt and pepper. Lay mushrooms gill side down on plate lined with 2 layers of coffee filters. Microwave mushrooms until they release their moisture and shrink in size, about 10 minutes. Flip caps gill side up and transfer to aluminum foil–lined rimmed baking sheet.

3. Cook bacon in 12-inch skillet over medium heat until crisp, 5 to 7 minutes. Using slotted spoon, transfer bacon to paper towel–lined bowl.

4. Add onion, 1 teaspoon salt, and ¼ teaspoon pepper to fat left in skillet and cook over medium heat until softened and lightly browned, 5 to 7 minutes. Stir in garlic, thyme, and pepper flakes and cook until fragrant, about 30 seconds. Stir in spinach, 1 handful at a time, and cook until wilted and dry, about 4 minutes; remove from heat.

5. Process boiled cashews and remaining 2 tablespoons oil in food processor until smooth, about 2 minutes, scraping down sides of bowl as needed. Add spinach mixture and pulse until spinach is coarsely chopped, about 10 pulses. Season with salt and pepper to taste.

6. Spoon spinach mixture into mushroom caps and sprinkle with crisp bacon and toasted cashews. (Stuffed mushrooms can be held at room temperature for up to 2 hours.) Bake mushrooms until heated through, 10 to 12 minutes. Serve.

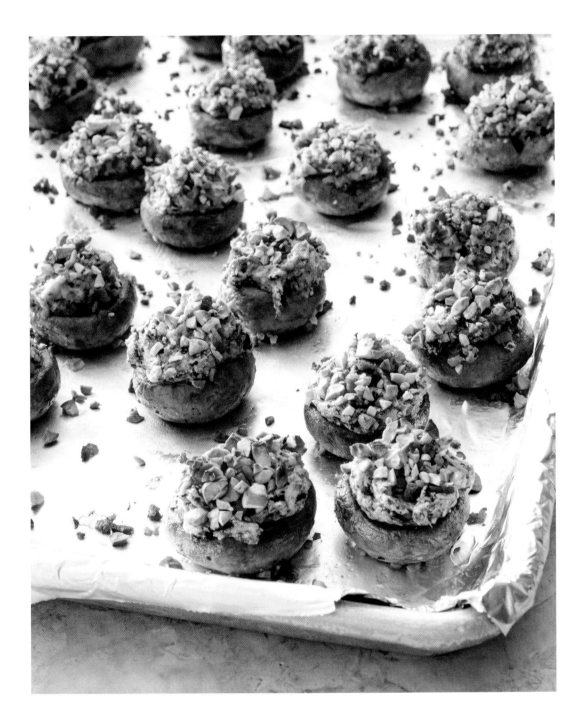

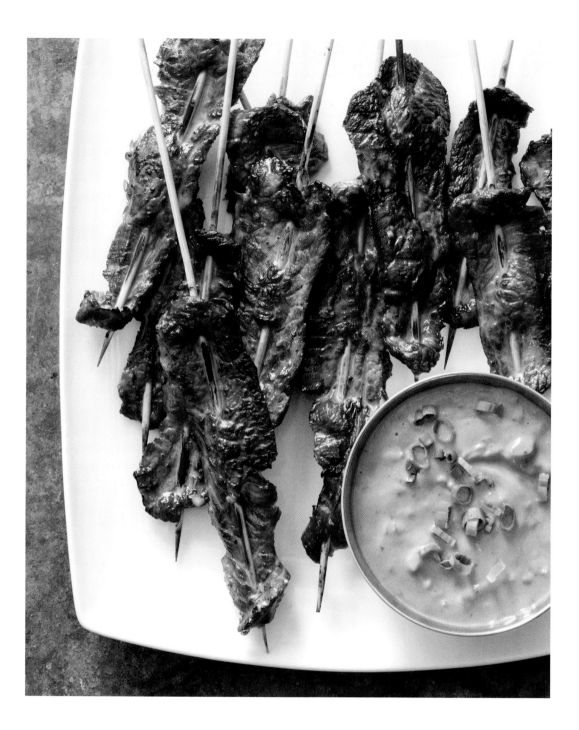

Beef Satay with Spicy Almond Sauce

Serves 6 to 8

✓ **WHY THIS RECIPE WORKS** Satay is a Southeast Asian dish in which slices of marinated meat (usually beef, chicken, or shrimp) are woven onto skewers and briefly grilled. With a few tweaks, we thought beef satay would make a perfect paleo-friendly appetizer—and, since we were already making changes to the recipe, we also decided to bring the cooking indoors to make it more convenient. We opted to use flank steak, as it is easy to slice into long, thin strips and has great beefy flavor. Slicing the meat against the grain and pounding it thin kept it tender. To replace the traditional (but nonpaleo) soy sauce in the marinade, we turned to coconut aminos, which has a similar flavor profile. A little minced garlic, salt, and pepper rounded out the flavor of our marinade. To cook the meat, we used the intense, direct heat of the broiler to approximate the heat of a grill. The only thing missing now was a great dipping sauce. Normally, satay is served with a flavorful peanut sauce, which isn't an option in a paleo kitchen. Instead, we used nutty almond butter as our sauce base, and added some coconut aminos, hot sauce, fresh cilantro, and scallions to boost the sauce's flavor. To make slicing the flank steak easier, freeze it for 15 minutes. For more information on coconut aminos, see page 11.

SKEWERS

1	(1½-pound) flank steak, trimmed
¼	cup coconut aminos
2	garlic cloves, minced
1	teaspoon kosher salt
½	teaspoon pepper
30	wooden skewers

DIPPING SAUCE

½	cup creamy almond butter
¼	cup hot tap water
2	tablespoons lime juice
1½	tablespoons hot sauce
1	tablespoon coconut aminos
2	scallions, sliced thin
1	tablespoon minced fresh cilantro
1	garlic clove, minced

1. FOR THE SKEWERS Slice steak in half with grain, then slice each piece against grain on bias into ¼-inch-thick slices. Lay pieces of meat in single layer between 2 sheets of plastic wrap and pound until roughly ⅛ inch thick.

2. Combine coconut aminos, garlic, salt, and pepper in large bowl. Stir in beef, cover, and refrigerate for at least 30 minutes or up to 1 hour.

3. FOR THE DIPPING SAUCE Whisk all ingredients together in serving bowl until smooth; set aside.

4. Set wire racks in 2 aluminum foil–lined rimmed baking sheets. Adjust oven rack 3 inches from broiler element and heat broiler. (If necessary, set upside-down rimmed baking sheet on oven rack to get closer to broiler element.) Pat beef dry with paper towels and weave onto wooden skewers, 1 piece per skewer. Lay skewers evenly on prepared racks with skewer ends facing center of sheet; cover skewer ends with strip of foil. Working with 1 sheet at a time, broil skewers until meat is browned, 8 to 10 minutes, flipping skewers halfway through broiling. Serve skewers with sauce.

TEST KITCHEN TIP
PREVENTING BURNT SKEWERS

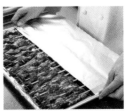

To prevent skewers from burning, use narrow strip of aluminum foil to cover exposed portion of skewers. Secure foil by crimping tightly at edges.

Oven-Baked Buffalo Wings

Serves 6 to 8

✓ **WHY THIS RECIPE WORKS** For this barroom classic, we set out to ditch the deep-fryer but still turn out wings with crunchy exteriors covered in a flavorful, spicy, paleo-friendly sauce. Patting the wings dry with paper towels helped to create a dry surface that crisped easily when roasted in a superhot oven; baking the wings on a wire rack let the rendered fat drip away. A quick stint under the broiler crisped the skin even further and ensured a flavorful char. As for the sauce, we used classic Frank's RedHot as our base. A spoonful of honey provided depth and mild sweetness, while ghee, rather than butter, added richness to our oven-baked Buffalo wings. We found that the flavor of Frank's RedHot Original Cayenne Pepper Sauce was crucial to the flavor of this dish; we don't suggest using another hot sauce here. If you buy chicken wings that are already split, with the tips removed, you will need only 3½ pounds.

4 pounds chicken wings, halved at joint and wingtips removed, trimmed
2 teaspoons kosher salt
½ cup hot sauce
¼ cup ghee, melted
1 tablespoon honey

1. Adjust oven rack to middle position and heat oven to 475 degrees. Set wire rack in aluminum foil–lined rimmed baking sheet. Pat wings dry with paper towels, then toss with salt. Arrange wings in single layer on prepared rack. Bake wings until golden on both sides, 45 minutes to 1 hour, flipping wings and rotating sheet halfway through baking.

2. Remove wings from oven. Adjust oven rack 6 inches from broiler element and heat broiler. Broil wings until golden brown on both sides, 6 to 8 minutes, flipping wings halfway through broiling.

3. Whisk hot sauce, melted ghee, and honey together in large bowl. Add wings to sauce and toss to coat. Serve.

VARIATION

Oven-Baked Honey-Mustard Wings

Substitute 6 tablespoons Dijon mustard for hot sauce and increase honey to 3 tablespoons.

TEST KITCHEN TIP **CUTTING UP CHICKEN WINGS**

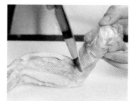

1. Using chef's knife, cut through joint between drumette and wingette.

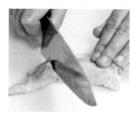

2. Cut off and discard wing tip.

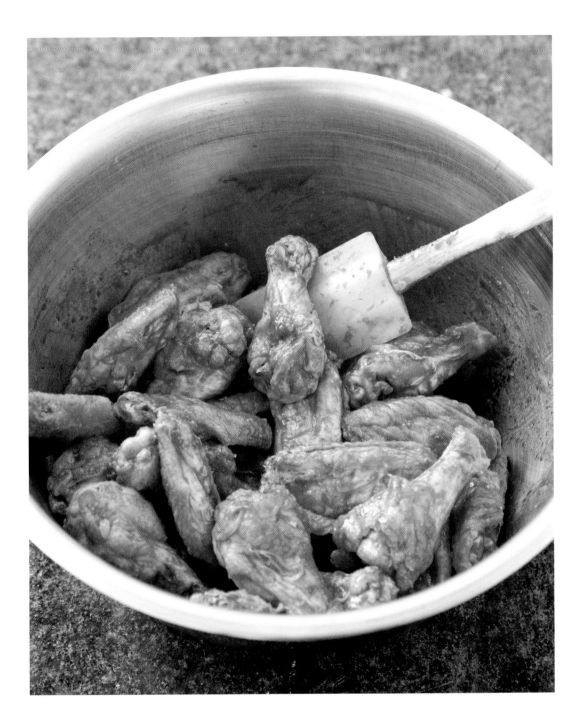

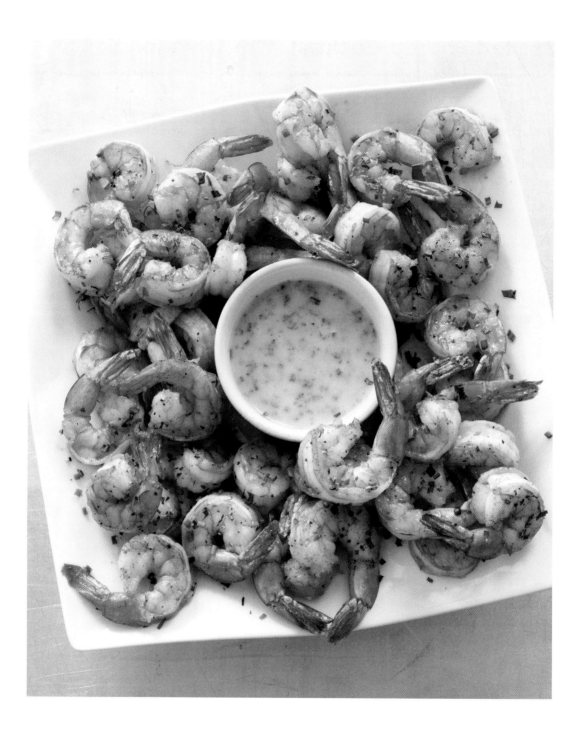

Broiled Shrimp Cocktail with Tarragon Sauce

Serves 10 to 12

☑ **WHY THIS RECIPE WORKS** For the easiest-ever version of shrimp cocktail, we bypassed the traditional method of poaching the shrimp in a work-intensive broth known as a court bouillon, and instead put the high heat of the broiler to work. A simple rub of salt, pepper, coriander, and cayenne infused the shrimp with flavor, while a little paleo-friendly coconut sugar helped the shrimp caramelize quickly under the broiler. Instead of a traditional cocktail sauce, we paired the shrimp with a creamy homemade aïoli. Chives provided a mild onion flavor, and lemon juice and fresh tarragon contributed brightness. Other fresh herbs such as dill, basil, or cilantro can be substituted for the tarragon.

SAUCE

- 6 tablespoons coconut oil, melted
- 6 tablespoons extra-virgin olive oil
- 4 teaspoons lemon juice
- 1 tablespoon water, plus extra as needed
- 1 large egg yolk
- 1 teaspoon Dijon mustard
- ½ teaspoon honey
  Kosher salt and pepper
- 3 tablespoons minced fresh tarragon
- 2 tablespoons minced fresh chives

SHRIMP

- 2 tablespoons extra-virgin olive oil
- ¾ teaspoon ground coriander
- ¾ teaspoon kosher salt
- ¼ teaspoon pepper
- ½ teaspoon coconut sugar
- ⅛ teaspoon cayenne pepper
- 2 pounds extra-large shrimp (21 to 25 per pound), peeled and deveined
- 1 tablespoon minced fresh chives
- 1 teaspoon minced fresh tarragon

1. FOR THE SAUCE Combine melted coconut oil and olive oil in liquid measuring cup. Whisk lemon juice, water, egg yolk, mustard, honey, ¾ teaspoon salt, and ¼ teaspoon pepper together in large bowl until thoroughly combined. Whisking constantly, slowly drizzle oil into egg mixture. If pools of oil gather on surface as you whisk, stop addition of oil and whisk mixture until well combined, then resume whisking in oil in slow stream. Sauce should be thick and glossy with no pools of oil on its surface. Adjust sauce consistency with extra water as needed. Stir in tarragon and chives and season with salt and pepper to taste.

2. FOR THE SHRIMP Adjust oven rack 3 inches from broiler element and heat broiler. (If necessary, set upside-down rimmed baking sheet on oven rack to get closer to broiler element.) Combine oil, coriander, salt, pepper, sugar, and cayenne in large bowl. Pat shrimp dry with paper towels, add to spice mixture, and toss until evenly coated.

3. Spread shrimp in single layer on rimmed baking sheet. Broil shrimp until opaque and edges begin to brown, about 4 minutes. Transfer shrimp to serving platter and sprinkle with chives and tarragon. Serve shrimp with sauce.

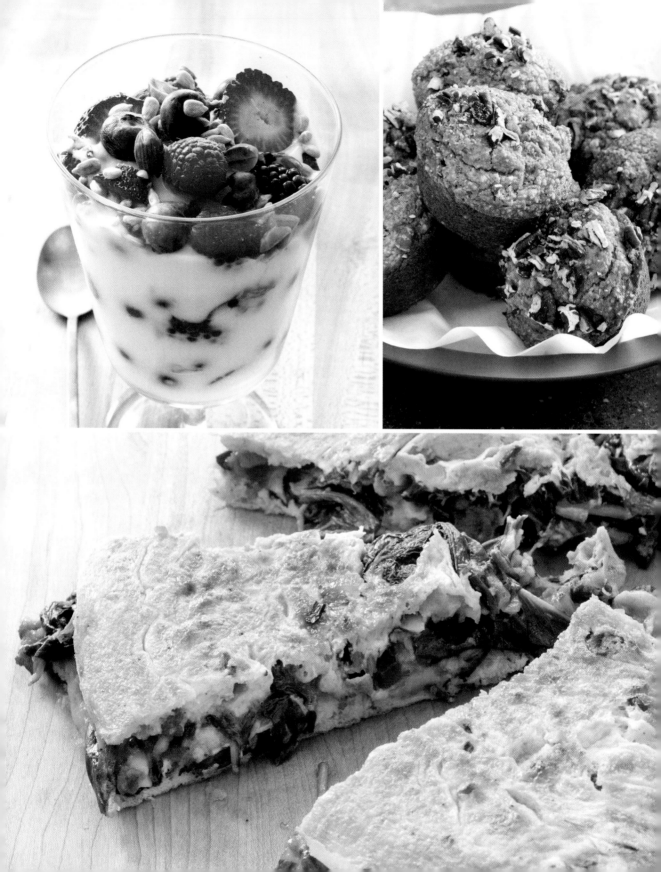

BREAKFAST FAVORITES

CHAPTER 2

Sweet Potato and Celery Root Hash with Fried Eggs

Serves 4

✔ **WHY THIS RECIPE WORKS** White potatoes are a staple of classic hash, but they're not allowed on the paleo diet. We set out to create a paleo hash with all the crispy, flavorful appeal of traditional versions. Our first move was to swap out the regular spuds for sweet potatoes. Unfortunately, our first attempts resulted in a very soft, mushy hash—sweet potatoes don't boast the same starchiness as russets, so they don't retain their shape as well once cooked. We got better results by adding some celery root to the sweet potatoes; not only did the celery root offer good textural contrast, but its earthy flavor was also a perfect complement to the sweet potatoes. To speed things up, we parcooked the veggies in the microwave until tender and then moved them to the skillet to brown and crisp. Smoky bacon added depth of flavor, and we used the bacon fat to cook our hash. A diced Golden Delicious apple added a hint of sweetness; as it cooked, it broke down and helped bind the hash together. We rounded out the flavor of the hash with onion, thyme, and a sprinkling of fresh chives. To make our hash a hearty meal, we fried some eggs in the same skillet we used to cook the hash. The tender whites and rich yolks paired perfectly with the earthy, comforting flavors in the hash. If you notice that the hash isn't getting brown in step 3, turn up the heat. You can also use a well-seasoned cast-iron skillet here; however, the eggs may stick slightly.

1   **pound sweet potatoes, unpeeled, cut into ½-inch pieces**
½   **celery root (7 ounces), peeled and cut into ½-inch pieces**
3   **tablespoons ghee, melted**
     Kosher salt and pepper
4   **slices bacon, chopped**
1   **onion, chopped fine**
1   **Golden Delicious apple, peeled, cored, and cut into ½-inch pieces**
1   **teaspoon minced fresh thyme or ¼ teaspoon dried**
8   **large eggs**
1   **tablespoon minced fresh chives**

1. Toss sweet potatoes, celery root, 1 tablespoon melted ghee, 1 teaspoon salt, and ¼ teaspoon pepper together in bowl. Cover and microwave until vegetables begin to soften, 5 to 8 minutes, stirring halfway through microwaving; drain vegetables.

2. Cook bacon in 12-inch nonstick skillet over medium heat until crisp, 5 to 7 minutes. Stir in onion and apple and cook until softened and lightly browned, about 8 minutes. Stir in thyme and microwaved vegetables.

3. Using back of spatula, gently pack hash into skillet and cook undisturbed for 2 minutes. Flip hash, 1 portion at a time, and lightly repack into skillet. Repeat flipping process every few minutes until hash is well browned, 6 to 8 minutes. Season with salt and pepper to taste. Transfer hash to bowl and cover to keep warm.

4. Wipe skillet clean with paper towels. Crack eggs into 2 small bowls (4 eggs per bowl) and season with salt and pepper. Heat remaining 2 tablespoons melted ghee in now-empty skillet over medium heat until shimmering. Working quickly, pour 1 bowl of eggs into 1 side of skillet and second bowl of eggs into other side. Cover and cook for 2 minutes.

5. Remove skillet from heat and let stand, covered, for about 2 minutes for runny yolks (white around edge of yolk will be barely opaque), about 3 minutes for soft but set yolks, and about 4 minutes for medium-set yolks. Divide hash onto warm plates. Separate eggs and slide on top of hash. Sprinkle with chives and serve immediately.

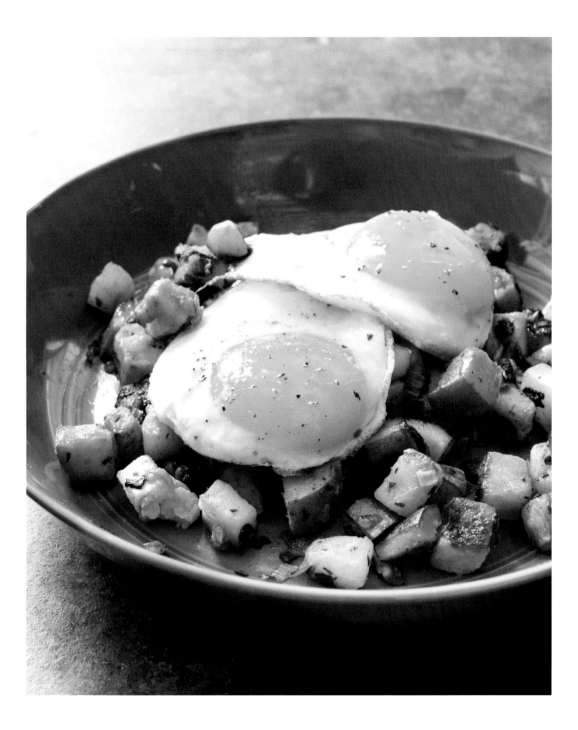

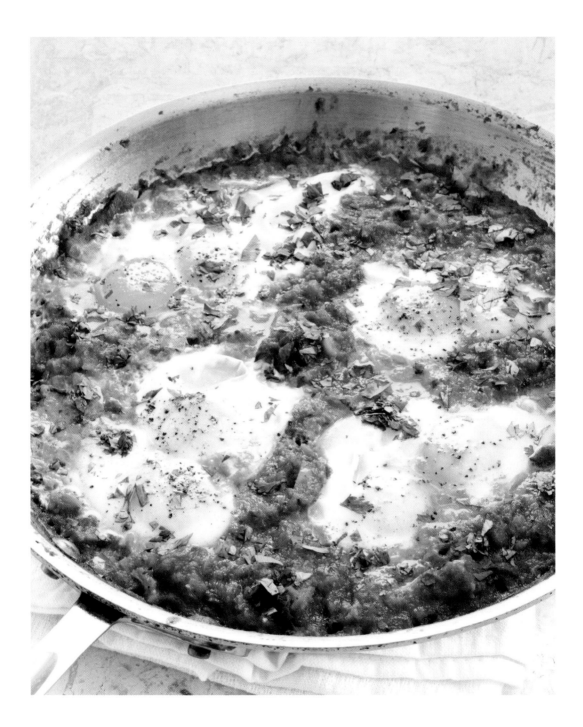

Poached Eggs in Spicy Tomato Sauce

Serves 4

WHY THIS RECIPE WORKS *Shakshuka*, a savory dish of eggs poached in a spicy tomato-pepper sauce, is a classic Tunisian breakfast dish. However, many recipes call for canned tomatoes and jarred piquillo peppers, both of which often contain ingredients that aren't paleo-friendly. We set out to create a version with the perfect balance of piquancy, acidity, richness, and sweetness—without the added sugar or preservatives. We started with fresh tomatoes and broiled them to give the backbone of our sauce a deep, roasted flavor. Roasting the onions with the tomatoes browned them and brought out their sweetness beautifully. Next, we needed to choose the right pepper to star in this dish; we landed on a combination of fresh yellow bell peppers and roasted red bell peppers, which created a vibrant, multidimensional sauce. Pureeing a portion of the sauce gave it a silky texture and helped to meld all the flavors together. Finally, we poached the eggs by simply nestling them into indentations we made in the sauce. A sprinkling of bright cilantro provided freshness and balance.

2	tomatoes, cored and halved
2	onions, chopped
3	tablespoons extra-virgin olive oil
2	yellow bell peppers, stemmed, seeded, and cut into ¼-inch pieces
4	garlic cloves, minced
2	teaspoons tomato paste
	Kosher salt and pepper
1	teaspoon ground cumin
1	teaspoon ground turmeric
⅛	teaspoon cayenne pepper
1½	cups jarred roasted red peppers, chopped coarse
½	cup water
2	bay leaves
⅓	cup chopped fresh cilantro
8	large eggs

1. Adjust oven rack 6 inches from broiler element and heat broiler. Toss tomatoes and onions with 1 tablespoon oil and spread onto aluminum foil–lined rimmed baking sheet; arrange tomatoes cut side down. Broil vegetables until softened and tomato skins are well charred, 8 to 10 minutes, rotating sheet halfway through broiling. Transfer vegetables to food processor and pulse until coarsely chopped, about 5 pulses.

2. Heat remaining 2 tablespoons oil in 12-inch skillet over medium heat until shimmering. Add bell peppers and cook until softened and lightly browned, 8 to 10 minutes. Stir in garlic, tomato paste, 2 teaspoons salt, ¼ teaspoon pepper, cumin, turmeric, and cayenne. Cook, stirring frequently, until tomato paste begins to darken, about 3 minutes.

3. Stir in processed tomato mixture, red peppers, water, and bay leaves. Bring to simmer and cook, stirring occasionally, until sauce is slightly thickened, about 10 minutes.

4. Off heat, discard bay leaves and stir in ¼ cup cilantro. Transfer 2 cups sauce to now-empty processor and process until smooth, about 60 seconds. Return puree to skillet and bring sauce to simmer over medium-low heat.

5. Off heat, make 4 shallow indentations (about 3 inches wide) in surface of sauce using back of spoon. Crack 2 eggs into each indentation and season eggs with salt and pepper. Cover and cook over medium-low heat until egg whites are just set and yolks are still runny, 5 to 10 minutes. Sprinkle with remaining cilantro and serve immediately.

Scrambled Eggs with Easy Homemade Sausage and Bell Pepper

Serves 4 to 6

☑ **WHY THIS RECIPE WORKS** Great scrambled eggs should be fluffy, light, and creamy, but achieving this while keeping the recipe paleo-friendly can be a challenge. Most scrambled egg recipes call for milk or cream, and there's an important reason: Dairy contains fat (which helps to keep the eggs tender) and water (which converts to steam and makes the eggs fluffier). Incorporating water into our eggs was easy, but we needed a replacement for the milk fat to ensure tender eggs. The solution turned out to be very simple: Since we were already using ghee to cook our eggs, we increased the amount by a couple of tablespoons. As we stirred and folded the mixture, the ghee became incorporated into the eggs and kept them perfectly tender. Next, we wanted to add some hearty meat and vegetables to our scramble. Since most store-bought sausage contains added sugar or preservatives, we made a quick homemade version with just ground pork and spices. To preserve the texture of the eggs, we sautéed the meat and vegetables first to eliminate as much moisture as possible. Once the eggs were cooked, we folded everything together for a fluffy and flavorful scramble. You can also use a well-seasoned cast-iron skillet here; however, the eggs may stick slightly.

- 8 ounces ground pork
- 1 garlic clove, minced
- 1 teaspoon minced fresh thyme or ¼ teaspoon dried
- 1 teaspoon minced fresh sage or ¼ teaspoon dried
  Kosher salt and pepper
  Pinch red pepper flakes
- 12 large eggs
- 2 tablespoons water
- 3 tablespoons ghee
- 1 red bell pepper, stemmed, seeded, and cut into ½-inch pieces
- 3 scallions, white and green parts separated and sliced thin

1. Mix ground pork, garlic, thyme, sage, ½ teaspoon pepper, ¼ teaspoon salt, and pepper flakes in bowl until thoroughly combined. In separate bowl, beat eggs, water, 1 teaspoon salt, and ¼ teaspoon pepper with fork until thoroughly combined and mixture is pure yellow; do not overbeat.

2. Heat 1 tablespoon ghee in 12-inch nonstick skillet over medium heat until shimmering. Add bell pepper and scallion whites and cook until softened and lightly browned, 5 to 7 minutes. Add pork mixture and cook, breaking up meat with wooden spoon, until no longer pink, about 3 minutes; transfer to bowl.

3. Wipe skillet clean with paper towels. Heat remaining 2 tablespoons ghee in now-empty skillet over medium heat until shimmering, swirling to coat skillet. Add egg mixture and, using heat-resistant rubber spatula, constantly and firmly scrape along bottom and sides of skillet until eggs begin to clump and spatula leaves trail on bottom of skillet, 1½ to 2½ minutes.

4. Reduce heat to low and gently but constantly fold eggs until clumped and slightly wet, 30 to 60 seconds. Off heat, gently fold in sausage mixture; if eggs are still underdone, return skillet to medium heat for no longer than 30 seconds. Sprinkle with scallion greens and season with salt and pepper to taste. Serve immediately.

VARIATION

Scrambled Eggs with Easy Homemade Sausage and Asparagus
Omit scallions. Substitute 8 ounces asparagus, trimmed and cut on bias into ½-inch lengths, for bell pepper. Sprinkle with 1 tablespoon chopped fresh parsley before serving.

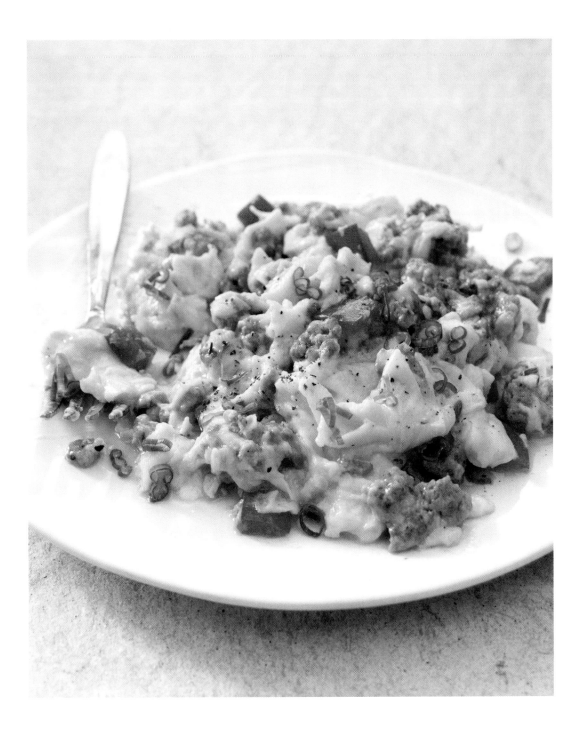

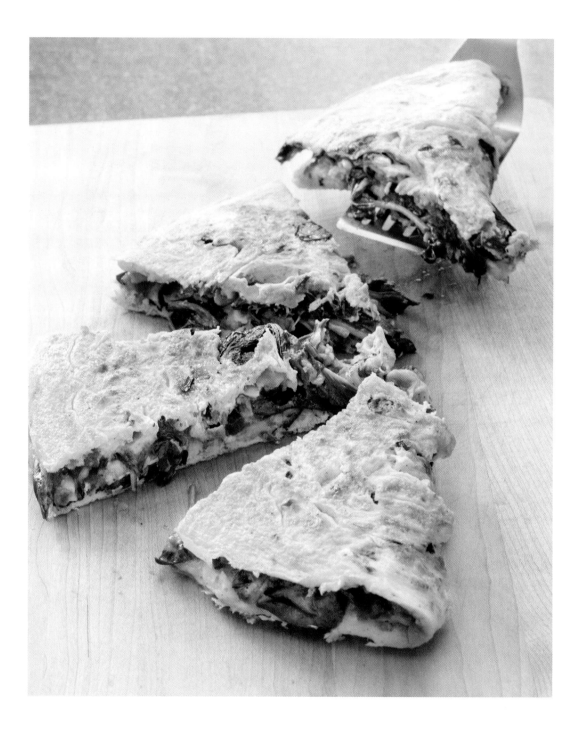

Family-Size Omelet with Bacon and Spinach

Serves 4

👌 **WHY THIS RECIPE WORKS** An omelet is a great breakfast or brunch dish, but cooking omelets one at a time for more than a couple of people is just not practical. We wanted to find a way to make an omelet that was big enough to serve four people and that would feature tender eggs and a rich, meaty filling. We knew we wanted to use two eggs and two slices of bacon per serving, plus a variety of sautéed vegetables. But flipping a huge eight-egg omelet was a nonstarter; we needed to find a way to cook the top of the omelet at the same time as the bottom. We first tried cooking the omelet longer over lower heat, but this resulted in an unpleasant texture. Next, we employed a stirring and tilting technique to help the uncooked eggs reach the bottom of the skillet. This worked better, but we were still having trouble getting the top of the omelet to set before the bottom turned tough. To solve this problem, we covered the pan once the bottom of the omelet was set but the top was still runny. The lid trapped heat and moisture, which steamed the top of the omelet without overcooking the rest. You can also use a well-seasoned cast-iron skillet here; however, the eggs may stick slightly.

8   **large eggs**
½   **teaspoon kosher salt**
¼   **teaspoon pepper**
8   **slices bacon, chopped fine**
1   **onion, chopped fine**
4   **ounces (4 cups) baby spinach**

1. Beat eggs, salt, and pepper with fork in bowl until thoroughly combined and mixture is pure yellow; do not overbeat. Cook bacon in 12-inch nonstick skillet over medium heat until crisp, 5 to 7 minutes. Using slotted spoon, transfer bacon to paper towel–lined plate.

2. Pour off all but 2 tablespoons fat from skillet, add onion, and cook over medium heat until softened, about 5 minutes. Stir in spinach, 1 handful at a time, and cook until wilted, about 1 minute.

3. Add egg mixture and crisp bacon to skillet and cook, stirring gently in circular motion, until mixture is slightly thickened, about 1 minute. Using heat-resistant rubber spatula, gently pull cooked eggs back from edge of skillet and tilt skillet, allowing any uncooked egg to run to cleared edge of skillet. Repeat this process, working your way around skillet, until bottom of omelet is just set but top is still runny, about 1 minute. Cover skillet, reduce heat to low, and cook until top of omelet begins to set but is still moist, about 5 minutes.

4. Using rubber spatula, slide half of omelet onto serving platter, then tilt skillet so remaining omelet flips over onto itself. Cut into wedges and serve immediately.

VARIATION

Family-Size Omelet with Bacon, Tomato, and Bell Pepper

Omit spinach. Add 1 finely chopped green bell pepper and 1 finely chopped tomato to skillet with onion and cook until vegetables are softened, about 8 minutes. Stir in 4 minced garlic cloves and cook until fragrant, about 30 seconds. Add egg mixture and crisp bacon and continue to cook omelet as directed.

TEST KITCHEN TIP
MAKING A FAMILY-SIZE OMELET

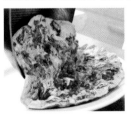 Use rubber spatula to loosen omelet. Slide half of omelet onto serving platter, then tilt skillet so remaining omelet flips over onto itself to make half-moon shape.

Leek and Prosciutto Frittata

Serves 6

✓ WHY THIS RECIPE WORKS For a hearty frittata to serve a crowd, we started with a dozen eggs and a hefty amount of leeks and prosciutto. To ensure that our frittata didn't turn out soggy, we precooked the leeks to drive off excess moisture before adding the prosciutto and eggs to the pan. Using a generous amount of ghee provided some richness and helped to keep the eggs tender as they cooked. Although frittatas often feature copious amounts of cheese, we found that the savory prosciutto, aromatic leeks, and earthy basil more than compensated for it—tasters didn't miss the cheese at all. Because broilers vary in intensity, watch the frittata carefully as it cooks. You can also use a well-seasoned cast-iron skillet here; however, the eggs may stick slightly.

12	large eggs
2	tablespoons water
	Kosher salt and pepper
4	ounces thinly sliced prosciutto, cut into ½-inch pieces
¼	cup chopped fresh basil or parsley
3	tablespoons ghee
1	pound leeks, white and light green parts only, halved lengthwise, sliced thin, and washed thoroughly

1. Adjust oven rack 6 inches from broiler element and heat broiler. Beat eggs, water, ½ teaspoon salt, and ¼ teaspoon pepper with fork in bowl until thoroughly combined and mixture is pure yellow; do not overbeat. Stir in prosciutto and basil.

2. Melt ghee in 10-inch ovensafe nonstick skillet over low heat. Add leeks and ½ teaspoon salt, cover, and cook, stirring occasionally, until softened, 8 to 10 minutes.

3. Add egg mixture and, using heat-resistant rubber spatula, constantly and firmly scrape along bottom and sides of skillet until large curds form and spatula leaves trail on bottom of skillet but eggs are still very wet, about 2 minutes. Shake skillet to distribute eggs evenly and continue to cook, without stirring, for 30 seconds to let bottom set.

4. Transfer skillet to oven and broil until frittata has risen and surface is puffed and spotty brown, 3 to 4 minutes; when cut into with paring knife, eggs should be slightly wet and runny.

5. Let frittata rest for 5 minutes. Carefully run spatula around skillet edge to loosen frittata, then slide it out onto serving platter. Cut frittata into wedges and serve warm or at room temperature.

TEST KITCHEN TIP **PREPARING LEEKS**

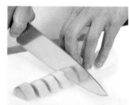

1. Trim and discard root end and dark green leaves. Cut trimmed leek in half lengthwise, then slice it crosswise as directed in recipe.

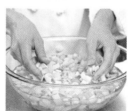

2. Submerge cut leeks in bowl of water and rinse thoroughly to remove dirt and sand. Drain washed leeks.

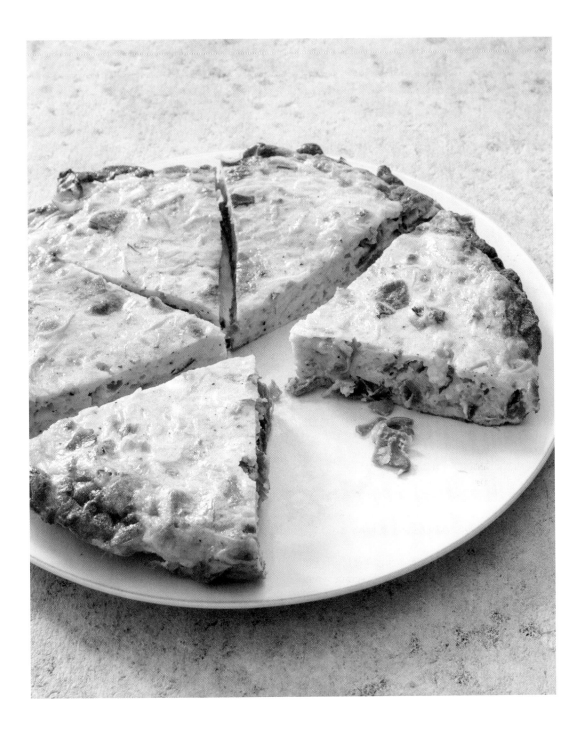

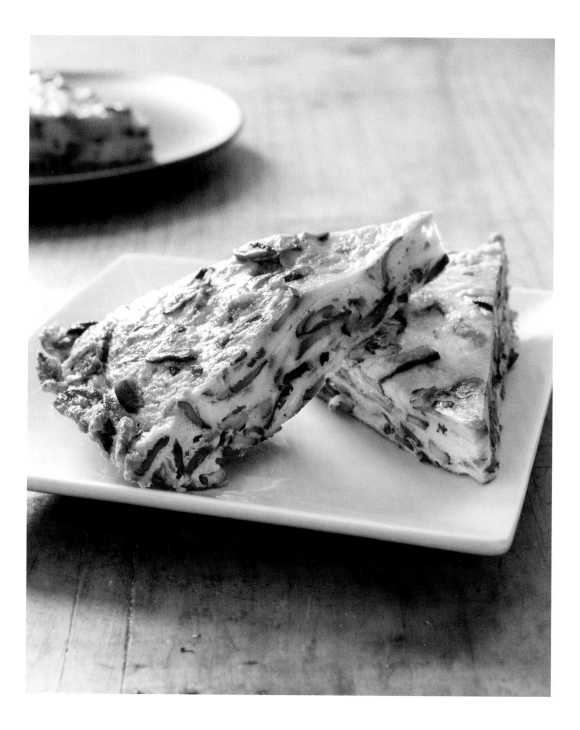

Wild Mushroom Frittata

Serves 6

✓ WHY THIS RECIPE WORKS We wanted a recipe for a meatless frittata that would still be substantial and flavorful. First, we needed to choose our stir-ins. Earthy, hearty mushrooms were a good choice; we used a generous amount to ensure mushroom flavor in every bite. Using two types of mushrooms, earthy cremini and smoky shiitakes, provided multidimensional flavor and textural contrast. We cooked the mushrooms before adding them to the eggs, which rid them of excess moisture and allowed them to brown nicely. Cooking an onion along with the mushrooms contributed background sweetness, while some minced garlic provided more aromatic depth. A brief stint under the broiler helped our frittata to puff up and finish cooking. Because broilers vary in intensity, watch the frittata carefully as it cooks. You can also use a well-seasoned cast-iron skillet here; however, the eggs may stick slightly.

12   **large eggs**

2   **tablespoons water**

    Kosher salt and pepper

¼   **cup minced fresh chives**

3   **tablespoons extra-virgin olive oil**

12   **ounces cremini mushrooms, trimmed and sliced thin**

8   **ounces shiitake mushrooms, stemmed, halved, and sliced thin**

1   **onion, chopped fine**

2   **garlic cloves, minced**

1. Adjust oven rack 6 inches from broiler element and heat broiler. Beat eggs, water, ½ teaspoon salt, and ¼ teaspoon pepper with fork in bowl until thoroughly combined and mixture is pure yellow; do not overbeat. Stir in chives.

2. Heat oil in 10-inch ovensafe nonstick skillet over medium-high heat until shimmering. Add cremini mushrooms, shiitake mushrooms, onion, and 1 teaspoon salt. Cover and cook until mushrooms have released their liquid, about 5 minutes. Uncover and continue to cook, stirring occasionally, until vegetables are dry and lightly browned, 5 to 10 minutes. Stir in garlic and cook until fragrant, about 30 seconds.

3. Add egg mixture and, using heat-resistant rubber spatula, constantly and firmly scrape along bottom and sides of skillet until large curds form and spatula leaves trail on bottom of skillet, but eggs are still very wet, about 2 minutes. Shake skillet to distribute eggs evenly and continue to cook, without stirring, for 30 seconds to let bottom set.

4. Transfer skillet to oven and broil until frittata has risen and surface is puffed and spotty brown, 3 to 4 minutes; when cut into with paring knife, eggs should be slightly wet and runny.

5. Let frittata rest for 5 minutes. Carefully run spatula around skillet edge to loosen frittata, then slide it out onto serving platter. Cut frittata into wedges and serve warm or at room temperature.

TEST KITCHEN TIP
REMOVING FRITTATA FROM SKILLET

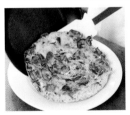

Run spatula around skillet edge to loosen frittata, then carefully slide it out onto serving platter.

Spiced Breakfast Casserole with Tomatoes and Swiss Chard

Serves 4 to 6

✓ **WHY THIS RECIPE WORKS** Our ideal egg casserole had to have a creamy, custardy egg base and a healthy dose of perfectly cooked vegetables. We knew we would have to make our custard without dairy, so we set out to find a substitute. We first tried mixing coconut and almond flours with water and whipping the mixtures into our eggs, but the resulting casseroles turned out spongy or grainy. Next we decided to try incorporating a paste made from softened and pureed cashews, which had made a perfect creamy element in recipes like our Spinach and Bacon–Stuffed Mushrooms (page 48). We tested varying amounts of the cashew puree and found that just ½ cup provided the perfect amount of creaminess and structure. Now our custard-like base could easily support an abundance of hearty vegetables. We packed our casserole with plump, sweet pan-roasted cherry tomatoes and earthy Swiss chard, and added more flavor with onion, garlic, and curry powder for deep, nutty richness. Chicken broth also added a savory note to the dish that complemented the flavors better than water. To ensure that our casserole was fully cooked but not overdone, we baked it until the center was fully puffed and just set, with a lightly browned top. You can substitute an equal amount of slivered almonds for the cashews. We prefer to use homemade chicken broth; however, you can substitute your favorite store-bought brand.

½ cup raw cashews

3 tablespoons ghee, melted

1 large onion, chopped

Kosher salt and pepper

1 pound cherry tomatoes

2 garlic cloves, minced

2 teaspoons curry powder

1 pound Swiss chard, stemmed and cut into ½-inch pieces

½ cup Paleo Chicken Broth (page 16)

8 large eggs

1. Bring 4 cups water to boil in medium saucepan over medium-high heat. Add cashews and cook until softened, about 15 minutes. Drain and rinse well.

2. Adjust oven rack to middle position and heat oven to 350 degrees. Grease 8-inch square baking dish. Heat 1 tablespoon melted ghee in 12-inch skillet over medium heat until shimmering. Add onion, ½ teaspoon salt, and ¼ teaspoon pepper and cook until softened, about 5 minutes. Add tomatoes and cook until tomatoes begin to break down and release their liquid, 3 to 5 minutes; transfer to prepared dish.

3. Wipe skillet clean with paper towels. Heat 1 tablespoon melted ghee in now-empty skillet over medium-high heat until shimmering. Add garlic and curry powder and cook until fragrant, about 30 seconds. Stir in chard, cover, and cook until wilted but still bright green, about 2 minutes. Uncover and continue to cook, stirring frequently, until chard is dry, about 1 minute. Spread chard evenly over tomato mixture in dish.

4. Process boiled cashews, ¼ cup broth, remaining 1 tablespoon melted ghee, and 1½ teaspoons salt in food processor until smooth, about 2 minutes, scraping down sides of bowl as needed. Add eggs and remaining ¼ cup broth and process until thoroughly combined, about 1 minute. Pour egg mixture over layered vegetables. Bake until casserole is risen, center is set but soft, and surface is lightly browned, 30 to 35 minutes, rotating dish halfway through baking. Let casserole rest for 5 minutes. Serve.

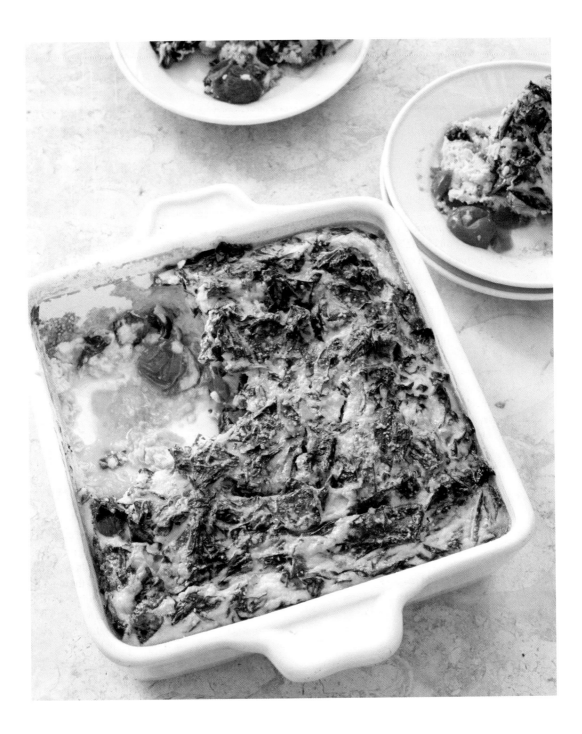

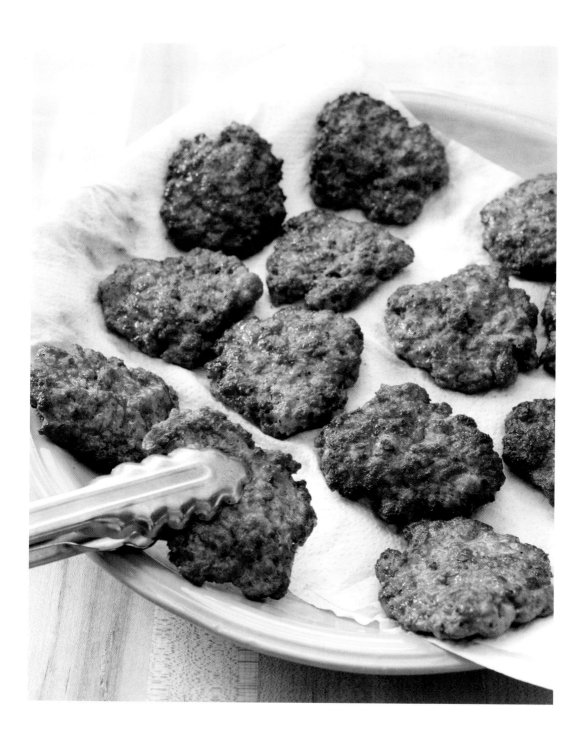

Homemade Breakfast Sausage

Makes 24 patties

✓ WHY THIS RECIPE WORKS Store-bought breakfast sausage patties are far from paleo-friendly; they usually contain added sugar, sodium, and preservatives. By making our own, we could ensure high-quality ingredients and great flavor. Since the pork would be playing a starring role, we skipped preground pork and opted to "grind" our own meat instead. To ensure that the meat was evenly ground but not pasty, we cut it into chunks, froze it until just firm, and then processed it in batches in a food processor. Many recipes for homemade sausage call for pork butt, a well-marbled, flavorful cut. However, the pork butts we found were inconsistent in their fat content, and roasts that were too lean produced tough, dry patties. To ensure the right ratio of meat to fat, we decided to fully trim the pork butt and then add in a measured amount of ghee. The melted ghee solidified as it hit the cold meat, creating small particles of rich, savory fat throughout the patties. Finally, we added classic breakfast sausage flavorings: garlic, dried sage and thyme, and cayenne for a touch of heat. A small amount of maple syrup rounded out the flavor of the patties. Pork butt roast is often labeled Boston butt in the supermarket. You should get 2½ to 2¾ pounds of trimmed pork from the pork butt.

1   **(3-pound) boneless pork butt roast, pulled apart at seams, trimmed and cut into ½-inch pieces**

½   **cup plus 1 tablespoon ghee, melted**

1½   **tablespoons maple syrup**

1   **tablespoon kosher salt**

2½   **teaspoons dried sage**

2   **teaspoons pepper**

1½   **teaspoons garlic powder**

1   **teaspoon dried thyme**

⅛   **teaspoon cayenne pepper**

1. Spread pork in single layer on rimmed baking sheet. Freeze meat until very firm and starting to harden around edges but still pliable, about 35 minutes.

2. Pulse one-quarter of meat in food processor until finely ground into 1/16-inch pieces, about 15 pulses, stopping and redistributing meat around bowl as necessary to ensure pork is evenly ground. Transfer meat to sheet and repeat grinding with remaining meat in 3 batches. Spread ground meat over sheet and inspect carefully, discarding any long strands of gristle or large chunks of hard meat or fat.

3. Combine ½ cup melted ghee, maple syrup, salt, sage, pepper, garlic powder, thyme, and cayenne in bowl. Drizzle ghee mixture over ground meat and gently toss with fork to combine. Divide meat evenly into 24 lightly packed balls, then gently flatten into ¼-inch-thick patties. (Patties can be refrigerated overnight or frozen for up to 1 month. To cook frozen patties, proceed with step 4, cooking patties for 7 to 9 minutes per side and adjusting heat as needed to prevent scorching.)

4. Heat 1 teaspoon melted ghee in 12-inch skillet over medium-high heat until just smoking. Place 8 patties in skillet and cook until well browned and cooked through, about 2 minutes per side. Transfer patties to paper towel–lined platter and tent loosely with aluminum foil. Wipe skillet clean with paper towels and repeat with remaining 2 teaspoons melted ghee and remaining 16 patties in 2 batches. Serve.

VARIATION

Homemade Apple-Fennel Breakfast Sausage

Substitute 2½ teaspoons ground fennel for sage. Sprinkle 1 peeled, cored, and grated Golden Delicious apple over ground meat before drizzling with ghee mixture in step 3.

Blueberry Muffins

Makes 12 muffins

✓ **WHY THIS RECIPE WORKS** Baking a great paleo muffin is a serious challenge, since traditional muffin recipes rely on wheat flour, sugar, and butter for structure and flavor. We set out to create a paleo-friendly recipe that would produce muffins with light, fluffy interiors and nicely browned, domed tops. Our first task was finding the right flours and starches to replace wheat flour. We chose neutral-flavored almond flour as our base, but its inability to absorb liquid meant that our muffins turned out dense and greasy. A small amount of coconut flour helped to absorb moisture and gave the muffins more structure, but they were still a bit heavy. Arrowroot flour lightened the texture considerably; combining the arrowroot with the liquid ingredients and letting the mixture rest for 30 minutes allowed the starch to fully hydrate and prevented a gritty texture in the muffins. To ensure that our muffins rose nicely, we put the stand mixer to work. While traditional muffins require gently folding the batter together, we used a stand mixer to incorporate air into the batter and lighten the mixture. A simple faux-streusel made with sliced almonds gave our muffins crunchy, attractive tops. If using frozen blueberries, rinse them gently after thawing to remove excess juice, then spread out on paper towels to absorb excess moisture before using. For more information on coconut sugar, see page 11.

¼	cup sliced almonds, toasted
2	tablespoons coconut sugar, plus ⅔ cup (3⅓ ounces)
1	tablespoon lemon zest plus 1 tablespoon juice
1	cup (4 ounces) arrowroot flour
3	large eggs
½	cup water
3	tablespoons coconut oil, melted and cooled
1	tablespoon vanilla extract
1	teaspoon kosher salt
3	cups (9 ounces) almond flour
3	tablespoons coconut flour
1½	teaspoons baking soda
¼	teaspoon cream of tartar
⅛	teaspoon ground nutmeg
7½	ounces (1½ cups) fresh or thawed frozen blueberries

1. Adjust oven rack to middle position and heat oven to 325 degrees. Grease 12-cup muffin tin. Combine almonds, 2 tablespoons sugar, and lemon zest in bowl; set aside.

2. Using stand mixer fitted with whisk, whip arrowroot flour, eggs, water, melted coconut oil, vanilla, salt, remaining ⅔ cup sugar, and lemon juice together on medium speed until thoroughly combined, about 1 minute. Let mixture rest in mixer bowl for 30 minutes.

3. Whisk almond flour, coconut flour, baking soda, cream of tartar, and nutmeg together in bowl. With mixer set to low speed, add flour mixture and mix until incorporated, about 30 seconds. Increase speed to high and whip batter until light and fluffy, about 1 minute, scraping down sides of bowl as needed. Using rubber spatula, fold in blueberries.

4. Divide batter evenly among prepared muffin cups (cups will be filled to top) and sprinkle with almond mixture. Bake until muffins are golden brown and toothpick inserted in center comes out clean, about 25 minutes, rotating muffin tin halfway through baking.

5. Let muffins cool in muffin tin for 10 minutes, then transfer to wire rack and let cool for 15 minutes before serving. (Muffins are best eaten warm on day they are made, but they can be cooled and immediately transferred to zipper-lock bag and stored at room temperature for up to 1 day. To serve, warm in 300-degree oven for 10 minutes. Muffins can also be wrapped individually in plastic wrap, transferred to zipper-lock bag, and frozen for up to 3 weeks. To serve, remove plastic and microwave muffin for 20 to 30 seconds, then warm in 350-degree oven for 10 minutes.)

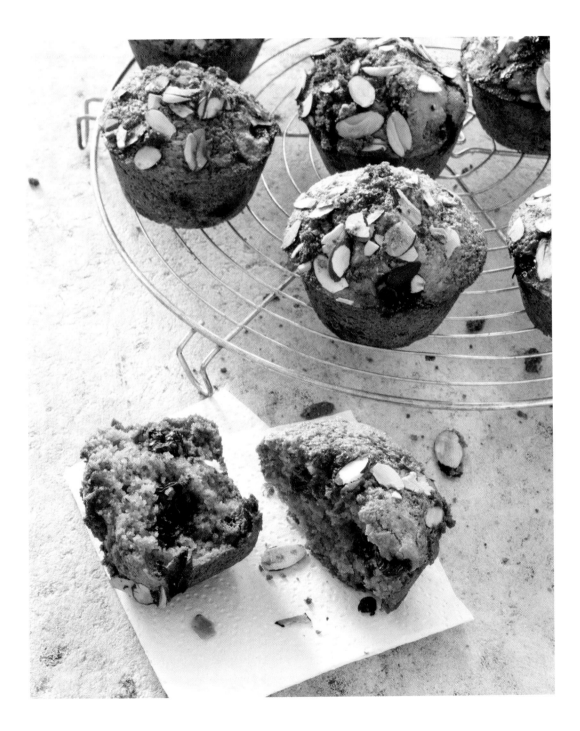

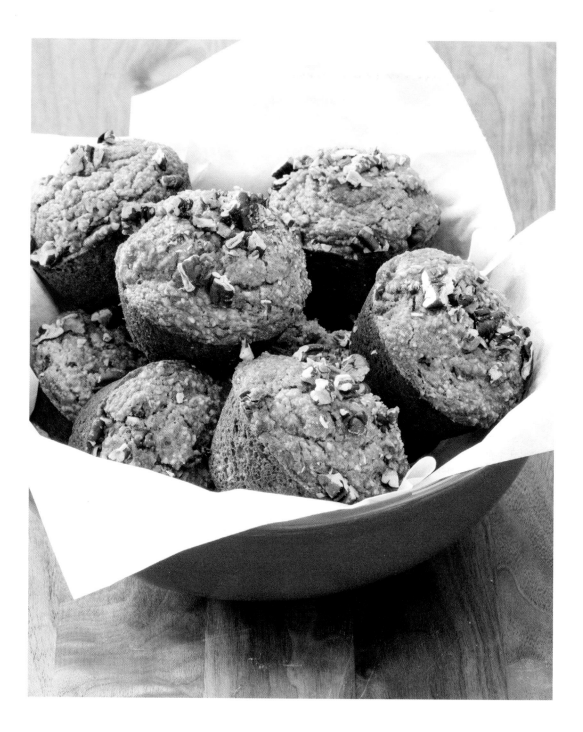

Applesauce-Spice Muffins

Makes 12 muffins

✓ **WHY THIS RECIPE WORKS** Building on the success of our Blueberry Muffins (page 74), we decided to create a second muffin with a different flavor profile. We chose apple, hoping that we could use unsweetened applesauce as our liquid and replace the blueberries with juicy chunks of apple. In an initial test, we found that applesauce worked well: It provided the right amount of moisture as well as some flavor and sweetness. But the chunks of apple produced too much steam as they baked, and turned the interior of the muffins gummy. Instead, we turned to raisins, which didn't add any moisture but provided pleasant bursts of sweetness in the finished muffins. Next, we turned our focus to leavening agents. In our Blueberry Muffins, we used cream of tartar, which is acidic, to activate the baking soda, and found that this strategy worked perfectly in these muffins as well. To get the sweetness of our muffins just right, we tested honey, maple syrup, and coconut sugar, a natural sugar made from the sap of the coconut plant. Although honey gave the muffins a beautiful golden color, tasters found the flavor overpowering. Maple syrup tasted better, but muffins made with it didn't brown at all, leaving us with pale, unattractive muffins. In the end, coconut sugar gave the muffins just the right amount of sweetness as well as nicely browned exteriors. For more information on coconut sugar, see page 11.

1⅓	cups unsweetened applesauce
1	cup (4 ounces) arrowroot flour
3	large eggs
⅓	cup (1⅔ ounces) coconut sugar
3	tablespoons coconut oil, melted and cooled
1¼	teaspoons vanilla extract
1	teaspoon kosher salt
3	cups (9 ounces) almond flour
3	tablespoons coconut flour
1½	teaspoons baking soda
1	teaspoon ground cinnamon
1	teaspoon ground ginger
¾	teaspoon ground cardamom
¼	teaspoon cream of tartar
1	cup raisins
⅓	cup pecans, toasted and chopped (optional)

1. Adjust oven rack to middle position and heat oven to 325 degrees. Grease 12-cup muffin tin.

2. Using stand mixer fitted with whisk, whip applesauce, arrowroot flour, eggs, sugar, melted coconut oil, vanilla, and salt on medium speed until thoroughly combined, about 1 minute. Let mixture rest in mixer bowl for 30 minutes.

3. Whisk almond flour, coconut flour, baking soda, cinnamon, ginger, cardamom, and cream of tartar together in bowl. With mixer set to low speed, add flour mixture and mix until incorporated, about 30 seconds. Increase speed to high and whip batter until light and fluffy, about 1 minute, scraping down sides of bowl as needed. Using rubber spatula, fold in raisins.

4. Divide batter evenly among prepared muffin cups (cups will be filled to top) and sprinkle with pecans, if using. Bake until muffins are golden brown and toothpick inserted in center comes out clean, about 25 minutes, rotating muffin tin halfway through baking.

5. Let muffins cool in muffin tin for 10 minutes, then transfer to wire rack and let cool for 15 minutes before serving. (Muffins are best eaten warm on day they are made, but they can be cooled and immediately transferred to zipper-lock bag and stored at room temperature for up to 1 day. To serve, warm in 300-degree oven for 10 minutes. Muffins can also be wrapped individually in plastic wrap, transferred to zipper-lock bag, and frozen for up to 3 weeks. To serve, remove plastic and microwave muffin for 20 to 30 seconds, then warm in 350-degree oven for 10 minutes.)

Pancakes

Serves 4 to 6

⊘ **WHY THIS RECIPE WORKS** Perfect pancakes should be fluffy, tender, lightly sweet, and simple to make. For a paleo recipe that would stand up to its traditional counterparts, we started by choosing the flours that would be the base of our recipe. We knew from previous testing that a combination of almond and arrowroot flours would give our pancakes volume and structure; we determined that a 5:1 ratio of almond to arrowroot worked best. Next, we focused our attention on achieving the fluffy, light texture that is characteristic of great pancakes. Some baking soda and cream of tartar provided good lift, but the batter needed an even bigger boost. Although an extra egg white helped, tasters thought the batter could be lighter still. The blender turned out to be the simple solution: We processed all of the liquid ingredients until the mixture was frothy, then added the dry ingredients and processed the batter for a minute longer. Mixing everything in the blender had multiple benefits: It streamlined the recipe, incorporated air into the batter to make fluffier pancakes, and ensured that the batter was perfectly smooth and pourable. To give our pancakes a hint of sweetness, we tried incorporating a little maple syrup since we'd likely be topping our pancakes with it anyway. Unfortunately, those pancakes cooked up with pale exteriors. Switching to honey gave our pancakes a beautiful golden hue and just enough sweetness, which we accented with a hint of vanilla extract. For our blueberry variation, we found that it worked better to stir the blueberries right into the batter; when we added them to the pancakes as they cooked, the berries left large craters in the pancakes. This recipe calls for a 12-inch nonstick skillet; however, a well-seasoned cast-iron skillet can be used instead.

⅔ cup water
2 large eggs plus 1 large white
¼ cup ghee, melted and cooled
2 tablespoons honey
1 teaspoon vanilla extract
2½ cups (7½ ounces) almond flour
½ cup (2 ounces) arrowroot flour
1 teaspoon cream of tartar
½ teaspoon baking soda
½ teaspoon kosher salt

1. Adjust oven rack to middle position and heat oven to 200 degrees. Grease wire rack set in rimmed baking sheet.

2. Process water, eggs and white, 3 tablespoons melted ghee, honey, and vanilla in blender until light and frothy, about 30 seconds. Add almond flour, arrowroot flour, cream of tartar, baking soda, and salt and process until thoroughly combined, about 1 minute.

3. Heat 1 teaspoon melted ghee in 12-inch nonstick skillet over medium-low heat until shimmering.

Using paper towels, carefully wipe out ghee, leaving thin film of ghee on bottom and sides of skillet. Using ¼ cup batter per pancake, portion batter into skillet in 3 places. Cook until edges are set and first side is golden, 2 to 4 minutes.

4. Flip pancakes and continue to cook until second side is golden, 2 to 3 minutes. Serve immediately or transfer to prepared rack and keep warm in oven. Repeat with remaining batter, using remaining 2 teaspoons melted ghee as necessary.

VARIATION

Blueberry Pancakes

Small, wild blueberries work best here because they allow the pancakes to cook through more evenly. Frozen blueberries can be substituted for fresh; thaw and rinse the berries gently to remove excess juice, then spread out on paper towels to absorb excess moisture before using.

After blending pancake batter, transfer to bowl and stir in 1 cup small blueberries; cook as directed.

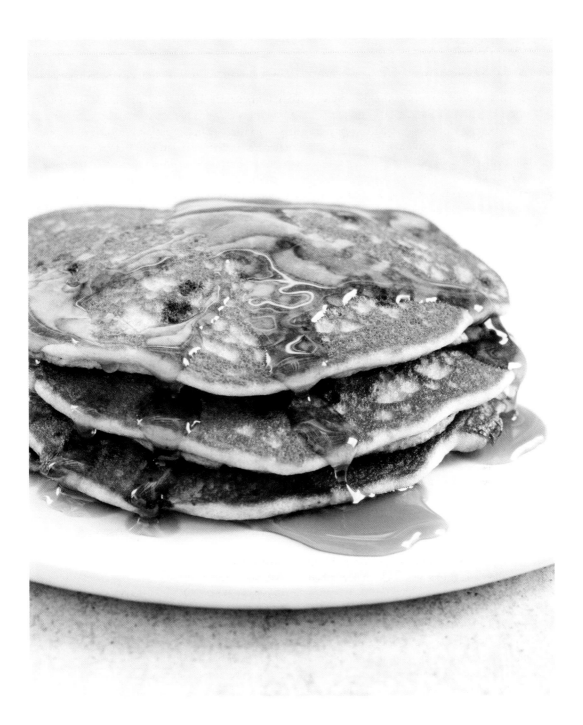

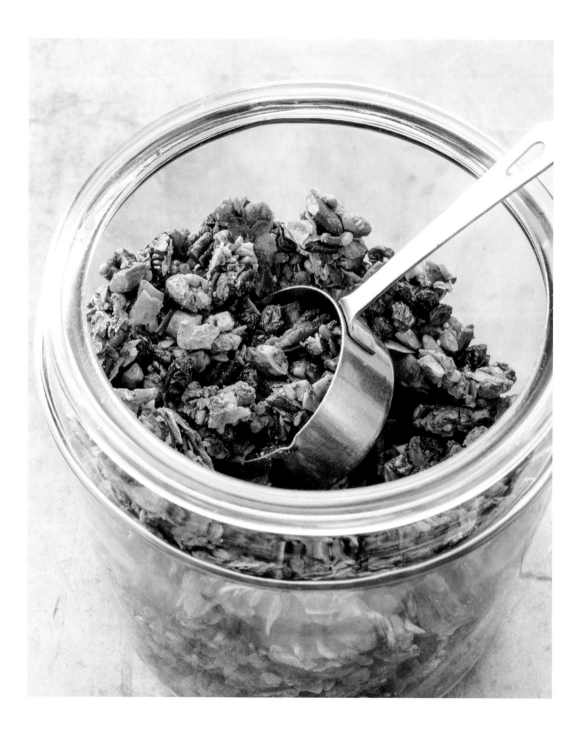

Nut and Seed Granola

Makes about 10 cups

✓ **WHY THIS RECIPE WORKS** Oats and sugar, key ingredients in most granolas, are not part of the paleo diet, so we set out to find a way to make crave-worthy granola without them. We replaced the oats with a combination of nuts and seeds, choosing different sizes and textures for lots of crunchy contrast. We also added unsweetened flaked coconut for its sweet, toasty crunch. To sweeten our granola without refined sugar, we tried combinations of maple syrup, coconut sugar, and honey; tasters preferred the clean-tasting sweetness of maple syrup. Since the nuts and coconut were high in fat, we found that just ¼ cup of coconut oil was enough to ensure that our granola crisped nicely as it baked. Although many paleo recipes call for processing some nuts and seeds into a mealy substance, or adding fruit puree or egg whites to hold the granola together, we found this step was unnecessary; the maple syrup and coconut oil provided the perfect amount of liquid "glue" to help bind the chunks of granola. When it came time to bake the mixture, we turned to a tried-and-true test kitchen method for making super-chunky granola: We used a sturdy spatula to press the mixture into a rimmed baking sheet, then baked it gently at 325 degrees without stirring. This produced granola "bark" that we could break into beautiful chunks of whatever size we wanted. All it needed now was some dried fruit, which we added at the very end so it would stay plump (it tended to turn leathery and overly sticky in the oven). Chopping the nuts by hand is our first choice for superior texture and crunch.

½	cup maple syrup
¼	cup coconut oil, melted
1	tablespoon vanilla extract
1½	teaspoons ground cinnamon
1	teaspoon ground ginger
1	teaspoon kosher salt
½	teaspoon pepper
½	teaspoon ground allspice
¼	teaspoon ground nutmeg
2	cups (10 ounces) whole almonds, chopped
2	cups (8 ounces) pecans, chopped
2	cups unsweetened flaked coconut
½	cup raw sunflower seeds
1½	cups raisins

1. Adjust oven rack to upper-middle position and heat oven to 325 degrees. Whisk maple syrup, melted coconut oil, vanilla, cinnamon, ginger, salt, pepper, allspice, and nutmeg together in large bowl. Add almonds, pecans, coconut, and sunflower seeds and toss until thoroughly coated.

2. Transfer nut mixture to parchment paper–lined rimmed baking sheet and spread into thin, even layer. Using stiff metal spatula, compress mixture until very compact. Bake granola until lightly browned, 25 to 35 minutes, rotating sheet halfway through baking.

3. Remove granola from oven and let cool on wire rack to room temperature, about 1 hour. Break cooled granola into pieces of desired size. Stir in raisins. (Granola can be stored at room temperature for up to 2 weeks.) Serve.

VARIATION

Tropical Nut and Seed Granola

Omit cinnamon and allspice. Reduce vanilla to 1 teaspoon and increase ginger to 1½ teaspoons and nutmeg to ¾ teaspoon. Substitute 2 cups macadamia nuts for pecans, ¼ cup sesame seeds for sunflower seeds, and 1½ cups chopped dried mango or pineapple for raisins.

All-Morning Energy Bars

Makes 10 bars

✔ **WHY THIS RECIPE WORKS** It can be hard to find granola bars that are paleo-friendly because so many are made with oats, grains, and refined sugars. We wanted a portable snack that was easy to make and contained only whole, nutritious ingredients. A hearty collection of healthy nuts and seeds provided the basis for our homemade bars. Toasting the nuts and seeds before pulsing them in the food processor gave our bars a pleasant roasted flavor, and the moderate heat of a 300-degree oven ensured that they all toasted evenly without burning. Dates and maple syrup not only added satisfying sweetness to the bars, but also aided in binding the bars together. We found that processing some of the dates with the maple syrup, warm water, and an egg white gave the bars a slight chew while still allowing the nuts and seeds to remain crisp. We stirred the remaining chopped dates into the mixture for textural contrast; tasters also liked the little bursts of sweetness. The final step in perfecting our homemade "granola" bars was to ensure they were evenly baked. After baking the nut and seed mixture in an 8-inch square baking pan, we cut it into bars while it was still warm (which made cutting clean lines much easier), spread the bars out on a baking sheet, and returned them to the oven to finish baking. The result: Evenly toasted bars with lots of crunch and a slight chew that made a perfect, energy-packed snack. Be sure not to overcook the nuts and seeds in step 2; they will continue to toast while the bars bake.

½	**cup whole raw almonds**
½	**cup raw cashews**
⅓	**cup raw pepitas**
¼	**cup raw sunflower seeds**
2	**tablespoons flax seeds**
1	**tablespoon sesame seeds**
3	**ounces pitted dates, chopped (½ cup)**
2	**tablespoons warm tap water**
2	**tablespoons maple syrup**
1	**large egg white**
¾	**teaspoon kosher salt**

1. Adjust oven rack to middle position and heat oven to 300 degrees. Make foil sling for 8-inch square baking pan by folding 2 long sheets of aluminum foil so each is 8 inches wide. Lay sheets of foil in pan perpendicular to each other, with extra foil hanging over edges of pan. Push foil into corners and up sides of pan, smoothing foil flush to pan, and grease foil.

2. Spread almonds, cashews, pepitas, sunflower seeds, flax seeds, and sesame seeds onto aluminum foil–lined rimmed baking sheet. Bake, stirring occasionally, until pale golden and fragrant, 15 to 20 minutes. Transfer nut mixture to food processor, let cool slightly, then pulse until coarsely chopped, about 5 pulses; transfer to large bowl.

3. Process ¼ cup dates, warm water, maple syrup, egg white, and salt in now-empty processor until smooth, about 30 seconds, scraping down sides of bowl as needed. Stir processed date mixture and remaining ¼ cup chopped dates into nut mixture until well combined. Spread mixture into prepared pan and press firmly into even layer using greased metal spatula. Bake bars until golden brown, 20 to 25 minutes, rotating pan halfway through baking. Do not turn off oven.

4. Let bars cool in pan for 15 minutes. Using foil sling, remove bars from pan, transfer to cutting board, and cut into 10 bars. Space bars evenly on parchment paper–lined baking sheet and bake until deep golden brown, 10 to 15 minutes. Let bars cool on wire rack to room temperature, about 1 hour. (Bars can be stored at room temperature for up to 1 week.) Serve.

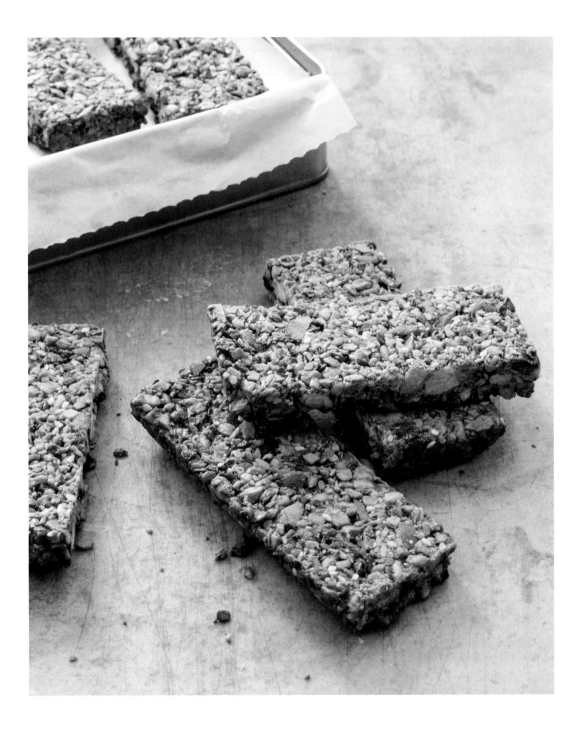

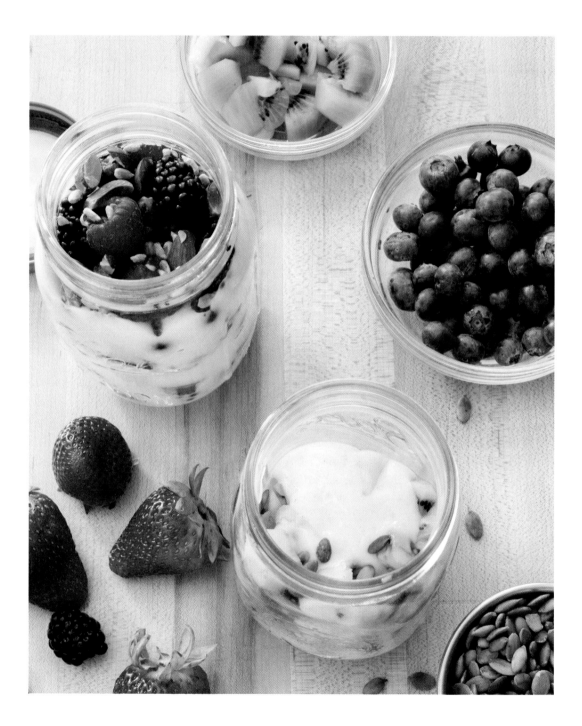

Almond Yogurt Parfaits

Serves 4

✓ **WHY THIS RECIPE WORKS** Creamy almond-milk yogurt, fresh fruit, and crunchy, toasted nuts make a delicious and wholesome start to the day—and layering them in a tall glass makes a simple breakfast feel like a special occasion. We used our homemade Paleo Almond Yogurt and sweetened it naturally with honey. The bright flavor of fresh berries perfectly complemented the rich, creamy yogurt. We also added almonds and sunflower seeds, which we toasted to bring out their flavor and crunch. For an easy variation, we substituted lively tropical pineapple and kiwi for the berries, and grassy pepitas for the sunflower seeds. We also created a version using juicy oranges and sweet bananas, and rounded out their flavors with some dried dates and warm spices. Almost any combination of fruits, nuts, and seeds will work well here. Do not substitute frozen fruit. Serve the parfaits within 15 minutes after assembling or the nuts and seeds will begin to turn soggy. We prefer to use homemade almond yogurt; however, you can substitute your favorite unsweetened store-bought brand.

3 cups Paleo Almond Yogurt (page 23)
2 tablespoons honey
1 cup almonds or walnuts, toasted and chopped
½ cup raw sunflower seeds, toasted
20 ounces (4 cups) blackberries, blueberries, raspberries, and/or sliced strawberries

Whisk yogurt and honey together in bowl until thoroughly combined. In separate bowl, combine almonds and sunflower seeds. Using four 16-ounce glasses, spoon ¼ cup yogurt-honey mixture into each glass, then top with ⅓ cup berries, followed by 2 tablespoons nut mixture. Repeat layering process 2 more times with remaining yogurt, berries, and nut mixture. Serve.

VARIATIONS

Almond Yogurt Parfaits with Pineapple and Kiwi

Add 1 teaspoon ground ginger to yogurt with honey. Substitute ½ cup toasted pepitas for sunflower seeds and 3 cups ½-inch pineapple pieces and 3 kiwis, peeled and cut into ½-inch pieces, for mixed berries.

Almond Yogurt Parfaits with Dates, Oranges, and Bananas

Microwave 1 cup chopped dried dates with 1 cup water in bowl for 30 seconds; drain and let cool. Cut away peel and pith from 2 oranges. Quarter oranges, then slice crosswise into ¼-inch-thick pieces. Add ½ teaspoon ground cinnamon and ¼ teaspoon ground nutmeg to yogurt with honey. Substitute softened dates, orange pieces, and 3 thinly sliced bananas for mixed berries.

TEST KITCHEN TIP TOASTING NUTS AND SEEDS

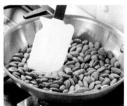

To toast 1 cup or less of nuts or seeds, toast in dry skillet over medium heat, stirring occasionally, until fragrant, 3 to 8 minutes.

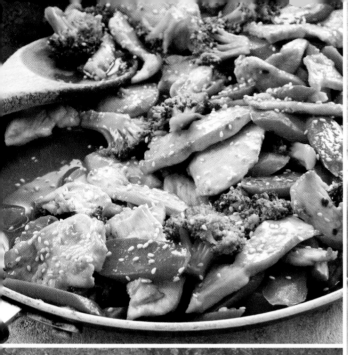

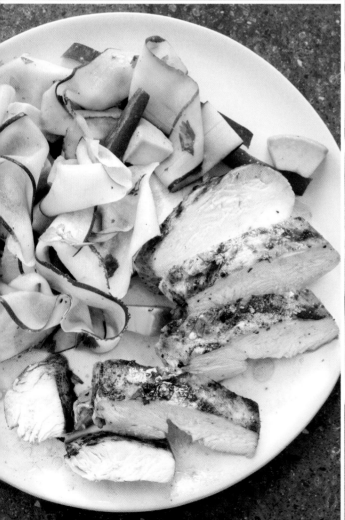

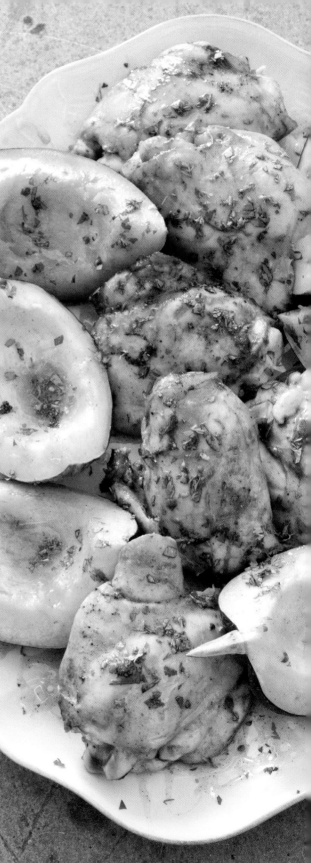

POULTRY

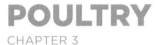

CHAPTER 3

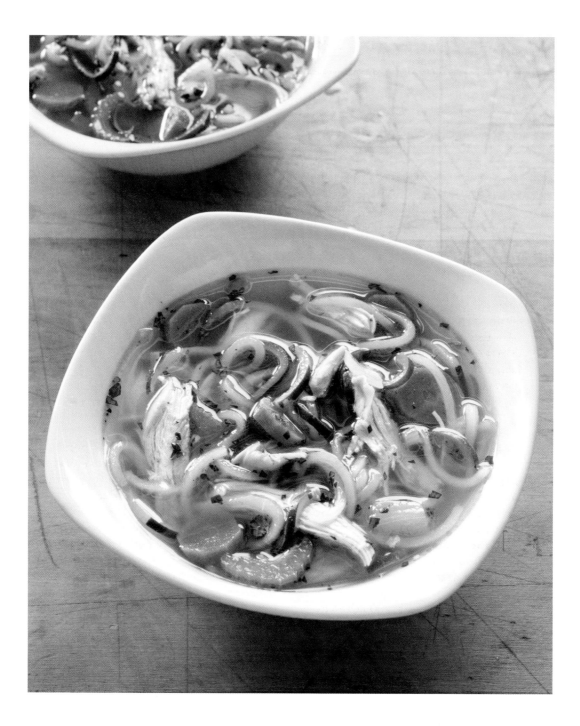

Chicken "Noodle" Soup

Serves 6 to 8

✔ **WHY THIS RECIPE WORKS** For a full-flavored paleo chicken soup recipe, we began by making our own broth using a whole chicken. We built a flavorful base by cooking aromatics in ghee, then placed the entire chicken in the pot with plenty of water, eliminating the need to hack up the chicken into parts. To keep the recipe cost-effective and streamlined, we wanted to use the chicken for more than just the broth; we also wanted to use the meat in our soup. To make this work, we needed to take the chicken out partway through cooking so that we wouldn't end up with inedibly overcooked meat. We shredded the meat off the bones and set it aside for later, then returned just the carcass to the broth to fortify it with rich chicken flavor. For paleo-friendly "noodles," we turned to mild zucchini and used a spiralizer to quickly turn the squash into thin strands. You can substitute 2 tablespoons ghee for the reserved chicken fat in step 5. Use a Dutch oven that holds 7 quarts or more for this recipe. If possible, use smaller, in-season zucchini, which have thinner skins and less seeds. For more information on spiralizing, see page 14.

STOCK

- 1 tablespoon ghee
- 2 onions, chopped
- 1 tablespoon kosher salt
- 1 (3½- to 4-pound) whole chicken, giblets discarded
- 3½ quarts water
- 2 bay leaves

SOUP

- 1 pound zucchini, trimmed
- 4 carrots, peeled and sliced ¼ inch thick
- 3 celery ribs, sliced ¼ inch thick
- 1 onion, chopped
  Kosher salt and pepper
- 1 tablespoon tomato paste
- 1 tablespoon minced fresh thyme or 1 teaspoon dried
- ¼ cup minced fresh parsley

1. FOR THE STOCK Heat ghee in Dutch oven over medium heat until shimmering. Add onions and salt and cook until softened and lightly browned, about 8 minutes. Place chicken breast side up in pot, then add water and bay leaves and bring to boil. Reduce heat to medium-low, partially cover, and simmer until breast registers 160 degrees and thighs register 175 degrees, 30 to 40 minutes.

2. Transfer chicken to carving board, let cool slightly, then shred meat into bite-size pieces using 2 forks; reserve bones and discard skin.

3. Add reserved bones to broth and return to simmer over medium heat. Cook, uncovered, until broth is deeply flavored, about 30 minutes.

4. Remove large bones from pot, then strain broth through fine-mesh strainer. Let broth settle for 5 to 10 minutes, then defat using wide, shallow spoon or fat separator, reserving 2 tablespoons fat. (Shredded chicken, strained broth, and reserved fat can be refrigerated in separate containers for up to 2 days; return broth to simmer before proceeding.)

5. FOR THE SOUP Using spiralizer, cut zucchini into ⅛-inch-thick noodles, then cut noodles into 2-inch lengths. Heat reserved fat in now-empty pot over medium heat until shimmering. Add carrots, celery, onion, and 1 teaspoon salt and cook until softened and lightly browned, 8 to 10 minutes. Stir in tomato paste and thyme and cook until fragrant, about 1 minute. Stir in strained broth, scraping up any browned bits. Bring to simmer and cook until vegetables are tender, about 5 minutes.

6. Stir in zucchini noodles and shredded chicken and cook until zucchini is just tender, 6 to 8 minutes. Stir in parsley and season with salt and pepper to taste. Serve.

Slow-Cooker Southwestern Chicken Soup

Serves 6 to 8

✓ **WHY THIS RECIPE WORKS** This turbocharged, south-of-the-border chicken soup features a spicy, tomatoey broth overflowing with tender shredded chicken and fresh, bright garnishes. Typically, this broth acquires its deep, smoky flavor from charred vegetables. To replicate these flavors in a slow cooker, we browned some of the vegetables in a skillet before adding them to the slow cooker. Using a combination of fresh jalapeño and chipotle chile powder ensured balanced spice in every bite. The gentle heat of the slow cooker kept our bone-in chicken breasts tender and moist through cooking. Zucchini added heartiness to the dish without making it heavy, and stirring it in at the end kept it from getting too mushy. Don't omit the garnishes; the flavor of the soup depends heavily on them. For a spicier soup, reserve, mince, and add the ribs and seeds from the jalapeño. We prefer to use homemade chicken broth; however, you can substitute your favorite store-bought broth. You will need a 4- to 7-quart slow cooker for this recipe.

3 tablespoons extra-virgin olive oil
2 onions, chopped fine
1 jalapeño chile, stemmed, seeded, and minced
  Kosher salt and pepper
3 tablespoons tomato paste
4 garlic cloves, minced
1 tablespoon minced fresh oregano or 1 teaspoon dried
1 tablespoon ground cumin
1½ teaspoons chipotle chile powder
8 cups Paleo Chicken Broth (page 16)
3 (12-ounce) bone-in split chicken breasts, trimmed
1 zucchini, quartered lengthwise and sliced ¼ inch thick
2 tomatoes, cored and chopped
2 avocados, halved, pitted, and cut into ½-inch pieces
4 radishes, trimmed and sliced thin
½ cup fresh cilantro leaves
  Lime wedges

1. Heat oil in 12-inch skillet over medium heat until shimmering. Add onions, jalapeño, and 1 tablespoon salt and cook until softened, about 5 minutes. Stir in tomato paste, garlic, oregano, cumin, and chile powder and cook until fragrant, about 1 minute. Stir in 1 cup broth, scraping up any browned bits; transfer to slow cooker.

2. Stir remaining 7 cups broth into slow cooker. Season chicken with salt and pepper and nestle into slow cooker. Cover and cook until chicken is tender, 3 to 5 hours on low.

3. Transfer chicken to cutting board, let cool slightly, then shred into bite-size pieces using 2 forks; discard skin and bones.

4. Using wide, shallow spoon, skim excess fat from surface of soup. Stir in zucchini, cover, and cook on high until tender, about 30 minutes.

5. Stir in shredded chicken and let sit until heated through, about 5 minutes. Season with salt and pepper to taste. Top individual portions with tomatoes, avocados, radishes, and cilantro and serve with lime wedges.

TEST KITCHEN TIP **SEEDING CHILES**

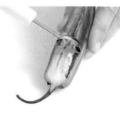

Cut chile in half lengthwise, then gently scrape out seeds and ribs using melon baller or teaspoon. Use sharp edge of melon baller to cut off stem.

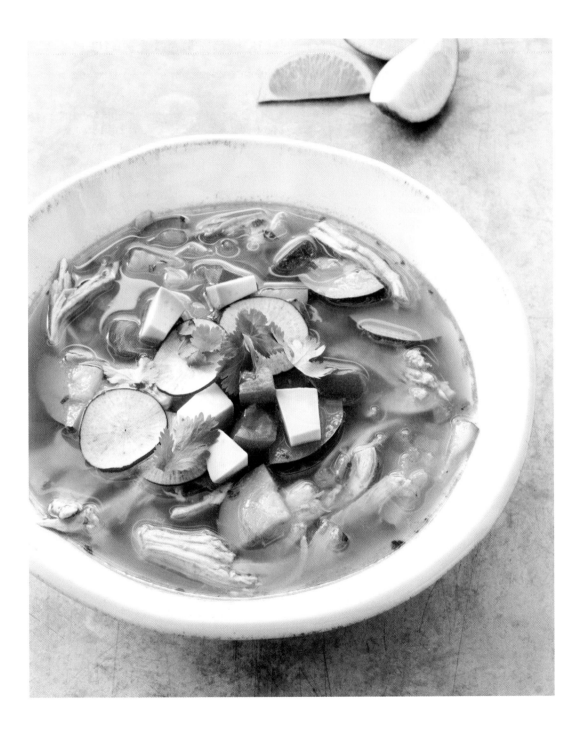

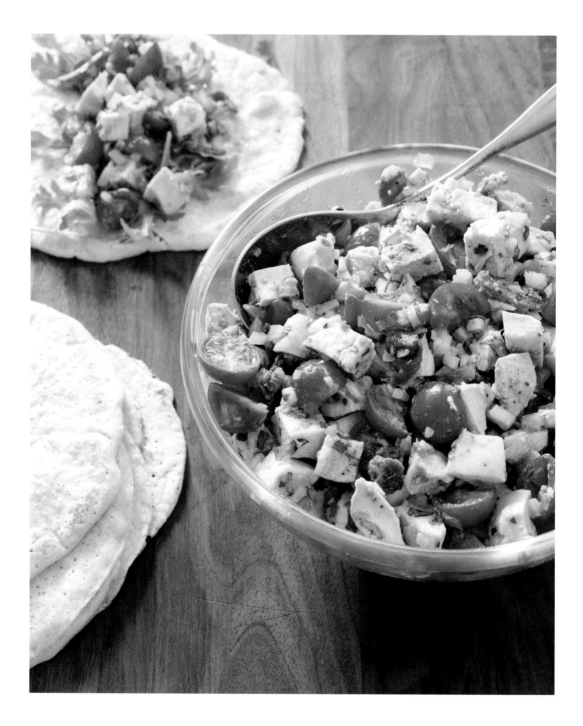

Chicken Salad with Bacon and Tomatoes

Serves 4 to 6

✓ **WHY THIS RECIPE WORKS** Most chicken salads are made with creamy, mayonnaise-based dressings. But store-bought mayo isn't part of the paleo diet, so we decided to take a different approach for our recipe and make a flavorful, vinaigrette-style dressing and incorporate some simple paleo-friendly mix-ins. Bacon seemed like a good place to start; its smoky, savory depth complemented the mild chicken breasts perfectly. We used the bacon in two ways: We cut it into small pieces, which we crisped and added to the salad for a crunchy textural element, and we used the bacon fat as a base for our dressing. Mixing the bacon fat with some extra-virgin olive oil lent the dressing a silkier texture. Aromatic shallot and garlic as well as some tangy apple cider vinegar and Dijon mustard rounded out our vinaigrette. Finally, we stirred fresh cherry tomatoes into the salad for acidity and mild sweetness. For perfectly tender, juicy meat, we poached chicken breasts in 6 cups of salted water, which acted as a brine to keep our chicken moist as the water slowly heated to 170 degrees. We then removed the pot from the heat and let it stand covered for about 15 minutes, allowing the chicken to cook through slowly and gently. To ensure that the chicken cooks through, use breasts that weigh no more than 8 ounces and pound them until they are 1 inch thick. Make sure to start with cold water in step 1. Serve in Paleo Wraps (page 24), pictured, or in lettuce leaves, or spoon over leafy greens.

Kosher salt and pepper

4 (6- to 8-ounce) boneless, skinless chicken breasts, trimmed

4 slices bacon, cut into 1-inch pieces

1 shallot, minced

2 garlic cloves, minced

3 tablespoons extra-virgin olive oil, plus extra as needed

2 teaspoons cider vinegar

2 teaspoons Dijon mustard

Pinch cayenne pepper

12 ounces cherry tomatoes, quartered

2 celery ribs, minced

¼ cup chopped fresh basil

1. Dissolve ¼ cup salt in 6 cups cold water in Dutch oven. Cover chicken with plastic wrap and pound to even 1-inch thickness.

2. Submerge chicken in water. Heat pot over medium heat until water registers 170 degrees. Turn off heat, cover, and let sit until chicken registers 165 degrees, 15 to 17 minutes. Transfer chicken to paper towel–lined baking sheet. Refrigerate until chicken is cool, about 30 minutes.

3. Cook bacon in 12-inch skillet over medium heat until crisp, 8 to 10 minutes. Using slotted spoon,

transfer bacon to paper towel–lined plate; set aside. (You should have about 3 tablespoons fat in skillet; if not, add extra oil as needed to equal 3 tablespoons.)

4. Add shallot to fat left in skillet and cook over medium heat until softened, about 2 minutes. Stir in garlic and cook until fragrant, about 30 seconds. Transfer mixture to large bowl and let cool slightly. Whisk in oil, vinegar, mustard, cayenne, and ¼ teaspoon salt until combined.

5. Pat chicken dry with paper towels and cut into ½-inch pieces. Add chicken, tomatoes, celery, basil, and crisp bacon to dressing and toss to combine. Season with salt and pepper to taste. Serve. (Salad can be refrigerated for up to 2 days. Let sit at room temperature for 30 minutes before serving.)

TEST KITCHEN TIP **POUNDING CHICKEN**

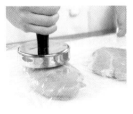

To ensure that chicken breasts cook evenly, lay breasts between 2 sheets of plastic and pound with meat pounder or rolling pin to desired even thickness.

Thai Chicken Lettuce Wraps

Serves 4

✅ **WHY THIS RECIPE WORKS** Flavorful ground chicken wrapped in crunchy lettuce leaves seems like a perfect paleo dinner option, but most recipes for this Thai-inspired dish aren't paleo-friendly since the sauce includes ingredients like soy sauce and cornstarch. And, to make matters worse, the chicken often turns out stringy and tasteless. For our recipe, we decided to skip store-bought ground chicken and "grind" flavorful chicken thighs ourselves. To ensure that we ended up with tender, distinct pieces of chicken, we placed the thighs in the freezer to firm up before we pulsed them in the food processor. We then marinated the chicken in a flavorful mixture of coconut aminos, fish sauce, and lime juice, easily avoiding ingredients such as soy sauce and sugar. We also added a bit of tapioca flour to the mixture, which coated the chicken and helped it retain moisture during cooking. Red bell pepper and shallots further boosted the chicken mixture's flavor. Finally, we added a vibrant, simple sauce to the skillet and cooked it briefly to meld the flavors. The sauce helped to keep the chicken moist and tender during the final stage of cooking and brightened the flavor of the dish. A combination of mint and cilantro provided welcome notes of freshness. For more information on coconut aminos, see page 11. This recipe calls for a 12-inch nonstick skillet; however, a well-seasoned cast-iron skillet can be used instead.

1 pound boneless, skinless chicken thighs, trimmed and cut into 1-inch pieces

2 tablespoons fish sauce, plus extra for seasoning

2 tablespoons lime juice, plus extra for seasoning

4 teaspoons coconut aminos

2½ teaspoons tapioca flour

½ teaspoon red pepper flakes
  Kosher salt and pepper

2 teaspoons honey

1 tablespoon coconut oil

1 red bell pepper, stemmed, seeded, and cut into ½-inch pieces

2 shallots, sliced thin

3 tablespoons chopped fresh mint

3 tablespoons chopped fresh cilantro

1 head Bibb lettuce (8 ounces), leaves separated

1. Spread chicken on large plate and freeze until firm and starting to harden around edges but still pliable, about 25 minutes.

2. Whisk 2 teaspoons fish sauce, 1 teaspoon lime juice, 1 teaspoon coconut aminos, 2 teaspoons flour, pepper flakes, ½ teaspoon salt, and ¼ teaspoon pepper together in large bowl. Pulse half of chicken in food processor until finely ground into ¼- to ⅛-inch pieces, 6 to 10 pulses. Transfer chicken to bowl with fish sauce mixture and repeat with remaining chicken. Toss chicken to coat and refrigerate for 15 minutes.

3. Whisk honey, remaining 4 teaspoons fish sauce, remaining 5 teaspoons lime juice, remaining 1 tablespoon coconut aminos, and remaining ½ teaspoon flour together in bowl.

4. Heat oil in 12-inch nonstick skillet over medium-high heat until just smoking. Add bell pepper, shallots, and chicken mixture and cook, breaking up any large pieces of chicken with wooden spoon, until chicken is no longer pink, 5 to 7 minutes.

5. Whisk honey mixture to recombine, then add to skillet. Cook, stirring constantly, until sauce is slightly thickened, about 15 seconds. Off heat, stir in mint and cilantro and season with fish sauce and lime juice to taste. Spoon mixture into lettuce leaves and serve.

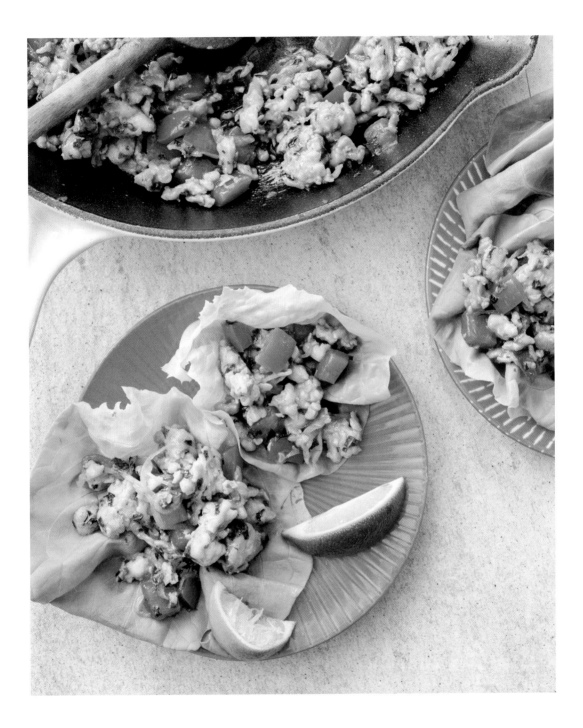

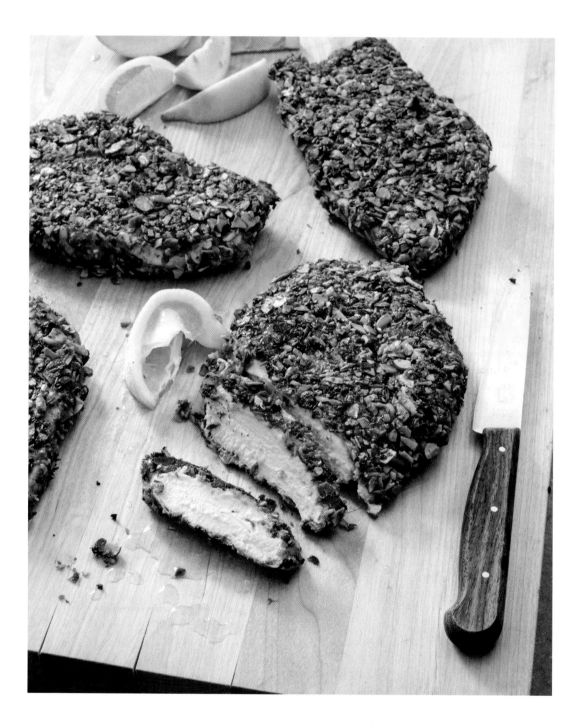

Nut-Crusted Chicken Breasts

Serves 4

☑ **WHY THIS RECIPE WORKS** A crunchy bread-crumb coating is a great way to add flavor and texture to lean, mild chicken breasts—unless you're on the paleo diet. Both the bread crumbs and the flour often used to create a bound breading aren't paleo-friendly. Instead, we set out to create a crunchy coating using chopped nuts. But nut coatings are often dense and leaden, and the rich flavor of the nuts rarely comes through. We discovered that chopped and toasted sliced almonds worked well, but were too heavy on their own. Some toasted shredded coconut ensured that the coating stayed crisp. To replace the all-purpose flour, we dredged the chicken in tapioca flour. For our liquid component, two eggs and a bit of water provided moisture and structure. We also found that scoring the chicken before dredging helped the coating adhere and not flake off when the chicken was cut. Once cooked, all the chicken needed was a spritz of tangy lemon juice. This recipe calls for a 12-inch nonstick skillet; however, a well-seasoned cast-iron skillet can be used instead.

6 tablespoons ghee
1 shallot, minced
 Kosher salt and pepper
2 garlic cloves, minced
1½ cups sliced almonds, chopped
½ cup unsweetened shredded coconut
1 tablespoon finely grated lemon zest, plus lemon wedges for serving
1 tablespoon minced fresh thyme
¼ teaspoon cayenne pepper
¾ cup tapioca flour
2 large eggs
3 tablespoons water
1 tablespoon Dijon mustard
4 (6- to 8-ounce) boneless, skinless chicken breasts, trimmed

1. Adjust oven rack to middle position and heat oven to 200 degrees. Set wire rack in rimmed baking sheet.

2. Heat 2 tablespoons ghee in 12-inch nonstick skillet over medium heat until shimmering. Add shallot and ¾ teaspoon salt and cook until softened and lightly browned, about 3 minutes. Stir in garlic and cook until fragrant, about 30 seconds. Stir in almonds and coconut and cook, stirring often, until golden brown, about 4 minutes.

3. Transfer almond mixture to shallow dish and stir in lemon zest, thyme, and cayenne. Spread flour in

second shallow dish. Lightly beat eggs, water, mustard, and ¼ teaspoon pepper together in third shallow dish.

4. Cover chicken with plastic wrap and pound to even ½-inch thickness. Pat chicken dry with paper towels and, with sharp knife, cut 1⁄16-inch-deep slits on both sides of breasts, spaced ½ inch apart, in crosshatch pattern. Season chicken with salt and pepper. Working with 1 breast at a time, dredge in flour, dip in egg mixture, and then coat with almond mixture, pressing gently to adhere; transfer to plate.

5. Wipe skillet clean with paper towels. Heat 2 tablespoons ghee in skillet over medium heat until shimmering. Place 2 chicken breasts in skillet and cook until deep golden brown and crisp and chicken registers 160 degrees, 3 to 5 minutes per side.

6. Drain chicken briefly on paper towels, then transfer to prepared rack and keep warm in oven. Wipe skillet clean with paper towels and repeat with remaining 2 tablespoons ghee and remaining chicken. Serve with lemon wedges.

TEST KITCHEN TIP **SCORING CHICKEN BREASTS**

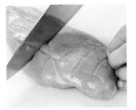

To ensure that coating clings to chicken, use sharp knife to cut 1⁄16-inch-deep slits on both sides of breasts, spaced ½ inch apart, in crosshatch pattern.

Chicken with Mexican Pumpkin Seed Sauce

Serves 4

♨ **WHY THIS RECIPE WORKS** Pumpkin seed sauce is unapologetically bold, tangy, nutty, and, best of all, naturally paleo. It's traditionally made by blending pumpkin seeds, tomatillos, jalapeños, and aromatics into a thick, hearty sauce. But most recipes are fairly time-consuming, making this otherwise versatile sauce unsuitable for a weeknight meal. We wanted to maintain the classic flavor profile while minimizing the work. Our first move was to toast sesame seeds and pepitas to deepen their flavor and bring out their inherent nuttiness. Onion, garlic, and thyme gave the sauce an aromatic base, while fresh jalapeño gave it lively spice. We chopped the tomatillos so they would soften evenly and quickly. Cooking bone-in chicken breasts in with the vegetables infused the sauce with meaty, savory flavor. Once the chicken was done, we pureed the sauce in the blender; lime juice, cilantro, and a dab of honey added at this point brightened the sauce nicely. For a spicier sauce, reserve, mince, and add the ribs and seeds from the jalapeño.

⅓ cup raw pepitas

¼ cup sesame seeds

4 (12-ounce) bone-in split chicken breasts, trimmed

Kosher salt and pepper

1 tablespoon extra-virgin olive oil

1 onion, chopped fine

1 jalapeño chile, stemmed, seeded, and chopped

3 garlic cloves, minced

1 teaspoon minced fresh thyme or ¼ teaspoon dried

6 ounces fresh tomatillos, husks and stems removed, rinsed well and dried, chopped

½ cup water, plus extra as needed

1 cup fresh cilantro leaves, plus 2 tablespoons minced

1 tablespoon lime juice

½ teaspoon honey

1. Adjust oven rack to middle position and heat oven to 450 degrees. Toast pepitas and sesame seeds in 12-inch ovensafe skillet over medium heat, stirring often, until seeds are golden and fragrant, about 8 minutes; transfer to bowl. Measure out 1 tablespoon toasted seeds and set aside for garnish.

2. Pat chicken dry and season with salt and pepper. Heat oil in now-empty skillet over medium-high heat until just smoking. Brown chicken well, about 5 minutes per side; transfer to plate.

3. Add onion, ½ teaspoon salt, and pinch pepper to fat left in skillet and cook over medium heat until softened and lightly browned, 5 to 7 minutes. Stir in jalapeño, garlic, and thyme and cook until fragrant, about 1 minute. Stir in tomatillos.

4. Nestle chicken skin side up into vegetables along with any accumulated juices. Transfer skillet to oven and roast until chicken registers 160 degrees, 20 to 25 minutes.

5. Using potholder (skillet handle will be hot), remove skillet from oven. Transfer chicken to plate, tent loosely with aluminum foil, and let rest while finishing sauce.

6. Being careful of hot skillet handle, stir water into vegetables, scraping up any browned bits. Transfer vegetable mixture to blender, add toasted seeds, cilantro leaves, lime juice, and honey, and process until mostly smooth, about 1 minute. Adjust sauce consistency with extra hot water as needed. Season with salt and pepper to taste. Serve chicken with sauce, sprinkling individual portions with reserved toasted seeds and minced cilantro.

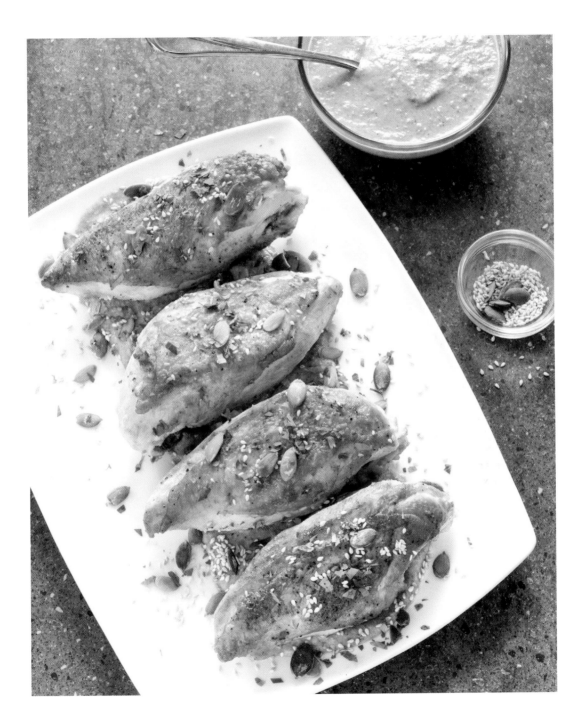

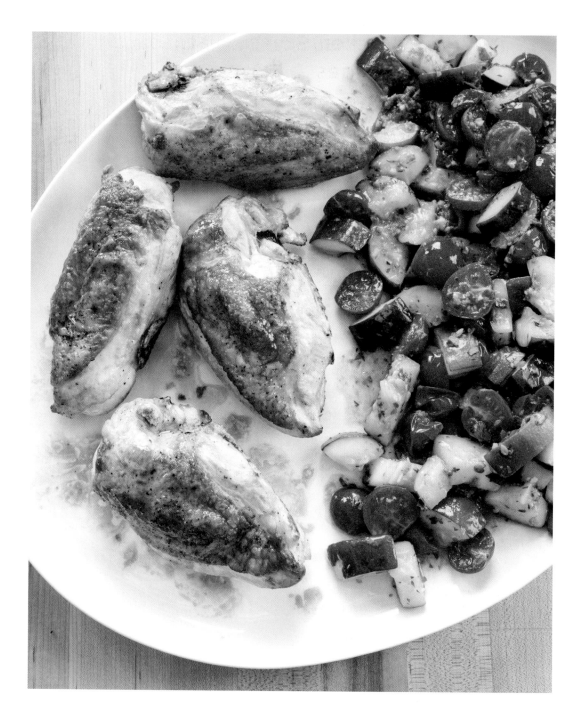

Pan-Roasted Chicken Breasts with Zucchini and Cherry Tomatoes

Serves 4

✓ **WHY THIS RECIPE WORKS** For a flavorful chicken dinner that could be made any night of the week (and that wouldn't leave a sinkful of dishes in its wake), we turned to flavorful bone-in chicken breasts, delicate zucchini, and juicy cherry tomatoes. First, we had to address a key challenge of cooking bone-in chicken: By the time the skin is crispy, the meat is often hopelessly overcooked. To solve this, we used a combined pan-searing and roasting method: We browned the chicken first in a skillet on the stovetop, which crisped the skin nicely, and then we let the chicken gently finish cooking in a baking dish in the even heat of the oven. This freed up the skillet, allowing us to cook our vegetables while the chicken was baking. After searing the zucchini quickly, we added the aromatics—garlic, thyme, and red pepper flakes—and then the tomatoes. As the tomatoes cooked, they released their flavorful juices, which brought all the flavors together. After cooking, we stirred in parsley for a burst of freshness, capers for some necessary brininess, and lemon zest and juice for added brightness. This recipe calls for a 12-inch nonstick skillet; however, a well-seasoned cast-iron skillet can be used instead.

4   (12-ounce) bone-in split chicken breasts, trimmed
     Kosher salt and pepper
3   tablespoons extra-virgin olive oil
1½   pounds zucchini, quartered lengthwise and sliced ½ inch thick
2   garlic cloves, minced
1   teaspoon minced fresh thyme or ¼ teaspoon dried
     Pinch red pepper flakes
1   pound cherry tomatoes, halved
1   tablespoon capers, rinsed and minced
1   tablespoon chopped fresh parsley
1   teaspoon grated lemon zest plus 1 teaspoon juice

1. Adjust oven rack to middle position and heat oven to 450 degrees. Pat chicken dry with paper towels and season with salt and pepper. Heat 1 tablespoon oil in 12-inch nonstick skillet over medium-high heat until just smoking. Brown chicken well, about 5 minutes per side.

2. Transfer chicken skin side up to 13 by 9-inch baking dish and roast until chicken registers 160 degrees, 20 to 25 minutes. Transfer chicken to serving platter.

3. Meanwhile, pour off all but 1 tablespoon fat from skillet and return to medium-high heat until just smoking. Add zucchini and cook, stirring occasionally, until just tender, 5 to 7 minutes. Stir in garlic, thyme, and pepper flakes and cook until fragrant, about 30 seconds. Stir in tomatoes and 1 teaspoon salt and cook until vegetables are softened and tomatoes begin to release their juices, about 4 minutes. Off heat, stir in capers, parsley, lemon zest and juice, and remaining 2 tablespoons oil. Season with salt and pepper to taste. Serve.

TEST KITCHEN TIP
TRIMMING BONE-IN CHICKEN BREASTS

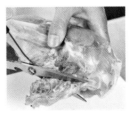

Using kitchen shears, trim off rib section from breast, following vertical line of fat from tapered end of breast to socket where wing was attached.

Grilled Greek-Style Chicken Kebabs

Serves 4

✔ **WHY THIS RECIPE WORKS** Chicken kebabs make a great quick paleo dinner option, so we set out to create a simple recipe with big flavor. To keep our boneless, skinless chicken breasts moist, we brined them briefly. We then tossed the chunks of chicken in a lemony, Greek-inspired vinaigrette before cooking. We also reserved some of the dressing to toss with the chicken after cooking for a boost of bright, vibrant flavor. To make sure the peppers and onions finished cooking at the same time as our chicken, we gave them a quick jump start in the microwave. You will need six 12-inch metal skewers for this recipe. Serve with Cauliflower Rice (page 288).

Kosher salt and pepper

2 pounds boneless, skinless chicken breasts, trimmed and cut into 1-inch pieces

½ cup extra-virgin olive oil

3 tablespoons minced fresh parsley

2 tablespoons minced fresh mint

3 garlic cloves, minced

2 teaspoons minced fresh oregano or ½ teaspoon dried

2 teaspoons honey

1½ teaspoons grated lemon zest plus ⅓ cup juice (2 lemons)

2 green bell peppers, stemmed, seeded, and cut into 1½-inch pieces

1 large red onion, cut into 1-inch pieces, 3 layers thick

1. Dissolve ¼ cup salt in 4 cups cold water in large container. Submerge chicken in brine, cover, and refrigerate for 30 minutes.

2. Combine 7 tablespoons oil, parsley, mint, garlic, oregano, honey, lemon zest and juice, and ½ teaspoon pepper in bowl. Transfer ⅓ cup of dressing to large bowl and stir in 1 teaspoon salt; set aside to toss with cooked chicken.

3. Microwave bell peppers, onion, and remaining 1 tablespoon oil in covered bowl, stirring occasionally, until just tender, 3 to 5 minutes. Remove chicken from brine and pat dry with paper towels. Toss chicken with remaining dressing. Thread chicken, bell peppers, and onion in alternating order onto six 12-inch metal skewers.

4A. FOR A CHARCOAL GRILL Open bottom vent completely. Light large chimney starter mounded with charcoal briquettes (7 quarts). When top coals are partially covered with ash, pour evenly over grill. Set cooking grate in place, cover, and open lid vent completely. Heat grill until hot, about 5 minutes.

4B. FOR A GAS GRILL Turn all burners to high, cover, and heat grill until hot, about 15 minutes. Leave all burners on high.

5. Clean and oil cooking grate. Place kebabs on grill. Cook (covered if using gas), turning as needed, until chicken and vegetables are well browned and chicken registers 160 degrees, 10 to 15 minutes. Using fork, push chicken and vegetables off skewers into bowl of reserved dressing. Toss to coat, cover, and let sit for 5 minutes. Serve.

TEST KITCHEN TIP

PREPARING ONIONS FOR KEBABS

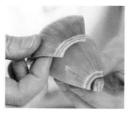
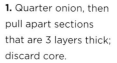

1. Quarter onion, then pull apart sections that are 3 layers thick; discard core.

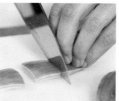

2. Cut each 3-layer section into 1-inch pieces.

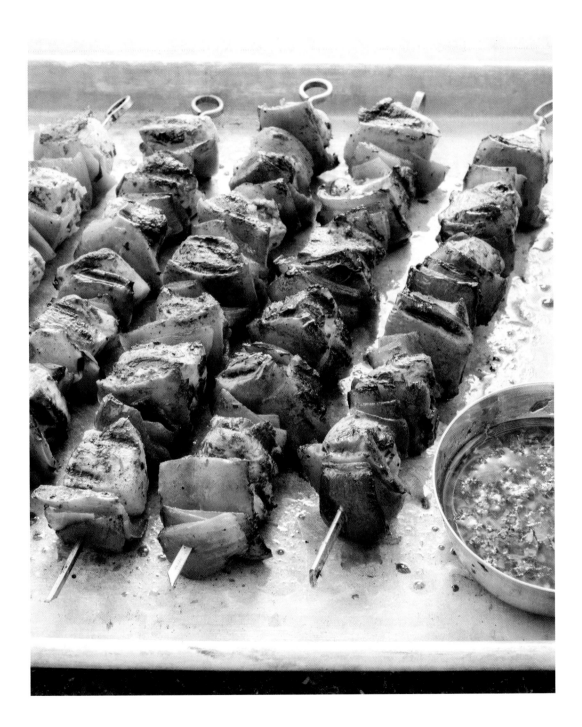

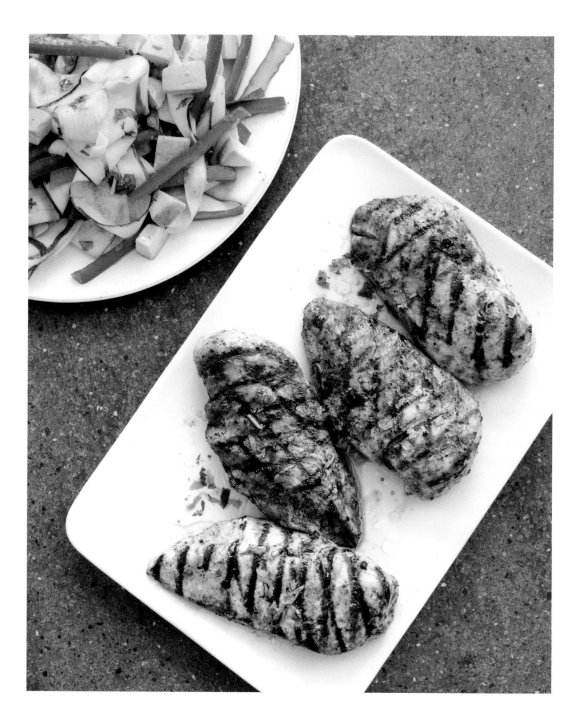

Grilled Chipotle-Lime Chicken Breasts with Shaved Zucchini and Avocado Salad

Serves 4

✓ **WHY THIS RECIPE WORKS** For a simple weeknight dinner off the grill, we paired boneless, skinless chicken breasts with a fresh zucchini salad. To ensure supremely flavorful and juicy chicken, we started by making a simple marinade with olive oil, lime juice, garlic, chile powder, and honey. Gently cooking the chicken breasts on the cooler side of the grill before quickly searing them on the hotter side ensured tender meat with a nicely charred exterior. For our salad, we combined thin ribbons of zucchini with creamy avocado and lightly sweet bell pepper. A subtle vinaigrette brought the chicken and salad together without masking the zucchini's delicate flavor. For more information on making zucchini ribbons, see page 307. If possible, use smaller, in-season zucchini, which have thinner skins and less seeds. Avoid marinating the chicken for more than 1 hour; it will turn the chicken mushy.

½ cup plus 1 tablespoon extra-virgin olive oil

¼ cup lime juice (2 limes)

2 tablespoons water

4 garlic cloves, minced

2 teaspoons chipotle chile powder
Kosher salt and pepper

1 teaspoon honey

4 (6- to 8-ounce) boneless, skinless chicken breasts, trimmed

1 pound zucchini, trimmed

4 teaspoons chopped fresh cilantro

1 avocado, halved, pitted, and cut into ½-inch pieces

1 red bell pepper, stemmed, seeded, and cut into ¼-inch-wide strips

1. Whisk ¼ cup oil, 1 tablespoon lime juice, water, garlic, chile powder, 1½ teaspoons salt, ½ teaspoon pepper, and honey together in bowl. Combine oil mixture and chicken in 1-gallon zipper-lock bag and toss to coat; press out as much air as possible and seal bag. Refrigerate for 30 minutes or up to 1 hour, flipping bag halfway through marinating. Remove chicken from marinade and let excess marinade drip off but do not pat dry.

2A. FOR A CHARCOAL GRILL Open bottom vent completely. Light large chimney starter filled with charcoal briquettes (6 quarts). When top coals are partially covered with ash, pour evenly over half of grill. Set cooking grate in place, cover, and open lid vent completely. Heat grill until hot, about 5 minutes.

2B. FOR A GAS GRILL Turn all burners to high, cover, and heat grill until hot, about 15 minutes. Leave primary burner on high and turn off other burner(s).

3. Clean and oil cooking grate. Place chicken on cooler side of grill, smooth side down, with thicker ends facing coals or flame. Cover and cook until bottom of chicken just begins to develop light grill marks and is no longer translucent, 6 to 9 minutes.

4. Flip chicken and rotate so that thinner ends face coals or flame. Cover and cook until chicken is opaque and firm to touch and registers 140 degrees, 6 to 9 minutes.

5. Slide chicken to hotter side of grill and cook, flipping as needed, until well browned on both sides and chicken registers 160 degrees, 2 to 6 minutes. Transfer chicken to serving platter, tent with aluminum foil, and let rest while making salad.

6. Using vegetable peeler, slice zucchini lengthwise into very thin ribbons. Whisk cilantro, remaining 5 tablespoons oil, remaining 3 tablespoons lime juice, 1 teaspoon salt, and ¼ teaspoon pepper together in large bowl. Drizzle chicken with 3 tablespoons dressing. Add avocado, bell pepper, and zucchini to remaining dressing and toss to combine. Season with salt and pepper to taste. Serve.

Grilled Lemon-Garlic Chicken Breasts with Fennel and Arugula Salad

Serves 4

✓ **WHY THIS RECIPE WORKS** A foolproof recipe for perfect grilled bone-in chicken breasts is a valuable thing to have in a paleo kitchen. We wanted to come up with a method that would produce great results every time, and make standard grilled chicken a little more interesting. A two-level grill fire, which has a hotter and a cooler side, ensured perfectly cooked meat and ultracrisp skin by allowing us to sear the skin over the hotter side before gently finishing the breasts on the cooler side. A vibrant marinade made with lemon zest and garlic infused the chicken with lots of flavor and helped to keep the meat moist on the grill. Since we already had the grill going, we decided to use it to create a quick side dish to accompany our chicken. We briefly grilled some aromatic fennel, infusing it with smoky flavor and softening it slightly. Peppery arugula and crunchy sliced almonds complemented the fennel nicely. Finally, we mixed up a bright vinaigrette of olive oil, lemon juice, chives, mustard, and honey, which brought the dish together perfectly.

6   **tablespoons extra-virgin olive oil**

3   **garlic cloves, minced**

1   **tablespoon grated lemon zest plus 4 teaspoons juice**
       Kosher salt and pepper

4   **(12-ounce) bone-in split chicken breasts, trimmed and halved crosswise**

2   **fennel bulbs, stalks discarded, bulbs cut vertically through base into ½-inch-thick slices**

¼   **cup minced fresh chives**

2   **teaspoons Dijon mustard**

1   **teaspoon honey**

4   **ounces (4 cups) baby arugula**

½   **cup sliced almonds, toasted**

1. Whisk 2 tablespoons oil, garlic, lemon zest, 1 teaspoon salt, and ½ teaspoon pepper together in large bowl. Add chicken and toss to coat. Cover and refrigerate for up to 30 minutes.

2. Microwave fennel, 1 tablespoon oil, ½ teaspoon salt, and ¼ teaspoon pepper in covered bowl, stirring occasionally, until softened, 6 to 8 minutes; drain well.

3A. FOR A CHARCOAL GRILL Open bottom vent completely. Light large chimney starter filled with charcoal briquettes (6 quarts). When top coals are partially covered with ash, pour evenly over half of grill. Set cooking grate in place, cover, and open lid vent completely. Heat grill until hot, about 5 minutes.

3B. FOR A GAS GRILL Turn all burners to high, cover, and heat grill until hot, about 15 minutes. Leave primary burner on high and turn off other burner(s).

4. Clean and oil cooking grate. Place chicken skin side down on hotter side of grill, cover, and cook until lightly browned, about 3 minutes per side.

5. Slide chicken to cooler side of grill with thicker ends facing hotter side of grill. Cover and cook, turning as needed, until well browned and chicken registers 160 degrees, 20 to 25 minutes. Transfer chicken to serving platter, tent loosely with aluminum foil, and let rest while finishing fennel.

6. As chicken finishes cooking, place fennel on hotter side of grill. Cook until tender and lightly browned, 2 to 4 minutes per side; transfer to cutting board and let cool slightly.

7. Cut fennel into 1-inch pieces. Whisk chives, mustard, honey, remaining 3 tablespoons oil, and lemon juice together in large bowl. Add arugula, almonds, and fennel to dressing and toss to coat. Season with salt and pepper to taste. Serve.

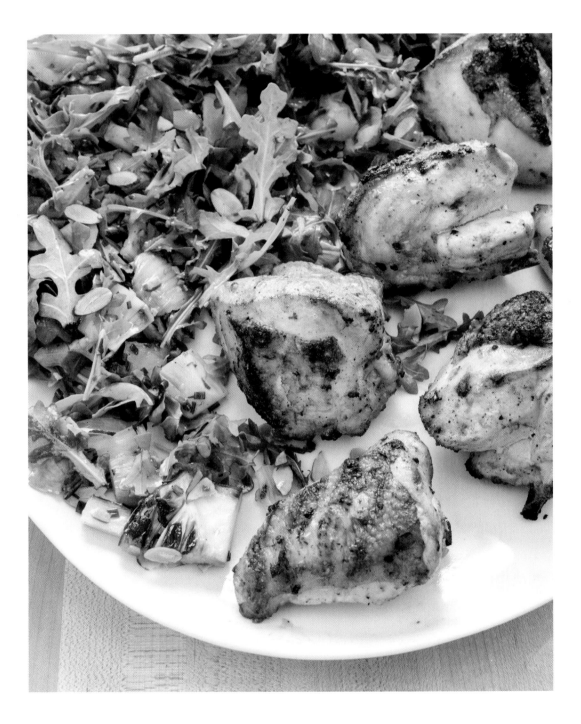

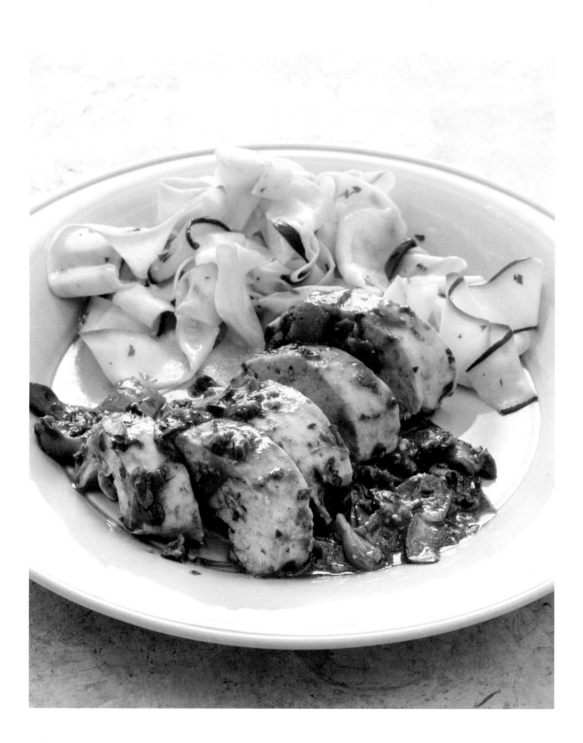

Rustic Braised Chicken with Mushrooms

Serves 4

☑ **WHY THIS RECIPE WORKS** We wanted to create a rustic, hearty chicken braise with complex flavor. We chose to build a savory base using bacon; we used the fat to brown our chicken and create flavorful fond. Sautéing cremini mushrooms and plenty of aromatics in the bacon fat deepened their flavors and gave the braise a well-rounded backbone. Tomato paste, rather than canned tomatoes, was a simple solution to creating great simmered tomato flavor. To the aromatics, we added a hefty amount of minced dried porcini. This served two purposes: It added a punch of bold mushroom flavor and also thickened the sauce so that it clung perfectly to the chicken. Once the chicken was cooked, we stirred the crisped bacon into the braising liquid to give the dish some crunchy contrast and extra meaty depth. A handful of fresh parsley and a splash of red wine vinegar provided bright notes that rounded out the warm, earthy flavors. Serve with Sautéed Summer Squash Ribbons (page 307), pictured.

- 4 slices bacon, chopped coarse
- 4 (12-ounce) bone-in split chicken breasts, trimmed
  Kosher salt and pepper
- 8 ounces cremini mushrooms, trimmed and sliced thin
- 1 onion, chopped
- ¼ cup tomato paste
- ¾ ounce dried porcini mushrooms, rinsed and minced
- 3 garlic cloves, minced
- 2 teaspoons minced fresh thyme or ½ teaspoon dried
- 1 cup water
- ¼ cup minced fresh parsley
- 1 tablespoon red wine vinegar

1. Cook bacon in Dutch oven over medium heat until crisp, 5 to 7 minutes. Using slotted spoon, transfer bacon to paper towel–lined plate; set aside. Pour off all but 1 tablespoon fat from pot.

2. Pat chicken dry with paper towels and season with salt and pepper. Heat fat left in pot over medium-high heat until just smoking. Brown chicken well, about 5 minutes per side; transfer to plate. Remove chicken skin.

3. Add cremini mushrooms and onion to fat left in pot and cook over medium heat until softened and lightly browned, about 8 minutes. Stir in tomato paste, porcini mushrooms, garlic, and thyme and cook until fragrant, about 1 minute. Stir in water, scraping up browned bits, and bring to simmer.

4. Nestle chicken into pot along with any accumulated juices. Reduce heat to medium-low, cover, and simmer gently until chicken registers 160 degrees, 10 to 15 minutes. Transfer chicken to serving platter. Stir crisp bacon, parsley, and vinegar into sauce and season with salt and pepper to taste. Spoon sauce over chicken and serve.

TEST KITCHEN TIP **STEMMING THYME**

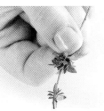

Run thumb and forefinger down stem to release leaves and smaller offshoots. Tender tips can be left intact and chopped along with leaves.

Slow-Cooker Curried Chicken Thighs with Acorn Squash

Serves 4

✅ **WHY THIS RECIPE WORKS** Meaty chicken thighs are a perfect match for the slow cooker, as they become ultratender in its moist heat environment and the risk of overcooking is slim. Here we opted to pair them with acorn squash, which is hearty enough to withstand a few hours in the slow cooker and still hold its shape. Arranging the squash along the bottom of the slow cooker ensured that the large wedges were perfectly tender by the end of cooking. To give this dish a distinct flavor profile, we rubbed the chicken with curry powder that we bloomed in the microwave with a little bit of oil. To finish, we created a quick dressing by combining minced cilantro, honey, and lime zest and juice, and then drizzled the mixture over the chicken and squash. This simple step tied together the flavors of this easy one-dish meal, perfect for a fall night. You will need a 5½- to 7-quart oval slow cooker for this recipe.

2	cinnamon sticks
6	tablespoons extra-virgin olive oil
1	tablespoon curry powder
⅛	teaspoon cayenne pepper
	Kosher salt and pepper
2	small acorn squashes (1 pound each), quartered pole to pole and seeded
8	(5- to 7-ounce) bone-in chicken thighs, trimmed
¼	cup minced fresh cilantro
1	tablespoon honey
½	teaspoon grated lime zest plus 2 tablespoons juice

1. Combine ½ cup water and cinnamon sticks in slow cooker. Microwave 2 tablespoons oil, curry powder, and cayenne in bowl until fragrant, about 30 seconds. Stir in 1½ teaspoons salt and 1 teaspoon pepper and let mixture cool slightly.

2. Season squash with salt and pepper and shingle cut side down into slow cooker. Rub chicken with oil mixture and place skin side up on top of squash. Cover and cook until chicken is tender, 4 to 5 hours on low.

3. Transfer chicken and squash to serving platter. Remove chicken skin and discard cooking liquid. Whisk cilantro, honey, lime zest and juice, and remaining ¼ cup oil together in bowl. Season with salt and pepper to taste. Drizzle chicken and squash with dressing and serve.

TEST KITCHEN TIP **PREPARING ACORN SQUASH**

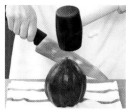

1. With squash set on damp dish towel, position chef's knife on top of squash and strike with mallet to drive it through squash.

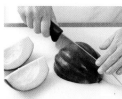

2. After scooping out seeds, place squash halves cut side down on cutting board and cut in half, pole to pole, using mallet if necessary.

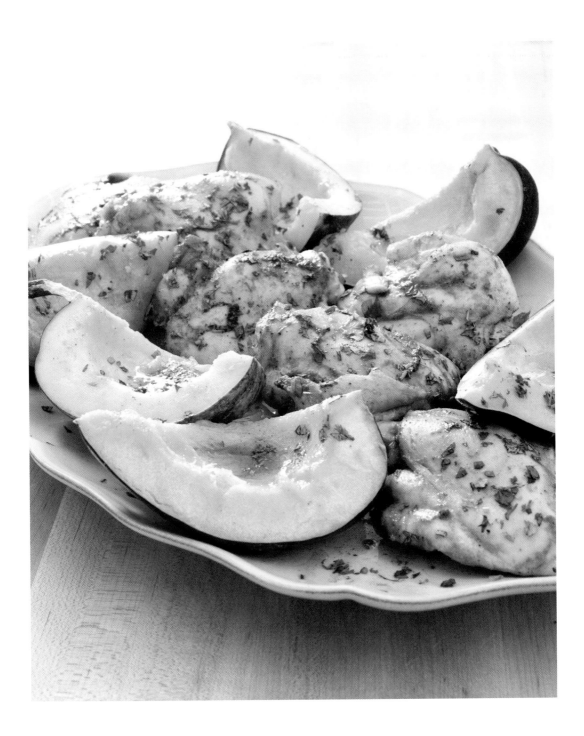

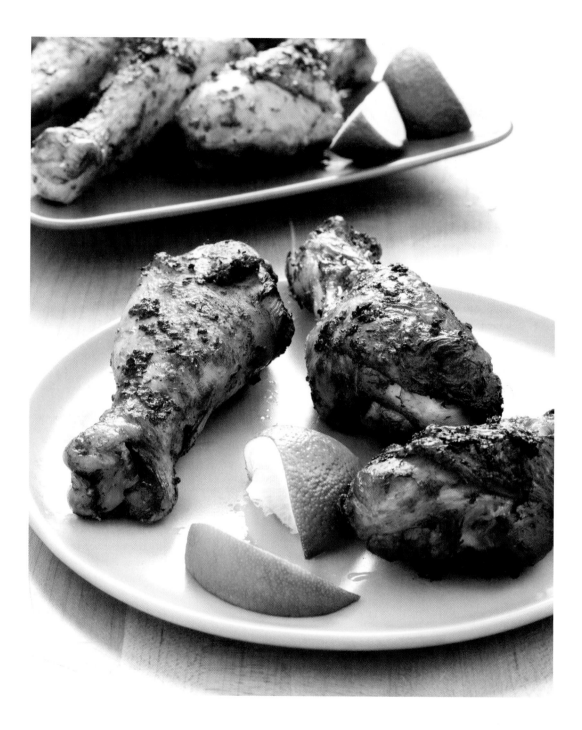

Slow-Cooker Caribbean Chicken Drumsticks

Serves 4 to 6

✓ **WHY THIS RECIPE WORKS** Meltingly tender, slow-cooked chicken drumsticks pair perfectly with bold, spicy flavors, so we set out to create a recipe for Caribbean jerk–style drumsticks. We started by building a flavorful jerk marinade using classic jerk ingredients such as habanero chile, garlic, and ginger. But once we got to the typical additions of molasses and brown sugar, we had to employ some creative techniques to replace these nonpaleo ingredients. A simple solution was to add raisins, which provided a subtle sweetness without giving themselves away. Once slow-cooked, our drumsticks were tender and flavorful, but tasters still wanted crisp skin. A quick stint under the broiler easily solved this problem; brushing the drumsticks twice with some reserved marinade while broiling ensured they stayed moist and contributed additional flavor. Try to buy drumsticks of similar size so that they will cook at the same rate. You can substitute a serrano chile for the habanero. Wear gloves when working with hot chiles. You will need a 5½- to 7-quart slow cooker for this recipe.

8	scallions, chopped coarse
3	tablespoons coconut oil
1	habanero chile, stemmed and seeded
1	(1-inch) piece ginger, peeled and sliced into ¼-inch-thick rounds
2	tablespoons raisins
2	tablespoons minced fresh thyme or 2 teaspoons dried
3	garlic cloves, peeled and smashed
1	tablespoon ground allspice
	Kosher salt and pepper
1	teaspoon ground coriander
4	pounds chicken drumsticks
	Lime wedges

1. Process scallions, oil, habanero, ginger, thyme, garlic, allspice, 2 teaspoons salt, ½ teaspoon pepper, and coriander in food processor until smooth, about 30 seconds, scraping down sides of bowl as needed. Transfer ½ cup paste to large bowl; transfer remaining paste to small bowl and set aside.

2. Add chicken to large bowl with paste and toss to coat; transfer to slow cooker. Cover and cook until chicken is tender, 3 to 4 hours on low.

3. Adjust oven rack 6 inches from broiler element and heat broiler. Set wire rack in aluminum foil–lined rimmed baking sheet. Transfer drumsticks to prepared rack; discard cooking liquid.

4. Microwave reserved paste until heated through, about 20 seconds. Brush chicken with half of paste and broil until lightly charred and crisp, about 15 minutes, flipping and brushing drumsticks with remaining paste halfway through broiling. Serve with lime wedges.

TEST KITCHEN TIP **PEELING GINGER**

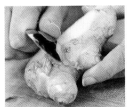

Hold knob of ginger firmly against cutting board and use edge of dinner spoon to scrape away thin brown skin. Grate or slice peeled ginger as directed.

Braised Chicken Thighs with Swiss Chard and Carrots

Serves 4

✔ **WHY THIS RECIPE WORKS** We wanted a one-pot meal loaded with flavor and replete with tender chicken and nourishing vegetables. We started with bone-in chicken thighs, which we browned on both sides to build flavor and help the skin crisp. We then took the chicken out of the pot and built our braising liquid. Plenty of aromatics provided depth of flavor, while a slightly unusual addition—anchovies—gave the dish a savory backbone without tasting fishy. Once our braising liquid was complete, we added carrots and our browned chicken thighs back to the pot. We encouraged the chicken skin to crisp up further by placing the thighs skin side up and leaving the pot uncovered, exposing the skin to the dry heat of the oven. While the chicken rested, we whisked a little arrowroot into the braising liquid to create a silky sauce and then quickly cooked the chard right in the sauce. Finally, a dab of mustard added a punch of flavor while lemon zest and juice added necessary brightness. Use carrots that measure ¾ inch to 1¼ inches at the thickest end.

8   (5- to 7-ounce) bone-in chicken thighs, trimmed
    Kosher salt and pepper
1   tablespoon extra-virgin olive oil
1   onion, chopped fine
6   garlic cloves, minced
1   tablespoon minced fresh thyme or 1 teaspoon dried
2   anchovy fillets, rinsed and minced
1   cup water
1   pound carrots, peeled and halved crosswise
1   tablespoon arrowroot flour
2   pounds Swiss chard, stemmed and sliced into ½-inch-wide strips
3   tablespoons whole-grain mustard
1   teaspoon grated lemon zest plus 2 teaspoons juice

1. Adjust oven rack to lower-middle position and heat oven to 325 degrees. Pat chicken dry with paper towels and season with salt and pepper. Heat oil in Dutch oven over medium-high heat until just smoking. Brown half of chicken well, about 5 minutes per side; transfer to plate. Pour off all but 1 tablespoon fat from pot and repeat with remaining chicken; transfer to plate.

2. Pour off all but 1 tablespoon fat from pot. Add onion and cook over medium heat until softened, about 5 minutes. Stir in garlic, thyme, and anchovies and cook until fragrant, about 30 seconds. Stir in water, scraping up any browned bits. Stir in carrots and bring to simmer.

3. Nestle chicken skin side up into pot (skin should be above surface of liquid) along with any accumulated juices. Transfer pot to oven and braise, uncovered, until chicken offers little resistance when poked with tip of paring knife but still clings to bones, 1 to 1¼ hours.

4. Transfer chicken to serving platter, tent with aluminum foil, and let rest while finishing vegetables.

5. Being careful of hot pot handles, whisk 2 tablespoons braising liquid and flour together in small bowl. Gently stir flour mixture into remaining braising liquid, bring to simmer over medium heat, and cook until slightly thickened, about 2 minutes. Stir in chard, 1 handful at a time, and cook until wilted and tender, about 5 minutes. Off heat, stir in mustard and lemon zest and juice. Season with salt and pepper to taste. Serve.

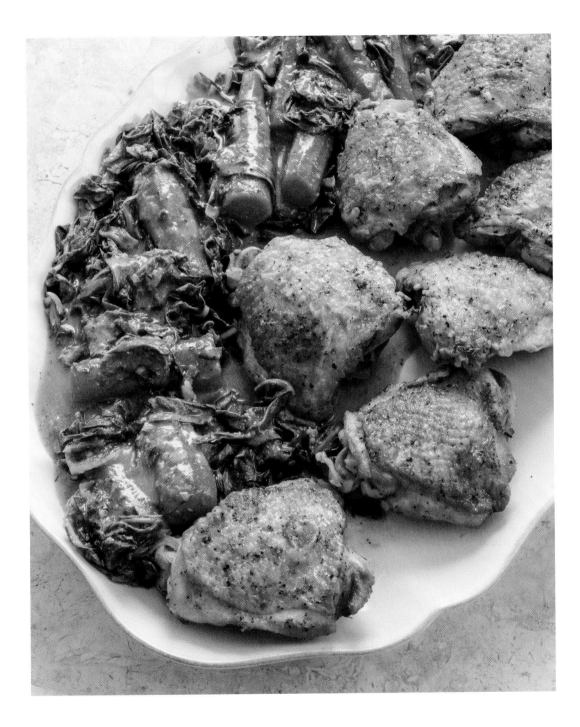

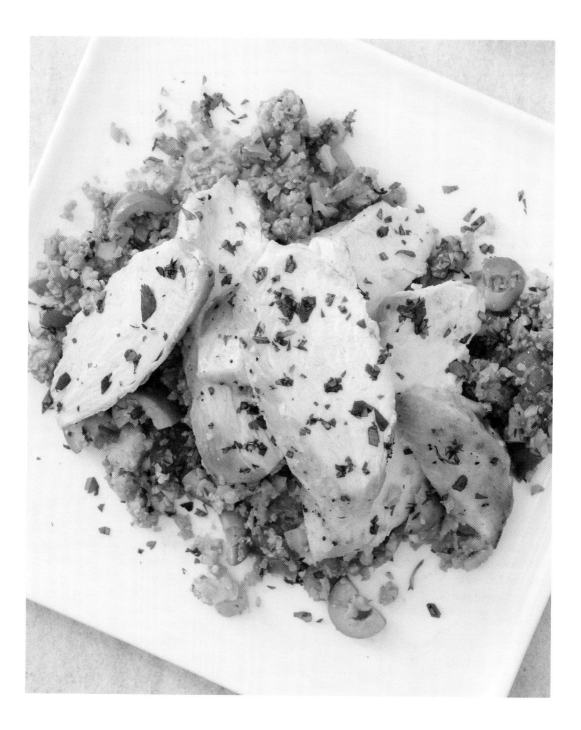

Latin-Style Chicken and Cauliflower Rice

Serves 4

✓ **WHY THIS RECIPE WORKS** We set out to create a variation on the classic combination of chicken and rice that paired flavorful chicken with paleo-friendly cauliflower rice. Since cauliflower is easy to break down into rice-size pieces and the granules cook up tender and distinct, it's a popular paleo substitute for rice. Chopping the cauliflower in the food processor was easy and produced a more even texture than chopping by hand. To keep the dish simple, we wanted to cook everything in one pan. Because the cauliflower rice cooked through quickly, our chicken had to as well. We settled on boneless, skinless chicken breasts, which we seared to jump-start the cooking and create flavorful browning. A bold, Latin-inspired flavor profile worked well with the mild chicken and cauliflower. We bloomed smoked paprika and cayenne with our aromatics to build a flavorful backbone, and added a little chicken broth to boost savory depth. We then stirred in our cauliflower rice and nestled in our browned chicken. Within minutes, the chicken and cauliflower were perfectly tender. As a finishing touch, we folded fresh tomatoes and briny olives into the rice, and finished the dish with a sprinkle of bright cilantro. We prefer to use homemade chicken broth; however, you can substitute your favorite store-bought broth. For more information on making cauliflower rice, see step photo on page 288.

1   **head cauliflower (2 pounds), cored and cut into 1-inch florets (6 cups)**
4   **(6- to 8-ounce) boneless, skinless chicken breasts, trimmed**
    Kosher salt and pepper
3   **tablespoons extra-virgin olive oil**
1   **onion, chopped fine**
1   **tablespoon tomato paste**
1   **tablespoon minced fresh oregano or 1 teaspoon dried**
2   **garlic cloves, minced**
2   **teaspoons smoked paprika**
⅛   **teaspoon cayenne pepper**
½   **cup Paleo Chicken Broth (page 16)**
1   **tomato, cored and chopped**
½   **cup pitted large green olives, chopped coarse**
3   **tablespoons minced fresh cilantro**

1. Working in 2 batches, pulse cauliflower in food processor until finely ground into ¼- to ⅛-inch pieces, 4 to 6 pulses, scraping down sides of bowl as needed; transfer to bowl.

2. Cover chicken with plastic wrap and pound to even thickness. Pat chicken dry with paper towels and season with salt and pepper. Heat 1 tablespoon oil in 12-inch skillet over medium-high heat until just smoking. Place chicken in skillet and cook until browned on 1 side, about 4 minutes; transfer to plate.

3. Add remaining 2 tablespoons oil to now-empty skillet and return to medium heat until shimmering. Add onion and 1 teaspoon salt and cook until softened, about 5 minutes. Stir in tomato paste, oregano, garlic, paprika, and cayenne and cook until fragrant, about 1 minute. Stir in broth, scraping up any browned bits, then stir in processed cauliflower. Nestle chicken browned side up into skillet along with any accumulated juices. Reduce heat to medium-low, cover, and cook until chicken registers 160 degrees, 10 to 12 minutes.

4. Transfer chicken to cutting board and let rest while finishing cauliflower rice. Stir tomato and olives into cauliflower rice and cook until cauliflower is tender and mixture is almost completely dry, about 5 minutes. Season with salt and pepper to taste. Transfer cauliflower rice to serving platter. Slice chicken into ½-inch-thick slices and arrange on top of cauliflower rice. Sprinkle with cilantro and serve.

Stir-Fried Chicken and Broccoli with Sesame-Orange Sauce

Serves 4

✓ **WHY THIS RECIPE WORKS** Traditional chicken stir-fries, surprisingly enough, are not paleo-friendly: Between the chicken itself, which is often coated in cornstarch (a process called velveting), and the sauce, which is usually laden with ingredients like soy sauce, sugar, Chinese wine, and more cornstarch, we had our work cut out for us. When velveting the chicken, we found that tapioca flour made a perfect replacement for cornstarch: It's a pure starch, and, when mixed with a bit of sesame oil, it clung to the chicken and protected it from the heat. Cooking the chicken in batches encouraged deep, flavorful browning. As for the sauce, a combination of coconut aminos and fish sauce replicated the savory flavor of soy sauce, while some fresh orange juice provided subtle sweetness and acidic notes. This recipe calls for a 12-inch nonstick skillet; however, a well-seasoned cast-iron skillet can be used instead. To make the chicken easier to slice, freeze it for 15 minutes. For more information on coconut aminos, see page 11. Serve with Cauliflower Rice (page 288).

SAUCE

- ¼ cup coconut aminos
- 2 tablespoons toasted sesame oil
- 2 teaspoons fish sauce
- 1½ teaspoons tapioca flour
- ½ teaspoon grated orange zest plus ½ cup juice

STIR-FRY

- 2 tablespoons plus 1 teaspoon toasted sesame oil
- 1½ teaspoons tapioca flour
- 1 teaspoon coconut aminos
- 1 pound boneless, skinless chicken breasts, trimmed and sliced thin into 2-inch-long pieces
- 3 garlic cloves, minced
- ¼ teaspoon red pepper flakes
- 2 tablespoons coconut oil
- 1 pound broccoli florets, cut into 1-inch pieces
- 4 carrots, peeled and sliced on bias ¼ inch thick
- 2 teaspoons sesame seeds, toasted

1. FOR THE SAUCE Whisk all ingredients together in bowl.

2. FOR THE STIR-FRY Whisk 2 tablespoons sesame oil, flour, and coconut aminos together in medium bowl until smooth, then stir in chicken. In separate bowl, combine garlic, pepper flakes, and remaining 1 teaspoon sesame oil.

3. Heat 2 teaspoons coconut oil in 12-inch nonstick skillet over high heat until just smoking. Add half of chicken, break up any clumps, and cook, without stirring, for 1 minute. Stir chicken and continue to cook until lightly browned, about 30 seconds; transfer to clean bowl. Repeat with 2 teaspoons coconut oil and remaining chicken; transfer to bowl.

4. Heat remaining 2 teaspoons coconut oil in now-empty skillet over medium-high heat until just smoking. Add broccoli and carrots and cook for 1 minute. Add ⅓ cup water, cover, and cook until vegetables are crisp-tender, about 2 minutes. Remove lid and continue to cook until vegetables are tender and most of liquid has evaporated, about 2 minutes.

5. Push vegetables to sides of skillet. Add garlic mixture to center and cook, mashing mixture into skillet, until fragrant, about 30 seconds. Stir mixture into vegetables.

6. Stir cooked chicken and any accumulated juices into vegetables. Whisk sauce to recombine, then add to skillet. Cook, stirring constantly, until sauce is thickened, about 30 seconds. Transfer to serving platter and sprinkle with sesame seeds. Serve.

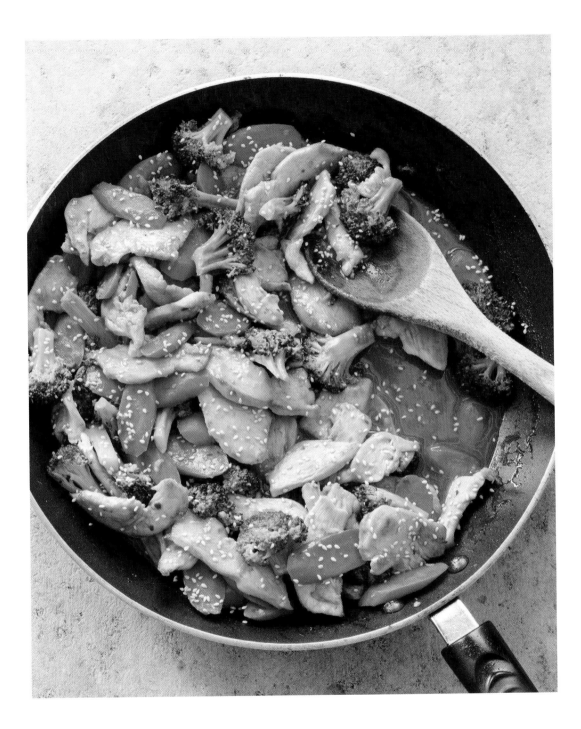

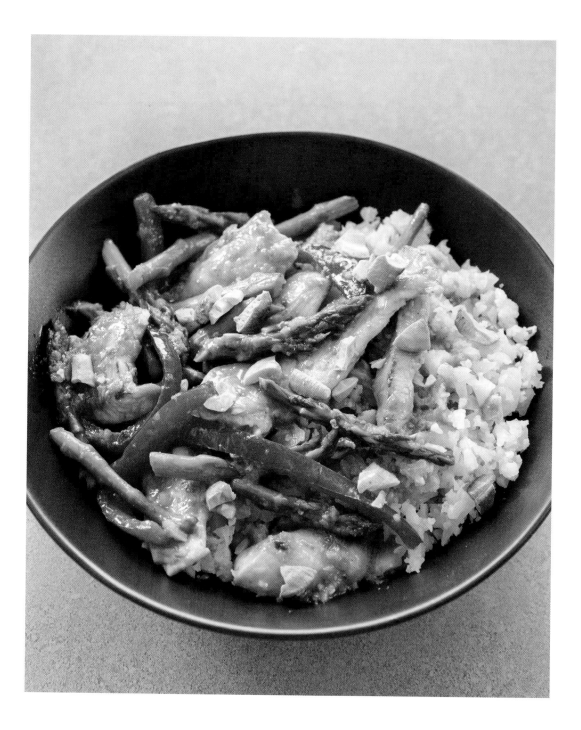

Gingery Stir-Fried Chicken with Asparagus and Bell Pepper

Serves 4

☑ **WHY THIS RECIPE WORKS** We wanted to explore the possibilities of paleo stir-fries and develop a chicken version with a punchy, spicy profile. First, we built our sauce. We made a base out of coconut aminos, a common paleo replacement for soy sauce; rice vinegar for tanginess; and chicken broth to round out the flavor. To ensure the sauce thickened enough to coat the chicken and vegetables, we swapped out the traditional cornstarch for paleo-friendly tapioca flour. But in early tastings, tasters thought the sauce lacked the depth that soy sauce–based stir-fry sauces usually have. Adding a bit of fish sauce easily solved this problem, providing savory notes without giving itself away. Next, we turned to the chicken. To ensure that the lean meat stayed tender through cooking, we coated it in a mixture of coconut aminos, tapioca flour, and sesame oil, which both gave the chicken a boost of flavor and created a barrier against the high heat. For the vegetables, we started with bok choy, but found its flavor and texture in the finished stir-fry lackluster. We turned instead to asparagus, which provided a welcome crisp texture and grassy flavor. Bell peppers offered a pop of color and a welcome sweetness. To give our stir-fry a distinctive backbone, we stirred in a whopping 2 tablespoons of grated fresh ginger toward the end of cooking. Although tasters liked the flavors of the stir-fry, they felt it needed an additional textural element. Cashews fit the bill perfectly; just ½ cup of the toasted and chopped nuts contributed a pleasant crunchy element and a nutty, buttery flavor. This recipe calls for a 12-inch nonstick skillet; however, a well-seasoned cast-iron skillet can be used instead. To make the chicken easier to slice, freeze it for 15 minutes. We prefer to use homemade chicken broth; however, you can substitute your favorite store-bought broth. For more information on coconut aminos, see page 11. Serve with Cauliflower Rice (page 288).

SAUCE
- ½ cup Paleo Chicken Broth (page 16)
- ¼ cup coconut aminos
- 2 teaspoons fish sauce
- 1½ teaspoons tapioca flour
- 1 teaspoon rice vinegar

STIR-FRY
- 2 tablespoons plus 1 teaspoon toasted sesame oil
- 2 teaspoons coconut aminos
- 1½ teaspoons tapioca flour
- 1 pound boneless, skinless chicken breasts, trimmed and sliced thin into 2-inch-long pieces
- 2 tablespoons grated fresh ginger
- 1 garlic clove, minced
- ¼ teaspoon red pepper flakes
- 2 tablespoons coconut oil
- 1 pound asparagus, trimmed and cut on bias into 2-inch lengths
- 2 red bell peppers, stemmed, seeded, and cut into ¼-inch-wide strips
- ½ cup raw cashews, toasted and chopped coarse

1. FOR THE SAUCE Whisk all ingredients together in bowl.

2. FOR THE STIR-FRY Whisk 2 tablespoons sesame oil, coconut aminos, and flour together in medium bowl until smooth, then stir in chicken. In separate bowl, combine ginger, garlic, pepper flakes, and remaining 1 teaspoon sesame oil.

3. Heat 2 teaspoons coconut oil in 12-inch nonstick skillet over high heat until just smoking. Add half of chicken, break up any clumps, and cook, without stirring, for 1 minute. Stir chicken and continue to cook until lightly browned, about 30 seconds; transfer to clean bowl. Repeat with 2 teaspoons coconut oil and remaining chicken; transfer to bowl.

4. Heat remaining 2 teaspoons coconut oil in now-empty skillet over medium-high heat until just smoking. Add asparagus and bell peppers and cook, stirring occasionally, until asparagus is spotty brown, 3 to 4 minutes. Push vegetables to sides of skillet. Add ginger mixture to center and cook, mashing mixture into skillet, until fragrant, about 30 seconds. Stir mixture into vegetables.

5. Stir cooked chicken and any accumulated juices into vegetables. Whisk sauce to recombine, then add to skillet. Cook, stirring constantly, until sauce is thickened, about 30 seconds. Transfer to serving platter and sprinkle with cashews. Serve.

TEST KITCHEN TIP **PREPARING CHICKEN FOR STIR-FRY**

Traditional stir-fry recipes often call for coating the chicken with a cornstarch mixture to keep the lean meat from drying out in the hot oil, a technique known as velveting. We had to find a way to make the coating paleo-friendly.

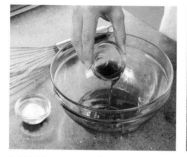

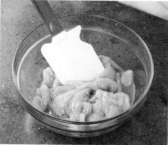

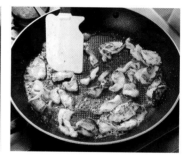

1. Whisk sesame oil, coconut aminos, and tapioca flour together in medium bowl until smooth. Tapioca flour and coconut aminos stand in for traditional cornstarch and soy sauce.

2. Stir in chicken. Make sure chicken is well coated to protect it from becoming dry during cooking.

3. Heat coconut oil in nonstick skillet until just smoking. Add half of chicken, break up clumps, and cook without stirring for 1 minute. Stir and continue to cook for 30 seconds; transfer to bowl and repeat with remaining chicken. Cooking in batches and not stirring for 1 minute encourages flavorful browning.

Batter-Fried Chicken Fingers

Serves 4 to 6

✓ **WHY THIS RECIPE WORKS** With their crispy, crunchy fried coating, chicken fingers are undeniably appealing to both kids and adults. But most batters rely heavily on nonpaleo ingredients like flour or cornstarch, and these recipes often call for 4 or more cups of frying oil—impractical when you're using paleo-friendly oils, which are more expensive than vegetable oils. We set out to solve these problems. We started with boneless, skinless chicken breasts, which we brined briefly to ensure that the meat stayed moist through cooking. For a coating that cooked up crisp, flavorful, and perfectly browned, we came up with a paleo version of a traditional batter, replacing the typical cornstarch and all-purpose flour with arrowroot and almond flours. The arrowroot's high starch content helped the batter to crisp up in the hot oil, while a small amount of almond flour prevented the batter from being too flaky. Taking a cue from other batter recipes, we lightened the batter by using seltzer in place of plain water. A 15-minute rest gave the flours time to absorb some liquid, thickening the batter nicely and preventing a gritty texture. Baking soda and cream of tartar ensured that the batter didn't become dense and encouraged flavorful browning. To fry our chicken, we decided to use coconut oil, which had a neutral flavor and performed well at the high temperature needed for frying. To avoid having to use copious amounts of the pricey oil, we switched from a large Dutch oven to a 10-inch skillet and fried the chicken in batches. We found that we could use a mere 1½ cups of oil and still achieve moist, tender chicken with a crisp, crunchy exterior. Do not substitute ghee for the coconut oil, as its flavor deteriorates during frying. Serve with dipping sauce (see recipes on page 124).

2	pounds boneless, skinless chicken breasts, trimmed
	Kosher salt and pepper
1	cup arrowroot flour
6	tablespoons almond flour
1½	teaspoons paprika
¾	teaspoon garlic powder
¼	teaspoon cayenne pepper
¾	cup seltzer
1½	teaspoons cream of tartar
¾	teaspoon baking soda
1½	cups coconut oil

1. Cover chicken with plastic wrap and pound to even thickness. Cut each chicken breast diagonally into 1-inch-thick pieces. Dissolve ¼ cup salt in 1½ quarts cold water in large container. Submerge chicken pieces in brine, cover, and refrigerate for 30 minutes.

2. Adjust oven rack to middle position and heat oven to 200 degrees. Line large plate with paper towels. Set wire rack in rimmed baking sheet.

3. Whisk arrowroot flour, almond flour, paprika, garlic powder, cayenne, ½ teaspoon salt, and ½ teaspoon pepper together in large bowl. Whisk in seltzer until thoroughly combined and smooth and let sit until thickened, about 15 minutes.

4. Whisk cream of tartar and baking soda into batter. Remove chicken from brine and pat dry with paper towels; discard brine. Add chicken to batter and toss to coat thoroughly.

5. Heat oil in 10-inch skillet over medium-high heat to 375 degrees. Remove one-quarter of chicken from batter, allowing excess batter to drip back into bowl, and carefully add chicken to hot oil. Fry chicken until deep golden brown on first side, about 3 minutes. Flip chicken and continue to fry until golden brown on second side, about 2 minutes.

Adjust burner, if necessary, to maintain oil temperature between 325 and 350 degrees. Drain chicken briefly on prepared plate, then transfer to prepared rack and keep warm in oven.

6. Return oil to 375 degrees. Toss remaining chicken to recoat in batter and repeat frying in 3 more batches. Serve.

Honey-Mustard Dipping Sauce
MAKES ABOUT 3/4 CUP

- ½ **cup honey**
- ⅓ **cup Dijon mustard**
  Kosher salt and pepper

Whisk honey and mustard together in bowl and season with salt and pepper to taste. Serve.

Ranch Dipping Sauce
MAKES ABOUT 3/4 CUP

We prefer to use homemade almond yogurt; however, you can substitute your favorite unsweetened store-bought brand.

- ¾ **cup Paleo Almond Yogurt (page 23)**
- 2 **tablespoons minced fresh cilantro**
- 1 **tablespoon minced fresh dill**
- 1 **tablespoon lemon juice**
- 1 **small garlic clove, minced**
  Kosher salt and pepper

Whisk almond yogurt, cilantro, dill, lemon juice, garlic, ½ teaspoon salt, and ¼ teaspoon pepper together in bowl. Season with salt and pepper to taste. Serve.

TEST KITCHEN TIP **MAKING PALEO BATTER**

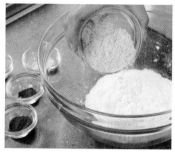

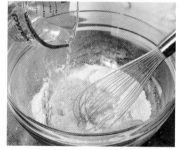

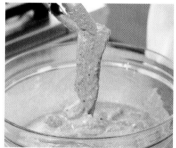

1. Whisk together arrowroot flour, almond flour, and seasonings in large bowl. Arrowroot flour allows batter to become crisp without being flaky.

2. To lighten batter, whisk in seltzer. Allow batter to rest until thickened, about 15 minutes, to ensure that flours are fully hydrated and not gritty. Add baking soda at this point so it does not activate too early.

3. Add chicken to batter and toss to coat thoroughly. To avoid doughy coating, let excess batter drip back into bowl before placing chicken in hot oil.

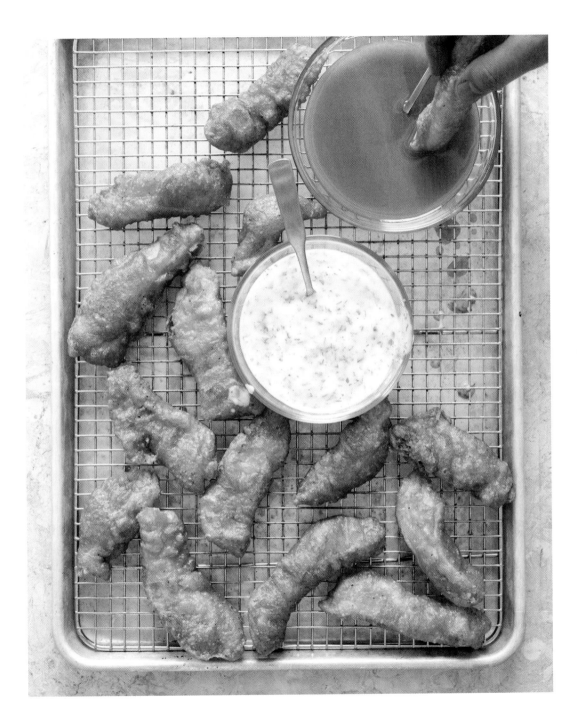

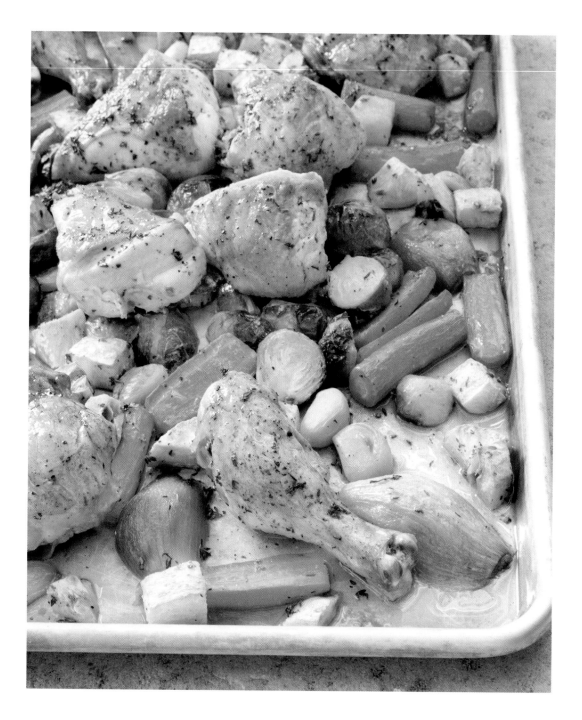

One-Pan Roast Chicken with Root Vegetables

Serves 4

☑ **WHY THIS RECIPE WORKS** Being able to cook flavorful chicken and a generous amount of vegetables together in one pan is a technique every cook should have in their arsenal, paleo or not. We wanted a fool-proof method to perfectly cook chicken and vegetables simultaneously. The key to a great finished dish was making sure that everything cooked at the same rate. To achieve this, we used chicken parts, which are smaller and cook faster than a whole bird. Placing the delicate chicken breasts in the center of a sheet pan with the thighs and drumsticks around the perimeter kept the white meat moist and tender while also allowing the dark meat to cook through. A similar treatment for the vegetables—leafy Brussels sprouts in the middle, hardier celery root and carrots on the outside—also proved effective. We were careful not to smother the vegetables underneath the chicken, which would have caused them to steam. Use Brussels sprouts no bigger than golf balls, as larger ones are often tough and woody.

12 ounces Brussels sprouts, trimmed and halved

1 celery root (14 ounces), peeled and cut into 1-inch pieces

4 carrots, peeled and cut into 2-inch lengths, thick ends halved lengthwise

8 shallots, peeled and halved

3 tablespoons ghee, melted

6 garlic cloves, peeled

4 teaspoons minced fresh thyme

1 teaspoon honey
Kosher salt and pepper

3½ pounds bone-in chicken pieces (2 split breasts cut in half crosswise, 2 drumsticks, and 2 thighs), trimmed

1. Adjust oven rack to upper-middle position and heat oven to 475 degrees. Toss Brussels sprouts, celery root, carrots, shallots, 1 tablespoon melted ghee, garlic, 2 teaspoons thyme, honey, 1 teaspoon salt, and ¼ teaspoon pepper together in bowl. In separate bowl, combine remaining 2 tablespoons melted ghee, remaining 2 teaspoons thyme, ¼ teaspoon salt, and ⅛ teaspoon pepper.

2. Pat chicken dry with paper towels and season with salt and pepper. Place vegetables in single layer on rimmed baking sheet, arranging Brussels sprouts in center. Place chicken skin side up on top of vegetables, arranging breast pieces in center and leg and thigh pieces around perimeter of sheet.

3. Brush chicken with herb mixture and roast until breasts register 160 degrees and drumsticks/thighs register 175 degrees, 35 to 40 minutes, rotating sheet halfway through roasting.

4. Transfer chicken to serving platter, tent with aluminum foil, and let rest for 5 to 10 minutes. Toss vegetables in pan juices and transfer to platter with chicken. Serve.

TEST KITCHEN TIP
HALVING BONE-IN CHICKEN BREASTS

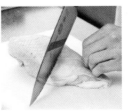

To make sure they cook in time, cut breasts in half. When knife hits bone, rock knife back and forth, applying pressure from heel of your other hand.

Roast Chicken with Mushroom Pan Sauce

Serves 4

✓ **WHY THIS RECIPE WORKS** Tender, moist chicken pairs perfectly with a bright, aromatic pan sauce, but most pan sauces are made with butter, wine, and other nonpaleo ingredients. We set out to bring pan sauce into the paleo kitchen. Focusing first on the chicken, we put a tried-and-true test kitchen technique to work: We roasted the bird using a preheated skillet, which gave the dark meat a jump start on cooking. Starting the chicken in a hot oven and then turning the oven off for the remainder of the cooking time allowed the chicken to cook through gently. Since this method uses a skillet to roast the chicken, we could easily make a pan sauce while the chicken rested. Unfortunately, our attempts to replace wine and butter with vinegar and ghee turned out pan sauces that were greasy, sour, or lackluster. Instead, we created a rounder, more balanced profile for our pan sauce by using earthy mushrooms as the base ingredient. Shallots, garlic, thyme, and tomato paste provided an aromatic backbone for the sauce. Deglazing with chicken broth melded all the flavors; but without the butter, this sauce was on the thin side. A little arrowroot flour thickened the sauce perfectly. Sherry vinegar, added at the end of cooking, brightened things up. You can substitute 2 tablespoons ghee for the reserved chicken fat in step 4. You will need a 12-inch ovensafe skillet for this recipe. We prefer to use homemade chicken broth; however, you can substitute your favorite store-bought broth. We recommend using a 3½- to 4-pound chicken for this recipe. If roasting a slightly larger bird, increase the time when the oven is on in step 2 to 35 to 40 minutes.

1   (3½- to 4-pound) whole chicken, giblets discarded
1   tablespoon ghee, melted
      Kosher salt and pepper
1½ cups Paleo Chicken Broth (page 16)
2   teaspoons arrowroot flour
8   ounces cremini mushrooms, trimmed and sliced thin
2   shallots, minced
2   teaspoons tomato paste
2   garlic cloves, minced
2   teaspoons minced fresh thyme or ½ teaspoon dried
½   teaspoon sherry vinegar

1. Adjust oven rack to middle position, place 12-inch ovensafe skillet on rack, and heat oven to 450 degrees. Pat chicken dry with paper towels, then rub entire surface with melted ghee and season with salt and pepper. Tie legs together with twine and tuck wingtips behind back.

2. Transfer chicken breast side up to hot skillet in oven. Roast chicken until breast registers 120 degrees and thighs register 135 degrees, 25 to 35 minutes. Turn oven off and leave chicken in oven until breast registers 160 degrees and thighs register 175 degrees, 25 to 35 minutes.

3. Using potholder (skillet handle will be hot), remove skillet from oven. Transfer chicken to carving board and let rest while finishing sauce. Carefully defat drippings using wide, shallow spoon or fat separator, reserving 2 tablespoons fat. Whisk defatted drippings, broth, and flour together in bowl.

4. Heat reserved fat in now-empty skillet over medium heat until shimmering. Add mushrooms, shallots, and ½ teaspoon salt and cook until softened and lightly browned, 8 to 10 minutes. Stir in tomato paste, garlic, and thyme and cook until fragrant, about 1 minute.

5. Whisk drippings mixture to recombine, then add to skillet. Cook, scraping up any browned bits, until sauce is thickened, about 8 minutes. Off heat, stir in vinegar and season with salt and pepper to taste. Carve chicken and serve, passing sauce separately.

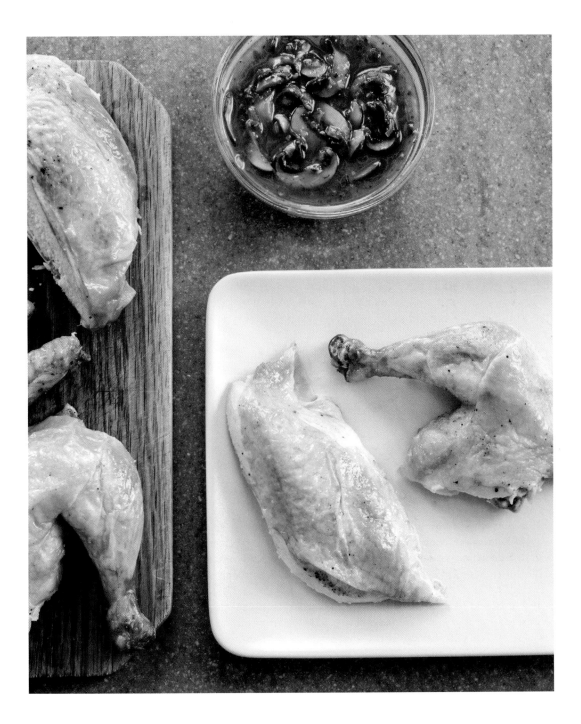

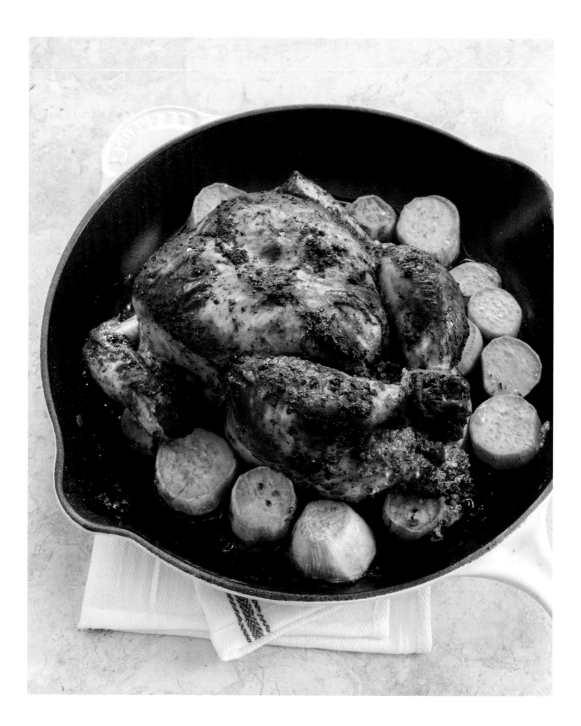

Peruvian Roast Chicken with Sweet Potatoes

Serves 4

☑ **WHY THIS RECIPE WORKS** For a distinctive new take on the everyday roast chicken, we found inspiration in a Peruvian preparation that boasts an evenly bronzed exterior, moist meat, and robust flavor. To replicate the traditional flavor profile, we started by applying a salty, oil-based paste made with garlic, fresh mint, habanero, and a myriad of spices. We rubbed the paste both underneath the skin and on the exterior of the bird to season the chicken thoroughly from skin to bone. We then let the bird marinate for at least 6 hours to ensure that the flavors had a chance to penetrate the meat. Since we were pan-roasting the bird, we decided to seize the opportunity and make a one-pan meal by adding a side dish to the pan. Potatoes seemed like a good choice; they're well suited to long roasting and would soak up the flavorful juices from the chicken. Since white potatoes aren't part of the paleo diet, we decided to use earthy sweet potatoes. We found that we could sear the potatoes in the pan and then place the chicken on top of them to bake. You can substitute 1 tablespoon of minced serrano chile for the habanero. Wear gloves when working with hot chiles. This recipe calls for a 12-inch ovensafe nonstick skillet; however, a well-seasoned cast-iron skillet can be used instead. If the top of the chicken starts to become too dark during roasting, place a piece of foil over the breast.

¼ cup fresh mint leaves

6 garlic cloves, chopped coarse

1 tablespoon plus 1 teaspoon extra-virgin olive oil

1 tablespoon ground cumin

1 tablespoon honey

2 teaspoons smoked paprika

2 teaspoons dried oregano

2 teaspoons grated lime zest plus ¼ cup juice (2 limes), plus lime wedges for serving
Kosher salt and pepper

1 teaspoon minced habanero chile

1 (3½- to 4-pound) whole chicken, giblets discarded

2 pounds sweet potatoes, peeled, ends squared off, and sliced into 1-inch-thick rounds

1. Process mint, garlic, 1 tablespoon oil, cumin, honey, paprika, oregano, lime zest and juice, 1 tablespoon pepper, 1½ teaspoons salt, and habanero in blender until smooth, 10 to 20 seconds.

2. Using your fingers, gently loosen skin covering breast and thighs of chicken. Spread half of paste under skin directly on meat of breast and thighs and spread remaining paste over exterior of chicken. Tie legs together with kitchen twine and tuck wingtips behind back. Place chicken in 1-gallon zipper-lock bag and refrigerate for at least 6 hours or up to 24 hours.

3. Adjust oven rack to lowest position and heat oven to 400 degrees. Heat remaining 1 teaspoon oil in 12-inch ovensafe nonstick skillet over medium heat until shimmering. Toss potatoes with ½ teaspoon salt and arrange, flat sides down, in single layer in skillet. Cook potatoes until browned on bottom, 6 to 10 minutes (do not flip).

4. Place chicken breast side up on top of potatoes, transfer skillet to oven, and roast until breast registers 160 degrees and thighs register 175 degrees, 1¼ to 1¾ hours. Using potholder (skillet handle will be hot), remove skillet from oven. Transfer chicken to carving board, tent loosely with aluminum foil, and let rest for 15 minutes. Carve chicken and serve with potatoes and lime wedges.

Roast Cornish Game Hens

Serves 4

✅ **WHY THIS RECIPE WORKS** Petite, tender Cornish game hens are a great paleo-friendly alternative to a whole roast chicken: Each diner gets their own bird, making for an attractive and impressive presentation. Plus, Cornish hens cook quickly, the breasts are less prone to drying out before the interiors cook through (a perennial hurdle when roasting regular chickens), and they have a high skin-to-meat ratio, which makes them both forgiving and flavorful. But because Cornish hens cook so quickly, the skin usually doesn't have time to become crisp. We wanted to change that. To start, we butterflied each hen to make sure the entire surface would be evenly exposed to the heat when placed in the oven, and cut them in half for easy handling. We then rubbed them with a flavorful herb-salt mixture and let them sit in the refrigerator, uncovered. This acted similar to a brine and helped keep the birds moist through cooking, and, with the addition of baking soda, also helped dry out the skin so that it would crisp in the short cooking time. We found that poking the hens with skewers helped to render the fat. We used a hot, 500-degree oven, and placed the hens skin side down on a preheated baking sheet, which gave the skin a jump start on cooking. Finishing the hens under the broiler ensured that the skin was perfectly crisp by the time the meat was cooked through.

4   (1¼- to 1½-pound) whole Cornish game
    hens, giblets discarded
    Kosher salt and pepper
1   teaspoon dried thyme
1   teaspoon dried marjoram
1   teaspoon dried rosemary, crushed
1   teaspoon extra-virgin olive oil
1   teaspoon baking soda

1. Working with 1 hen at a time, use kitchen shears to cut along both sides of backbone to remove it. Flatten hens and lay breast side up on counter. Using sharp chef's knife, cut through center of breast to make 2 halves.

2. Using your fingers, carefully separate skin from thighs and breast. Using metal skewer or tip of paring knife, poke 10 to 15 holes in fat deposits on top of breast halves and thighs. Tuck wing tips underneath hen. Pat hens dry with paper towels.

3. Combine 2 tablespoons salt, thyme, marjoram, and rosemary in bowl. Sprinkle half of salt mixture on underside (bone side) of hens. Stir oil into remaining salt mixture until mixture is evenly coated with oil. Add baking soda and stir until well combined. Turn hens skin side up and rub salt mixture evenly over surface. Transfer hens skin side up to wire rack set in rimmed baking sheet. Refrigerate, uncovered, for at least 4 hours or up to 24 hours.

4. Adjust oven racks to upper-middle and lower-middle positions, place rimmed baking sheet on lower rack, and heat oven to 500 degrees.

5. Once oven is fully heated, season hens with pepper and carefully transfer skin side down to heated sheet and roast for 10 minutes.

6. Remove hens from oven and heat broiler. Flip hens skin side up. Transfer sheet with hens to upper rack and broil until well browned and breasts register 160 degrees and thighs register 175 degrees, about 5 minutes, rotating sheet as necessary to promote even browning. Serve.

TEST KITCHEN TIP

BUTTERFLYING CORNISH GAME HENS

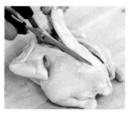

Using kitchen shears, cut along both sides of backbone; discard backbone. Then, flip bird breast side up and use heel of your hand to flatten breastbone.

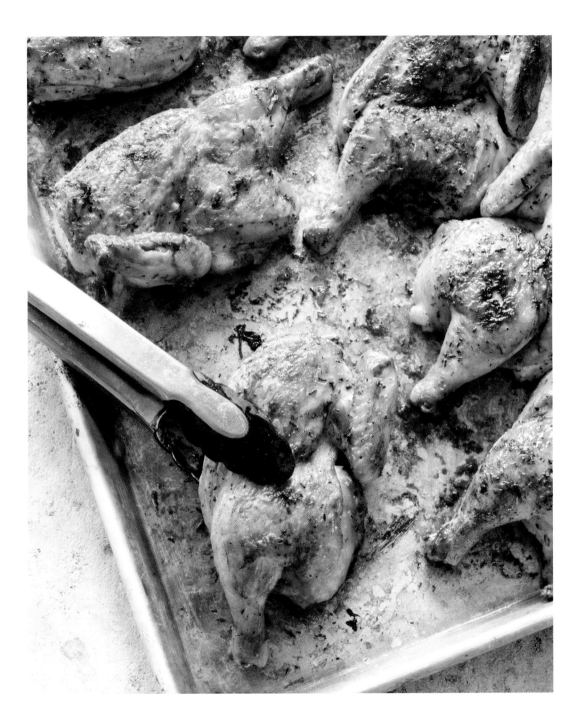

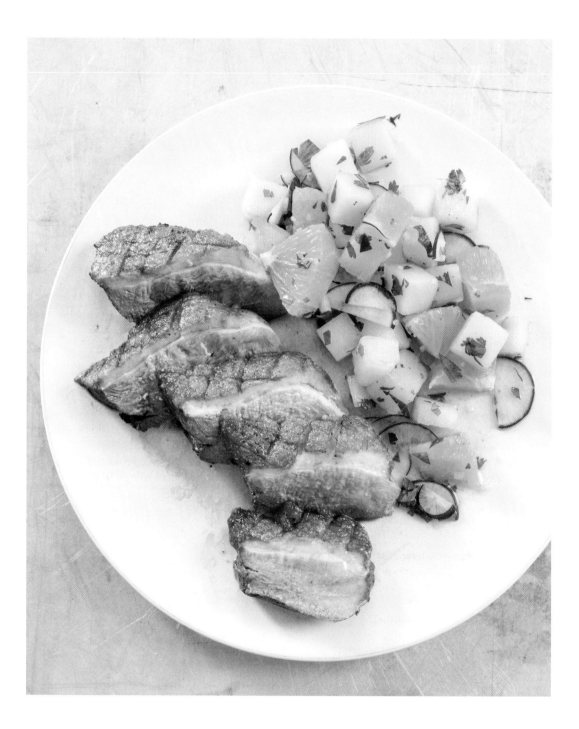

Pan-Seared Duck Breasts with Melon Relish

Serves 4

☑ **WHY THIS RECIPE WORKS** We wanted a recipe for perfect pan-seared duck, with beautifully crisp skin and tender, moist meat. We started by scoring the fat cap to encourage the fat to render and the skin to crisp. We preheated a dry skillet (no added fat was needed since the duck itself releases so much) for 3 full minutes and then added the duck breasts skin side down. Preheating the pan was essential, since it gave the skin a jump start on rendering; turning down the heat once we put the duck in the pan ensured that the meat didn't overcook. Cooking the duck skin side down for most of the cooking time thoroughly rendered the fat, creating the thin, crisp skin we were after. Next, we turned to creating a brightly flavored sauce to balance the rich meat. Although duck is often paired with a pan sauce, our attempts to make one with paleo ingredients were unsuccessful, resulting in sauces that were lackluster and overly sweet. We decided instead to create a vibrant, fruity relish. We used tangy oranges and sweet honeydew melon as the base of our relish, and balanced their flavors with fresh cilantro, aromatic shallot, citrusy coriander, and spicy, crunchy radishes. A bit of lime juice melded all the flavors. Ripe honeydew is important to the success of the relish. If you can't find ripe honeydew, you can substitute 1 small seedless English cucumber, cut into ½-inch pieces. We like this duck cooked to medium-rare, but if you prefer it more or less done, follow the guidelines in step 4.

2   oranges
2   cups ½-inch ripe honeydew pieces
4   radishes, trimmed, halved, and sliced thin
2   tablespoons lime juice
2   tablespoons chopped fresh cilantro
1   tablespoon minced shallot
1   tablespoon extra-virgin olive oil
¼   teaspoon ground coriander
    Kosher salt and pepper
4   (8-ounce) boneless split duck breasts, trimmed

1. Cut away peel and pith from oranges. Quarter oranges, then slice crosswise into ½-inch-thick pieces. Combine orange pieces, honeydew, radishes, lime juice, cilantro, shallot, oil, and coriander in bowl. Season with salt and pepper to taste. Set aside for serving.

2. Pat duck dry with paper towels and, with sharp knife, cut slits in fat cap of each breast, spaced ½ inch apart, in crosshatch pattern, being careful to cut down to but not into meat. Season duck with salt and pepper.

3. Heat 12-inch skillet over medium heat until hot, about 3 minutes. Place duck breasts skin side down in skillet, reduce heat to medium-low, and cook until fat begins to render, about 5 minutes. Continue to cook, adjusting heat as needed for fat to maintain constant but gentle simmer, until most of fat has rendered and skin is deep golden and crisp, 15 to 20 minutes.

4. Flip breasts and continue to cook until duck registers 120 to 125 degrees (for medium-rare), 2 to 5 minutes; 130 to 135 degrees (for medium), 4 to 7 minutes; or 140 to 145 degrees (for medium-well), 5 to 8 minutes. Transfer duck to cutting board and let rest for 5 minutes. Slice duck into ½-inch-thick slices and serve with relish.

TEST KITCHEN TIP **SCORING DUCK BREASTS**

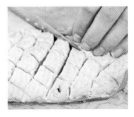

To help render fat, use sharp knife to cut slits in fat cap of breast, spaced ½ inch apart, in cross-hatch pattern, being careful to cut down to but not into meat.

Turkey Breast with Shallot-Porcini Gravy

Serves 6 to 8

✓ **WHY THIS RECIPE WORKS** No turkey dinner is complete without a rich, hearty gravy. But most gravies are thickened with a mixture of butter and flour called a roux—not an option in the paleo world. We wanted to create a paleo-friendly, deeply flavorful turkey gravy, and while we were at it, we wanted a foolproof method for cooking moist, juicy turkey. To make the recipe more versatile, we opted to use a turkey breast instead of a whole bird. To ensure moist, tender meat, we turned to a French technique called cooking *en cocotte*, in which the bird is cooked covered over very low heat with no added liquid, essentially braising the meat in its own flavorful juices. With our turkey settled, we turned our attention to the gravy. Usually, we add the flavorful drippings from the turkey to a roux-thickened broth to make gravy, but without the roux, all we had was thin drippings—and the shallots and celery we had added to the pot to create a flavorful backbone for our turkey. Could we use the contents of the pot to our advantage? The answer was yes: While the turkey rested, we transferred the aromatics and the turkey drippings to a blender and pureed the mixture until it was smooth. This made a decent, thick gravy, but tasters wanted even more flavor. Adding porcini mushrooms to the pot gave the gravy earthy depth and improved its color, while tomato paste further boosted savory flavor. Avoid "hotel-style" turkey breasts if possible; they still have the wings and rib cage attached. If this is the only type of breast you can find, remove the wings and cut away the rib cage with kitchen shears before proceeding with the recipe. Use a Dutch oven that holds 7 quarts or more for this recipe. Don't buy a turkey breast larger than 7 pounds; it won't fit in the pot. Serve with Celery Root Puree (page 291), pictured.

1   (6- to 7-pound) bone-in whole
    turkey breast, trimmed
    Kosher salt and pepper
2   tablespoons ghee
8   shallots, chopped
2   celery ribs, chopped
½   ounce dried porcini mushrooms,
    rinsed and minced
2   teaspoons tomato paste
4   sprigs fresh thyme
1   bay leaf
¼   cup water
1   tablespoon lemon juice

1. Adjust oven rack to lowest position and heat oven to 250 degrees. Pat turkey dry with paper towels and season with salt and pepper. Heat ghee in Dutch oven over medium-high heat until just smoking. Brown turkey on all sides, about 12 minutes; transfer to large plate.

2. Pour off all but 2 tablespoons fat from pot. Add shallots and celery and cook over medium heat until softened and lightly browned, 5 to 7 minutes. Stir in mushrooms, tomato paste, thyme sprigs, and bay leaf and cook until fragrant, about 1 minute. Off heat, return turkey breast side up to pot along with any accumulated juices.

3. Fit large piece of aluminum foil over pot, pressing to seal, then cover tightly with lid. Transfer pot to oven and cook until turkey registers 160 degrees, 2 to 2½ hours.

4. Transfer turkey to carving board, tent loosely with foil, and let rest for 20 minutes.

5. Meanwhile, being careful of hot pot handles, discard thyme sprigs and bay leaf. Transfer contents of pot, water, and lemon juice to blender and process until smooth, about 30 seconds. Transfer gravy to saucepan and set over low heat to keep warm. Season with salt and pepper to taste. Carve turkey and serve, passing gravy separately.

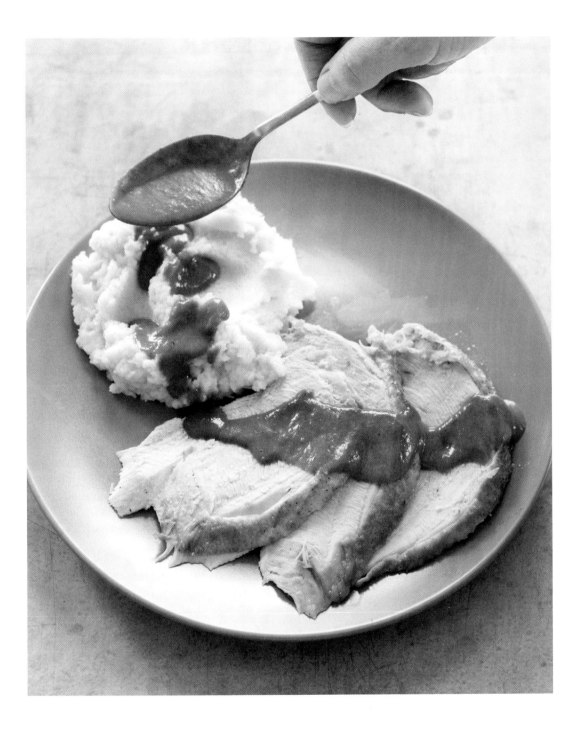

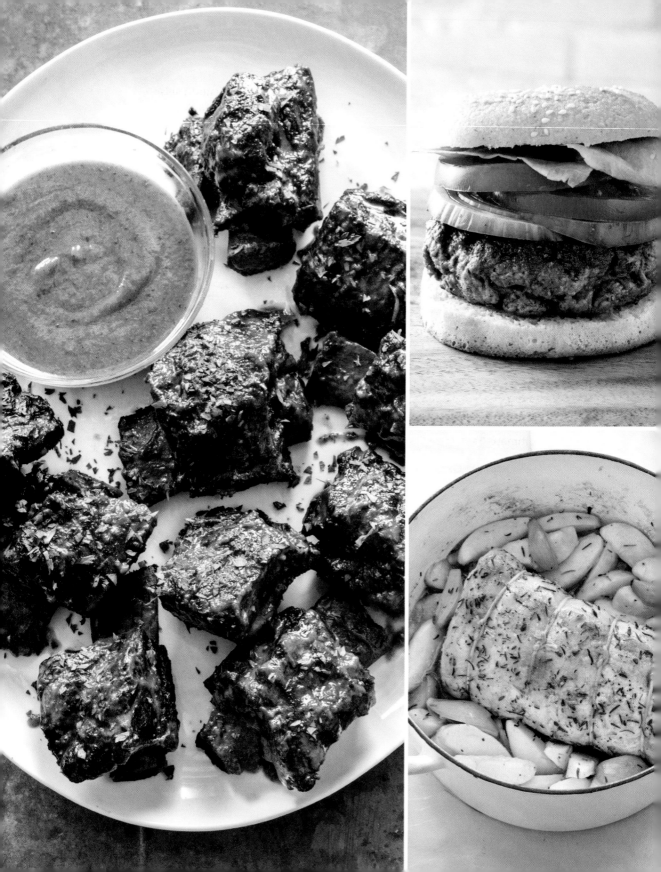

BEEF, PORK, LAMB, AND MORE

CHAPTER 4

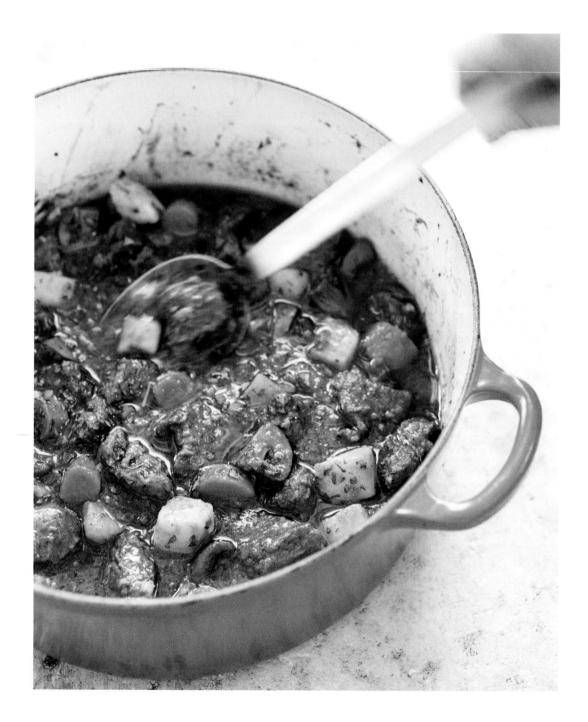

Ultimate Beef Stew

Serves 6 to 8

✓ **WHY THIS RECIPE WORKS** Few things are as soul-satisfying as a steaming bowl of beef stew, but many recipes rely on red wine, store-bought beef broth, potatoes, and flour as a thickener. We wanted a paleo beef stew with all the rich heartiness of traditional versions. We started with a chuck-eye roast, which turns meltingly tender with long, slow cooking. We browned half of the meat to create flavorful fond for our gravy. But without store-bought broth, we had to find a way to achieve the deeply savory flavor we expect of beef stew. We decided to create our own stock as part of the recipe. We made the base of our stock by cooking down beef bones, which gave our gravy a luxurious texture and meaty flavor, while tomato paste and porcini and cremini mushrooms contributed rounded savory flavor. To thicken our stew and create a hearty gravy, we mashed some of the cooked carrots and celery root (a great substitution for more traditional potatoes) with the soft marrow from the bones. Marrow bones (also sold as soup bones) can often be found in the freezer section of the grocery store; if using frozen bones, be sure to thaw them completely.

4 **pounds boneless beef chuck-eye roast, pulled apart at seams, trimmed, and cut into 1½-inch pieces**
  Kosher salt and pepper
1 **tablespoon extra-virgin olive oil**
1 **pound cremini mushrooms, trimmed and quartered**
1 **large onion, halved and sliced thin**
3 **tablespoons tomato paste**
½ **ounce dried porcini mushrooms, rinsed and minced**
1 **tablespoon minced fresh thyme or 1 teaspoon dried**
2 **garlic cloves, minced**
4 **cups water**
1 **pound marrow bones**
5 **carrots, peeled and cut into 1-inch pieces**
3 **bay leaves**
1 **celery root (14 ounces), peeled and cut into 1-inch pieces**
1 **tablespoon red wine vinegar**
¼ **cup chopped fresh parsley**

1. Adjust oven rack to lower-middle position and heat oven to 300 degrees. Pat beef dry with paper towels and season with salt and pepper. Heat oil in Dutch oven over medium-high heat until just smoking. Brown half of beef on all sides, about 8 minutes; transfer to bowl.

2. Add cremini mushrooms, onion, and 2 teaspoons salt to fat left in pot. Cover and cook over medium heat until mushrooms have released their liquid, about 5 minutes. Uncover and continue to cook until liquid has evaporated and vegetables are lightly browned, about 5 minutes. Add tomato paste, porcini mushrooms, thyme, and garlic and cook, stirring frequently, until fragrant, about 1 minute.

3. Stir in water, scraping up any browned bits, and bring to simmer. Stir in bones, carrots, bay leaves, browned beef and any accumulated juices, and remaining beef. Partially cover pot, transfer to oven, and cook for 1 hour.

4. Stir in celery root and vinegar, partially cover, and cook in oven until beef and vegetables are tender, 1 to 1½ hours.

5. Discard bay leaves. Transfer bones to cutting board and use end of spoon to extract marrow. Transfer marrow to medium bowl and discard spent bones. Using wide, shallow spoon, skim excess fat from surface of stew.

6. Being careful of hot pot handles, transfer 1 cup of vegetables to bowl with marrow and mash with potato masher until smooth. Stir marrow mixture and parsley into stew and season with salt and pepper to taste. Serve.

Slow-Cooker Oxtail Soup

Serves 6 to 8

✓ **WHY THIS RECIPE WORKS** Oxtails are prized for their richly flavored marrow, but they require a long simmering time to extract all their flavor and body. A slow cooker allows this process to occur with no supervision. To compensate for the lack of wine and store-bought broth (standard ingredients in this recipe), we browned the oxtails in a large skillet on top of the stove. This not only created flavorful fond but also rendered the fat, which we then used to brown mushrooms, onions, and aromatics. Once we transferred everything to the slow cooker, all that was left was to add the hearty vegetables that would transform our flavorful broth into oxtail soup. Since traditional potatoes weren't an option, we tried carrots, turnips, and parsnips. Tasters found that turnips were too bitter and detracted from the oxtails' flavor, but carrots and parsnips added some mild sweetness that nicely complemented the beefiness of the broth. After a long, slow simmer, this savory soup benefited from a fresh garnish of bright parsley. Tradition sometimes calls for placing a large oxtail in the center of each bowl, and, for an informal gathering, you can pick away at the meat and gnaw on the bones. We found this approach messy and prefer to serve the soup with shredded boneless meat. Try to buy oxtails that are approximately 2 inches thick and 2 to 4 inches in diameter; they will yield more meat for the soup. Oxtails can often be found in the freezer section of the grocery store; if using frozen oxtails, be sure to thaw them completely before using. You will need a 5½- to 7-quart slow cooker for this recipe.

4 pounds oxtails
    Kosher salt and pepper
1 tablespoon extra-virgin olive oil
1 pound cremini mushrooms, trimmed and quartered
2 onions, chopped
¼ cup tomato paste
4 garlic cloves, minced
1 tablespoon minced fresh thyme or 1 teaspoon dried
7 cups water
3 carrots, peeled and sliced ½ inch thick
3 parsnips, peeled and cut into ¾-inch pieces
3 bay leaves
2 tablespoons chopped fresh parsley

1. Pat oxtails dry with paper towels and season with salt and pepper. Heat oil in 12-inch skillet over medium-high heat until just smoking. Brown half of oxtails on all sides, 8 to 10 minutes; transfer to large bowl. Repeat with remaining oxtails; transfer to bowl.

2. Pour off all but 2 tablespoons fat from skillet. Add mushrooms, onions, and 1 tablespoon salt, cover, and cook over medium heat until mushrooms have released their liquid, 5 to 7 minutes. Uncover and continue to cook until liquid has evaporated and vegetables are lightly browned, about 5 minutes. Add tomato paste, garlic, and thyme and cook until fragrant, about 1 minute. Stir in 1 cup water, scraping up any browned bits; transfer to slow cooker.

3. Stir carrots, parsnips, bay leaves, and remaining 6 cups water into slow cooker. Nestle browned oxtails into slow cooker along with any accumulated juices. Cover and cook until beef is fully tender and sharp knife slips easily in and out of meat, 9 to 10 hours on low or 6 to 7 hours on high.

4. Transfer oxtails to cutting board, let cool slightly, then shred into bite-size pieces using 2 forks; discard excess fat and bones. Discard bay leaves. Using wide, shallow spoon, skim excess fat from surface of soup.

5. Stir shredded meat into soup and let sit until heated through, about 5 minutes. Stir in parsley and season with salt and pepper to taste. Serve.

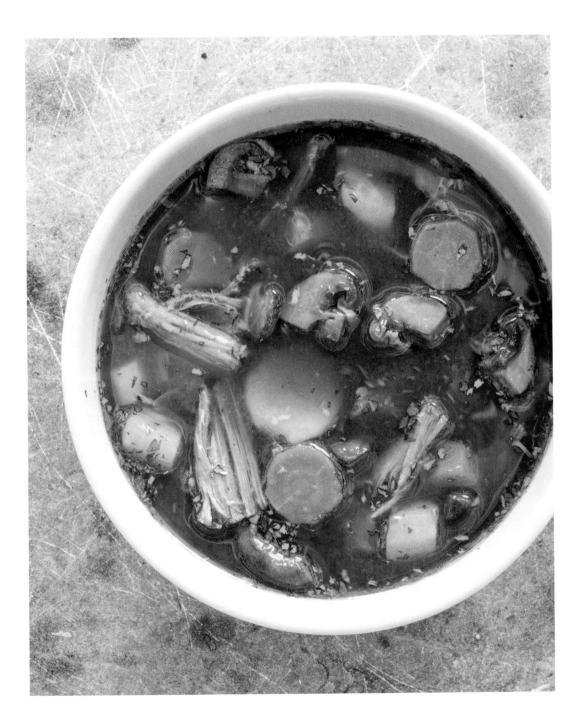

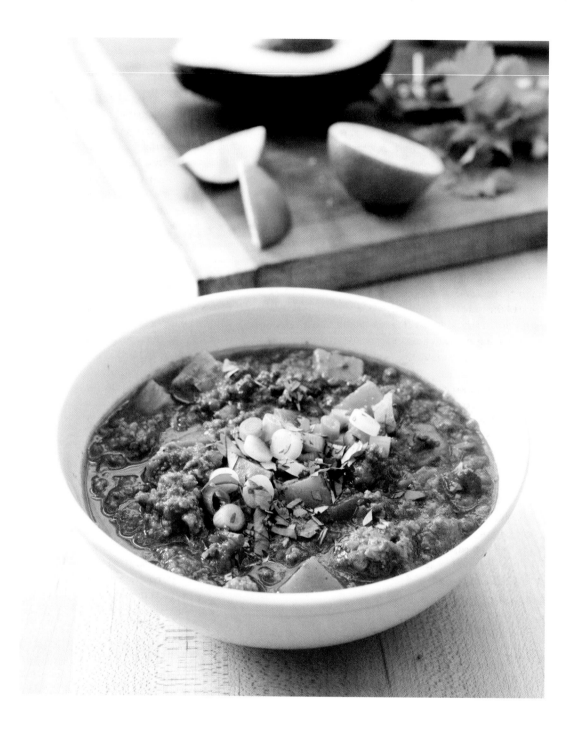

Bison Chili

Serves 6 to 8

✅ **WHY THIS RECIPE WORKS** While ground beef chili recipes are a dime a dozen, we decided that a chili made with ground bison would be a great way to incorporate a different protein into the paleo meal rotation. Bison has a much lower fat content than ground beef—about 2 percent compared to about 10 percent—which meant that we couldn't treat it like beef. To build flavor, we tried browning all of the meat before adding any liquid, but we found that the finished texture was a bit dry and grainy. Instead, we sautéed only half of the meat and added the rest in small pieces after the chili had simmered for an hour. The meat added at the beginning melted into the sauce, giving it a rich, meaty flavor, while the pieces added later stayed moist and tender. Next, we turned our attention to finding an alternative for the canned tomatoes that make up the backbone of many a chili recipe. Although some chili recipes forgo the tomatoes for a hearty, meat-based version, tasters thought that tomatoes provided balanced flavor. We pulsed a full 3 pounds of fresh tomatoes in a food processor to approximate canned diced tomatoes, and tomato paste provided a deep, cooked tomato flavor. Next, since beans weren't an option, we focused on additional veggies to round out our chili. Tasters liked red bell pepper and sweet potatoes for their bright and sweet notes that complemented the heat of the chili. Adding the sweet potatoes halfway through cooking ensured that they softened nicely but didn't fall apart. The sweet potatoes also absorbed some liquid and released a small amount of starch, giving the chili a hearty, thick consistency. You can substitute 90 percent lean ground beef for the bison. Serve with lime wedges, fresh cilantro, sliced scallions, minced onion, and/or diced avocado.

3 tablespoons chili powder

1 tablespoon ground cumin

Kosher salt and pepper

2 teaspoons ground coriander

1 teaspoon red pepper flakes

1 teaspoon dried oregano

⅛ teaspoon cayenne pepper

3 pounds tomatoes, cored and chopped

2 tablespoons extra-virgin olive oil

2 onions, chopped fine

1 red bell pepper, stemmed, seeded, and cut into ½-inch pieces

¼ cup tomato paste

6 garlic cloves, minced

2 pounds ground bison

1 cup water, plus extra as needed

1 pound sweet potatoes, peeled and cut into ½-inch pieces

1. Combine chili powder, cumin, 1 tablespoon salt, coriander, pepper flakes, oregano, and cayenne in bowl. Process tomatoes in food processor until smooth, about 30 seconds; set aside.

2. Heat oil in Dutch oven over medium heat until shimmering. Add onions and bell pepper and cook until softened, 8 to 10 minutes. Stir in spice mixture, tomato paste, and garlic and cook until fragrant, about 2 minutes.

3. Increase heat to medium-high, add half of ground bison, and cook, breaking up meat with wooden spoon, until no longer pink, 3 to 5 minutes. Stir in processed tomatoes and water and bring to simmer. Reduce heat to medium-low, cover, and simmer gently, stirring occasionally, for 1 hour.

4. Stir in sweet potatoes. Pat remaining ground bison together into ball, then pinch off teaspoon-size pieces of meat and stir into chili. Cover and continue to cook, stirring occasionally, until potatoes and bison are tender, about 45 minutes. (If chili begins to stick to bottom of pot or looks too thick, stir in extra water as needed.) Season with salt and pepper to taste. Serve.

Ultimate Burgers

Serves 4

✓ **WHY THIS RECIPE WORKS** We wanted to develop a recipe for perfectly tender, juicy burgers. But we faced a challenge: The quality of store-bought ground beef can be unreliable. We decided to "grind" our own grass-fed meat, and tested several different cuts; sirloin steak tips worked best. We cut the steak tips into small chunks and froze the pieces briefly before grinding them in the food processor. Freezing ensured that we ended up with distinct pieces of meat, not paste. Since the fat content of the meat varied widely from batch to batch, we trimmed the meat and then added a set amount of fat to ensure uniform results every time. We tested a variety of fats including ghee, coconut oil, olive oil, and rendered bacon fat. Melted ghee worked best: It solidified when it came into contact with the cold meat, creating small particles of fat throughout the patties. This improved the flavor and juiciness of the naturally lean meat. Finally, to make sure that our burgers were perfectly cooked, we seared them in a skillet using more ghee as our cooking medium. Sirloin steak tips, also known as flap meat, can be sold as whole steaks, cubes, and strips. When stirring the ghee, salt, and pepper into the ground meat and shaping the patties, do not overwork the meat or the burgers will become dense. We like these burgers cooked to medium-rare, but if you prefer them more or less done, see our guidelines on page 154. Serve in Paleo Sandwich Rolls (page 25), pictured, or lettuce leaves with your favorite toppings.

1½ **pounds sirloin steak tips, trimmed and cut into ½-inch pieces**

2 **tablespoons plus 1 teaspoon ghee, melted and cooled**

Kosher salt and pepper

1. Place beef pieces on rimmed baking sheet in single layer. Freeze until meat is very firm and starting to harden around edges but still pliable, about 35 minutes.

2. Place one-quarter of meat in food processor and pulse until finely ground into rice grain–size pieces (about 1/32 inch), 15 to 20 pulses, stopping and redistributing meat around bowl as necessary to ensure beef is evenly ground. Transfer meat to baking sheet. Repeat grinding with remaining meat in 3 batches. Spread mixture over sheet and inspect carefully, discarding any long strands of gristle or large chunks of hard meat or fat.

3. Drizzle 2 tablespoons melted ghee over ground meat and sprinkle with 1½ teaspoons salt and 1 teaspoon pepper. Gently toss meat with fork to combine. Divide meat into 4 balls. Toss each between your hands until uniformly but lightly packed. Gently flatten into patties ¾ inch thick and about 4½ inches in diameter.

4. Season 1 side of patties liberally with salt and pepper. Using spatula, flip patties and season other side. Heat remaining 1 teaspoon ghee in 12-inch skillet over high heat until just smoking. Using spatula, transfer burgers to skillet and cook, without moving them, for 3 minutes. Using spatula, flip burgers and continue to cook until burgers register 120 to 125 degrees (for medium-rare), about 3 minutes. Transfer burgers to plate and let rest for 5 minutes. Serve.

VARIATION

Ultimate Burgers with Caramelized Onions and Bacon

Cook 4 strips coarsely chopped bacon in medium saucepan over medium heat until fat is rendered, 3 to 5 minutes. Add 2 thinly sliced onions and ½ teaspoon minced fresh thyme, cover, and cook until onions are softened, about 5 minutes. Uncover and cook until onions are lightly browned and bacon is crisp, about 15 minutes. Stir in 1 tablespoon sherry vinegar and 1 tablespoon water, scraping up browned bits. Season with salt and pepper to taste. Serve topping with burgers.

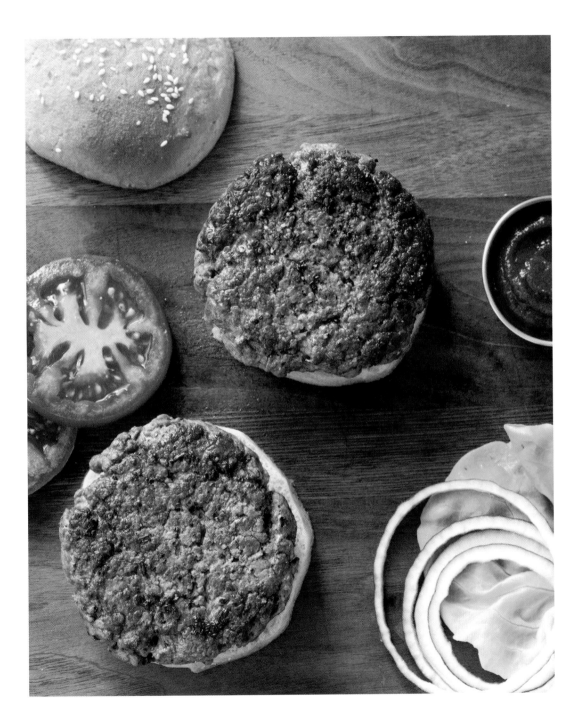

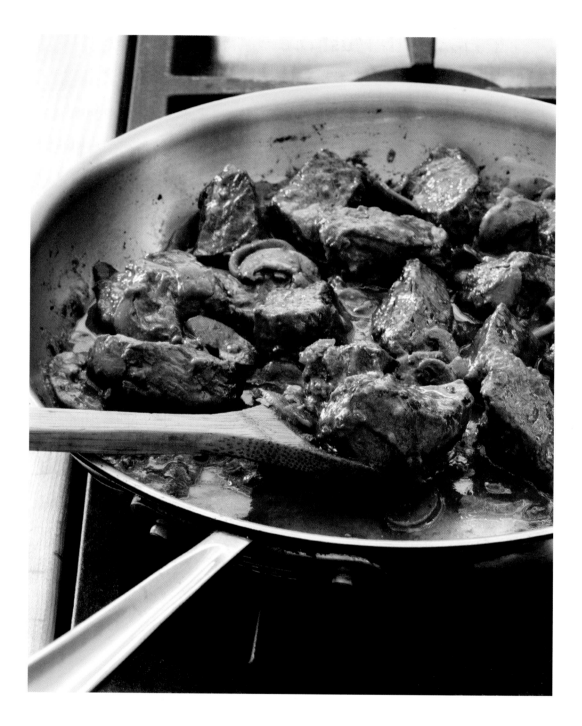

Steak Tips with Mushroom-Onion Gravy

Serves 4

✓ **WHY THIS RECIPE WORKS** Steak tips smothered in a savory, hearty mushroom and onion gravy are undeniably appealing, but making a paleo version required some problem solving: The gravy is usually thickened with flour and relies on store-bought beef broth for extra savory depth. We started by browning the beef to boost its flavor and create fond, then we removed it from the skillet and browned the mushrooms and onion so they could pick up all the savory browned bits from the pan. Since beef broth was not an option, we used water instead and enhanced the savory flavor of the dish by adding tomato paste and dried porcini mushrooms. The porcinis also intensified the mushroom flavor in our gravy. We also added minced garlic and woodsy thyme for a rounded, aromatic backbone. Although this gravy tasted good, it was still too thin. To thicken it without muddying the flavor we had worked so hard to create, we decided to puree some of the mushroom-onion mixture in a blender. We stirred the puree back into the pan to give our gravy a thick, rich consistency. Sirloin steak tips, also known as flap meat, can be sold as whole steaks, cubes, and strips. To ensure uniform pieces, we prefer to purchase whole steaks and cut them ourselves. We like these steak tips cooked to medium, but if you prefer them more or less done, see our guidelines on page 154. Serve with Celery Root Puree (page 291).

1½   **pounds sirloin steak tips, trimmed and cut into 1½-inch pieces**
      Kosher salt and pepper
2   **tablespoons extra-virgin olive oil**
1   **pound white mushrooms, trimmed and sliced thin**
1   **large onion, chopped**
¼   **ounce dried porcini mushrooms, rinsed and minced**
1   **tablespoon tomato paste**
2   **garlic cloves, minced**
½   **teaspoon minced fresh thyme or ⅛ teaspoon dried**
1¾   **cups water, plus extra as needed**
1   **tablespoon minced fresh parsley**

1. Pat beef dry with paper towels and season with salt and pepper. Heat 1 tablespoon oil in 12-inch skillet over medium-high heat until just smoking. Brown beef on all sides, about 8 minutes; transfer to plate.

2. Heat remaining 1 tablespoon oil in now-empty skillet over medium heat until shimmering. Add white mushrooms, onion, 1½ teaspoons salt, and ¼ teaspoon pepper. Cover and cook until mushrooms have released their liquid, about 5 minutes. Uncover and continue to cook until liquid has evaporated and vegetables are lightly browned, about 5 minutes. Stir in porcini mushrooms, tomato paste, garlic, and thyme and cook until fragrant, about 1 minute. Stir in 1 cup water, scraping up any browned bits.

3. Process ¾ cup of mushroom mixture and remaining ¾ cup water in blender until smooth, about 30 seconds. Stir processed mushroom mixture into skillet and bring to simmer over medium heat. Stir in browned beef and any accumulated juices and cook, stirring occasionally, until meat registers 130 to 135 degrees (for medium), 3 to 5 minutes. Adjust sauce consistency with extra hot water as needed. Stir in parsley and season with salt and pepper to taste. Serve.

Grilled Beef and Vegetable Kebabs

Serves 4

✓ **WHY THIS RECIPE WORKS** Grilled kebabs are a natural fit for the paleo diet—juicy pieces of meat and crisp-tender vegetables make for a flavorful complete meal. But most kebab recipes call for stringing the meat and vegetables on skewers together, resulting in uneven cooking. We solved this problem by cooking the meat and vegetables on separate skewers, allowing us to cook each element to perfection. Beefy steak tips worked great on the grill, and a punchy marinade ensured tender and flavorful meat. Sirloin steak tips, also known as flap meat, can be sold as whole steaks, cubes, and strips. To ensure uniform pieces, we prefer to purchase whole steaks and cut them ourselves. If you have long, thin pieces of meat, roll or fold them into approximate 2-inch pieces. We like these steak tips cooked to medium-rare, but if you prefer them more or less done, see our guidelines on page 154. You will need six 12-inch metal skewers for this recipe.

MARINADE

- 1 onion, chopped
- ⅓ cup water
- ⅓ cup extra-virgin olive oil
- 3 tablespoons tomato paste
- 6 garlic cloves, minced
- 2 tablespoons chopped fresh rosemary
- 1 tablespoon kosher salt
- 2 teaspoons grated lemon zest
- 1 teaspoon honey
- ¾ teaspoon pepper

BEEF AND VEGETABLES

- 2 pounds sirloin steak tips, trimmed and cut into 2-inch pieces
- 1 zucchini, halved lengthwise and sliced 1 inch thick
- 1 large red or green bell pepper, stemmed, seeded, and cut into 1½-inch pieces
- 1 large red onion, cut into 1-inch pieces, 3 layers thick

1. FOR THE MARINADE Process all ingredients in blender until smooth, about 45 seconds. Set aside ¾ cup marinade separately for vegetables.

2. FOR THE BEEF AND VEGETABLES Combine remaining marinade and beef in 1-gallon zipper-lock bag and toss to coat; press out as much air as possible and seal bag. Refrigerate for at least 1 hour or up to 2 hours, flipping bag every 30 minutes.

Gently combine zucchini, bell pepper, and onion with reserved marinade in bowl. Cover and let sit at room temperature for at least 30 minutes.

3. Remove beef from bag, pat dry with paper towels, and thread tightly onto two 12-inch metal skewers. Thread vegetables in alternating order onto four 12-inch metal skewers.

4A. FOR A CHARCOAL GRILL Open bottom vent completely. Light large chimney starter mounded with charcoal briquettes (7 quarts). When top coals are partially covered with ash, pour evenly over center of grill, leaving 2-inch gap between grill wall and charcoal. Set cooking grate in place, cover, and open lid vent completely. Heat grill until hot, about 5 minutes.

4B. FOR A GAS GRILL Turn all burners to high, cover, and heat grill until hot, about 15 minutes. Leave primary burner on high and turn other burner(s) to medium-low.

5. Clean and oil cooking grate. Place beef skewers on grill (directly over coals if using charcoal or over hotter side of grill if using gas). Place vegetable skewers on cooler side(s) of grill (near edge of coals if using charcoal). Cook (covered if using gas), turning as needed, until beef is well browned and registers 120 to 125 degrees (for medium-rare), 12 to 16 minutes.

6. Transfer beef skewers to platter; tent with aluminum foil. Continue cooking vegetable skewers until tender and lightly charred, about 5 minutes. Serve.

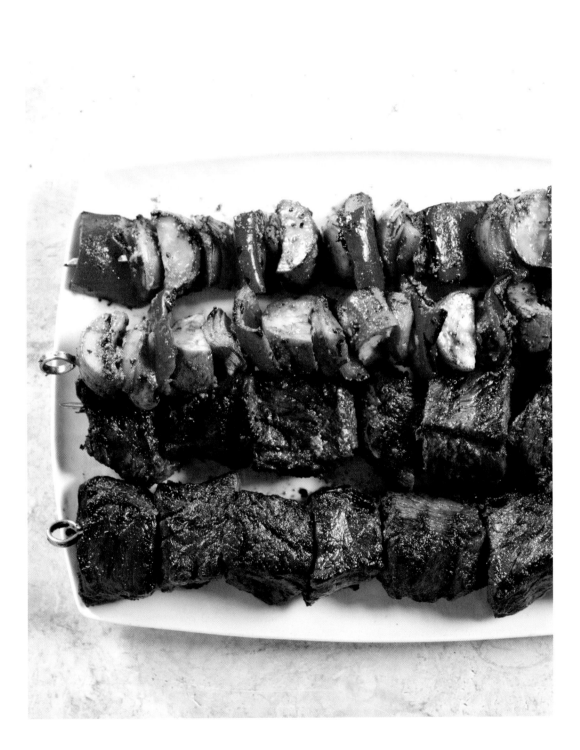

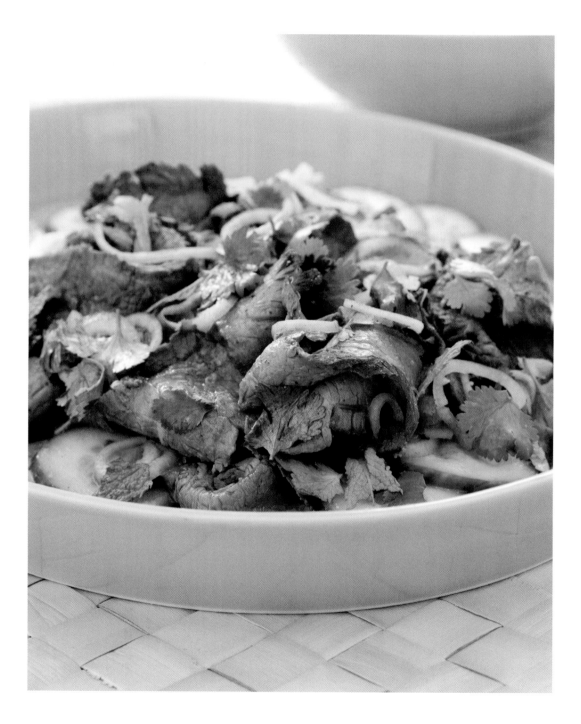

Spicy Thai Grilled Beef Salad

Serves 4

✓ **WHY THIS RECIPE WORKS** This bold-flavored salad brings Thai cuisine's five signature flavor elements—hot, sour, salty, sweet, and bitter—into balance, making for a light but satisfying dish. But many versions rely on nonpaleo ingredients like brown sugar, soy sauce, and rice, so we set out to create a paleo version. We tested a wide variety of cuts and landed on flank steak as our winner for its uniform shape, moderate price, and decent tenderness. Marinating the steak was unnecessary, since the dressing provided plenty of flavor after cooking. We grilled the steak over a half-grill fire, which concentrates the heat and allows the steak to char quickly before the interior can overcook. When creating our dressing, we needed to include sour, salty, sweet, and spicy elements to provide a counterpoint to the subtly bitter char of the meat. Lime juice, fish sauce, and honey fulfilled the sour, salty, and sweet notes. For our spicy element, a fresh Thai chile added a fruity, fiery hit to each bite, and some toasted cayenne pepper and paprika provided complexity. The salad is traditionally served with rice, but we decided to spread the salad on a bed of sliced cucumbers for a fresh, paleo-friendly presentation. If a fresh Thai chile is unavailable, substitute half of a serrano chile. This dish is traditionally quite spicy, but if you prefer a less spicy dish you can leave out the chile. We like this steak cooked to medium-rare, but if you prefer it more or less done, see our guidelines on page 154. Be sure to slice the cooked steak thin against the grain; otherwise, the meat will be tough and rubbery.

1 teaspoon paprika
1 teaspoon cayenne pepper
3 tablespoons lime juice (2 limes)
2 tablespoons fish sauce
2 tablespoons water
1 teaspoon honey
1 (1½- to 2-pound) flank steak, trimmed
  Kosher salt and pepper
1½ cups fresh mint leaves, torn
1½ cups fresh cilantro leaves
4 shallots, sliced thin
1 Thai chile, stemmed and sliced thin into rounds
1 seedless English cucumber, sliced ¼ inch thick on bias

1. Toast paprika and cayenne in 8-inch skillet over medium heat, stirring frequently, until fragrant, about 1 minute; transfer to bowl.

2. In large bowl, whisk lime juice, fish sauce, water, honey, and ¼ teaspoon toasted paprika mixture; set aside. Pat steak dry with paper towels and season with salt and pepper.

3A. FOR A CHARCOAL GRILL Open bottom vent completely. Light large chimney starter filled with charcoal briquettes (6 quarts). When top coals are partially covered with ash, pour evenly over half of grill. Set cooking grate in place, cover, and open lid vent completely. Heat grill until hot, about 5 minutes.

3B. FOR A GAS GRILL Turn all burners to high, cover, and heat grill until hot, about 15 minutes. Leave primary burner on high and turn off other burner(s).

4. Clean and oil cooking grate. Place steak on hotter side of grill. Cook (covered if using gas), turning as needed, until lightly charred on both sides and meat registers 120 to 125 degrees, 8 to 12 minutes.

5. Transfer steak to cutting board, tent with aluminum foil, and let rest for 5 to 10 minutes. Slice steak thin against grain, then transfer to bowl with lime juice mixture. Add mint, cilantro, shallots, and Thai chile and toss to combine. Line serving platter with cucumber slices and arrange steak mixture on top. Serve, passing remaining toasted paprika mixture separately.

Seared Flank Steak with Chimichurri Sauce

Serves 4

✓ **WHY THIS RECIPE WORKS** Topping a well-caramelized flank steak with a fresh herb sauce makes for a quick, easy, and impressive dinner. Flank steak is prized for its beefy flavor, but as a relatively thin cut it doesn't need very long to cook, and can be tough if not properly prepared. To make sure that the meat turned out tender, we heated oil in a skillet until it was smoking. The high heat created a flavorful browned crust on the exterior of the steak, and by the time both sides were well seared the center was approaching the right temperature. We rested the steak after cooking to allow the residual heat to continue cooking the meat to the perfect doneness. To ensure that the steak remained tender and juicy, we cut it against the grain into thin slices. Finally, all we needed was the perfect condiment to accompany this simple steak. Chimichurri sauce, a traditional Argentinian herb-based sauce, came to mind. The sharp, grassy flavors of the sauce were the perfect complement to the rich beefiness of the flank steak. Parsley, cilantro, oregano, garlic, red wine vinegar, red pepper flakes, and salt came together in a fruity extra-virgin olive oil. We like this steak cooked to medium-rare, but if you prefer it more or less done, see our guidelines below. Be sure to slice the cooked steak thin against the grain; otherwise, the meat will be tough and rubbery.

¼ cup hot water

2 teaspoons dried oregano

Kosher salt and pepper

1⅓ cups fresh parsley leaves

⅔ cup fresh cilantro leaves

6 garlic cloves, minced

½ teaspoon red pepper flakes

¼ cup red wine vinegar

½ cup plus 1 tablespoon extra-virgin olive oil

1 (1½- to 2-pound) flank steak, trimmed

1. Combine water, oregano, and 2 teaspoons salt in small bowl and let sit until oregano is softened, about 15 minutes. Pulse parsley, cilantro, garlic, and pepper flakes in food processor until coarsely chopped, about 10 pulses. Add water mixture and vinegar and pulse to combine. Transfer herb mixture to medium bowl and whisk in ½ cup oil until combined. Cover and let sit at room temperature for 1 hour.

2. Pat steak dry with paper towels and season with salt and pepper. Heat remaining 1 tablespoon oil in 12-inch skillet over medium-high heat until just smoking. Cook steak, turning as needed, until well browned on both sides and meat registers 120 to 125 degrees (for medium-rare), 8 to 12 minutes. Transfer steak to cutting board, tent loosely with aluminum foil, and let rest for 5 to 10 minutes. Slice steak thin against grain. Whisk sauce to recombine and serve with steak.

TEST KITCHEN TIP

KNOWING WHEN MEAT IS DONE

Note that the temperature will rise 5 to 10 degrees after resting.

TYPE OF MEAT	COOK UNTIL IT REGISTERS
Beef, Lamb, and Venison	
Rare	115°–120°
Medium-Rare	120°–125°
Medium	130°–135°
Medium-Well	140°–145°
Well-Done	150°–155°
Pork	
Chops and Tenderloin	145°
Loin Roasts	140°

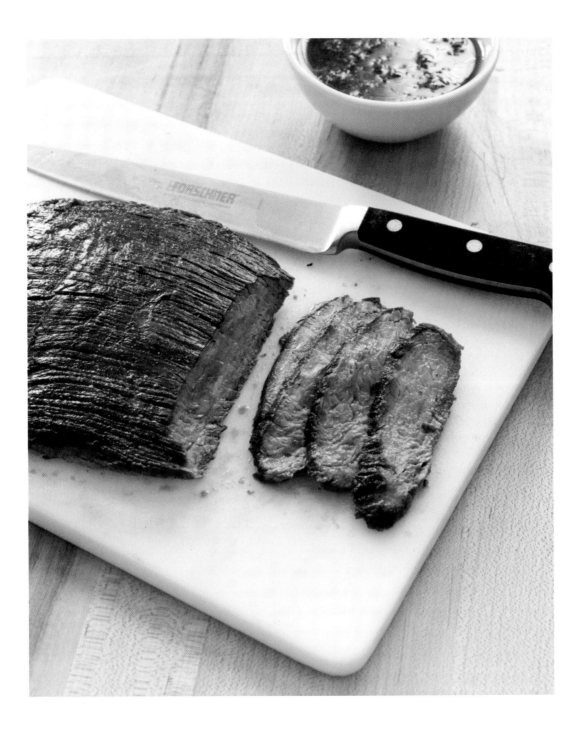

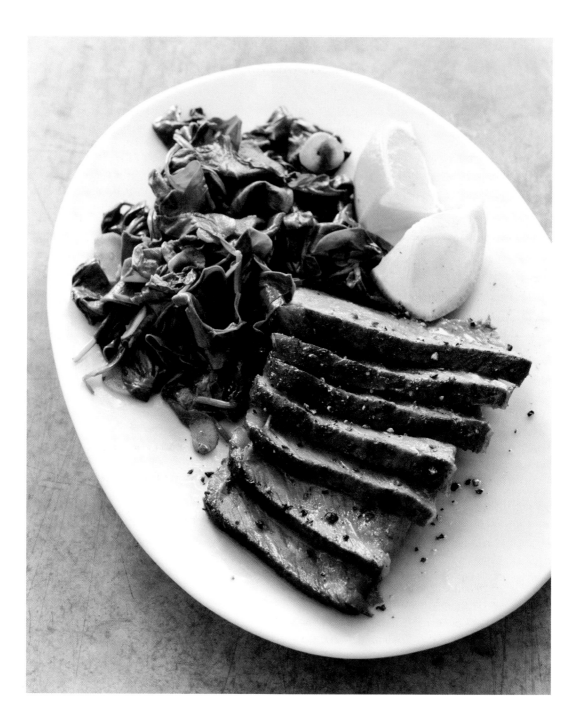

Tuscan-Style Steaks with Garlicky Spinach

Serves 4

✓ **WHY THIS RECIPE WORKS** What could be more suited to a paleo diet than a perfectly cooked, thick, juicy steak? We decided to develop a recipe that would not only produce a beautiful steak, but also a flavorful side dish. We took a cue from a simple and flavorful Italian preparation, in which steak is seasoned with olive oil and lemon, and decided to pair it with garlicky spinach. To keep things streamlined, we used just one skillet. We perfumed the meat with subtle garlic flavor by rubbing the steaks with a garlic clove; cooking over medium-high heat produced a well-browned crust and a medium-rare interior. Parcooking the spinach in the microwave helped rid it of excess liquid. If you don't have a microwave-safe bowl large enough to accommodate the entire amount of spinach, cook it in a smaller bowl in two batches; reduce the amount of water to 2 tablespoons per batch and the cooking time for each batch to about 1½ minutes. We like these steaks cooked to medium-rare, but if you prefer them more or less done, see our guidelines on page 154.

18   ounces (18 cups) baby spinach
2   (1¾-pound) porterhouse or T-bone steaks, 1 to 1½ inches thick, trimmed
5   garlic cloves (1 halved, 4 sliced thin)
     Kosher salt and pepper
¼   cup extra-virgin olive oil
¼   teaspoon red pepper flakes
     Lemon wedges

1. Microwave spinach and ¼ cup water in covered bowl, stirring occasionally, until spinach is beginning to wilt and has decreased in volume by half, about 4 minutes. Remove bowl from microwave and keep covered for 1 minute. Carefully uncover spinach, allowing steam to escape away from you, and transfer to colander. Squeeze spinach between tongs to release excess liquid; set aside.

2. Pat steaks dry with paper towels, rub halved garlic clove over bone and meat on each side, and season with salt and pepper. Heat 1 tablespoon oil in 12-inch skillet over medium-high heat until just smoking. Place steaks in skillet and cook, without moving, until well browned on first side, 5 to 7 minutes. Flip steaks, reduce heat to medium, and continue to cook until meat registers 120 to 125 degrees (for medium-rare), 5 to 12 minutes. Transfer steaks to carving board, tent loosely with aluminum foil, and let rest for 10 minutes.

3. Meanwhile, cook 1 tablespoon oil, pepper flakes, and sliced garlic in now-empty skillet over medium heat until fragrant, about 2 minutes. Add spinach and cook until heated through, about 2 minutes. Season with salt and pepper to taste.

4. Cut strip and tenderloin pieces off bones, then slice each piece crosswise into ¼-inch-thick slices. Transfer steak to serving platter and drizzle with remaining 2 tablespoons oil. Serve with spinach and lemon wedges.

TEST KITCHEN TIP

SLICING PORTERHOUSE AND T-BONE STEAKS

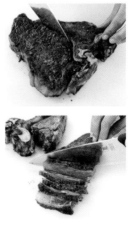

1. After meat has rested, cut along bone to remove large top loin, or strip, section.

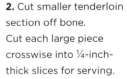

2. Cut smaller tenderloin section off bone. Cut each large piece crosswise into ¼-inch-thick slices for serving.

Pan-Seared Steaks with Tomato and Watercress Salad

Serves 4

🍴 **WHY THIS RECIPE WORKS** A well-caramelized exterior is key for great steak, but developing this flavorful crust indoors can be difficult. To ensure the best results, we relied on a threefold method. First, we made sure to use a very hot pan; we found that cooking the steaks in a pan that wasn't properly preheated caused the interior of the steaks to overcook before the exteriors developed a crust. We also made sure to pat the steaks dry before cooking, since excess moisture caused them to steam instead of brown. Finally, we used a 12-inch skillet to ensure that the steaks had enough room in the pan—crowding them in a smaller skillet resulted in subpar caramelization. With our indoor cooking method perfected, we decided to develop a fresh, flavorful accompaniment. Colorful, juicy cherry tomatoes and peppery watercress made a perfect base for a simple salad. Sliced red onion gave the salad some bite, and a bit of good olive oil and balsamic vinegar brought everything together. We found that it was important to wait until the steaks were resting to assemble the salad; once dressed, the tomatoes started to release their juices, wilting the delicate watercress and diluting the flavor of the salad. You can substitute strip steaks or rib-eye steaks for the top sirloin. We like these steaks cooked to medium-rare, but if you prefer them more or less done, see our guidelines on page 154.

2 **(1-pound) boneless top sirloin steaks, 1½ inches thick, trimmed**
   Kosher salt and pepper
3 **tablespoons extra-virgin olive oil**
1½ **pounds cherry tomatoes, halved**
½ **small red onion, sliced thin**
2 **ounces (2 cups) watercress**
1 **tablespoon balsamic vinegar**

1. Pat steaks dry with paper towels and season with salt and pepper. Heat 1 tablespoon oil in 12-inch skillet over medium-high heat until just smoking. Place steaks in skillet and cook, without moving, until well browned on first side, 5 to 7 minutes. Flip steaks, reduce heat to medium, and continue to cook until meat registers 120 to 125 degrees (for medium-rare), 5 to 10 minutes. Transfer steaks to carving board, tent loosely with aluminum foil, and let rest for 10 minutes.

2. Meanwhile, combine tomatoes, onion, and watercress in bowl. Drizzle with vinegar and remaining 2 tablespoons oil and toss to coat. Season with salt and pepper to taste. Slice steaks into ¼-inch-thick slices and serve with salad.

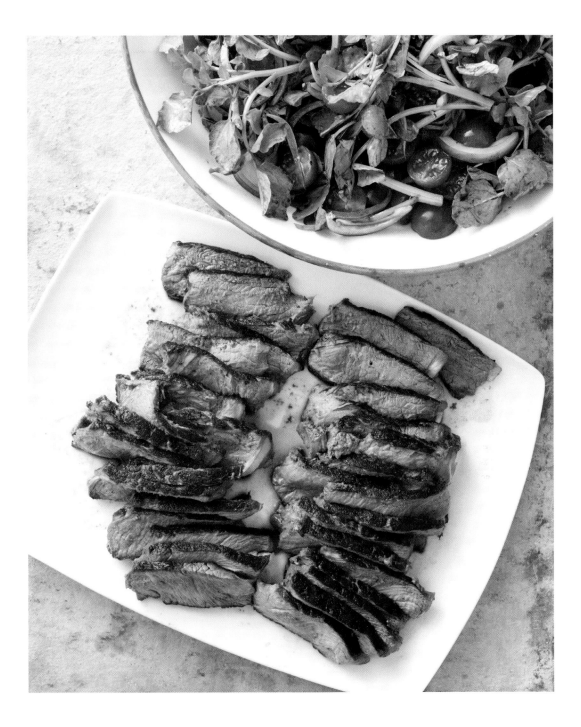

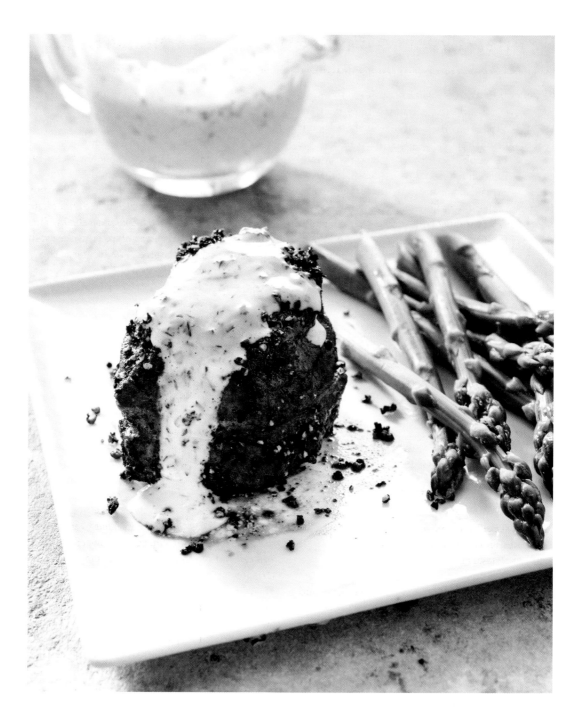

Pepper-Crusted Venison with Béarnaise Sauce

Serves 4

✓ **WHY THIS RECIPE WORKS** To expand our paleo menu options, we decided to develop a recipe for venison loin steaks, which are extremely tender and lean. A peppercorn crust allowed the prized cut to shine. We mellowed the peppercorns' heat by simmering them in olive oil, then made a paste from the cooked cracked peppercorns, salt, and oil and pressed it onto the exterior of the steaks. To ensure that the meat was perfectly cooked, we started by searing the steaks in a skillet to form a crunchy crust. We then let them finish cooking in a hot oven on a preheated baking sheet, which ensured that the steaks cooked evenly. A classic béarnaise made an impressive accompaniment to our steaks. In its most traditional form, creamy béarnaise relies on clarified butter, so ghee was a natural choice. Making our béarnaise in a blender kept the process streamlined and simple. You can substitute beef tenderloin steaks for the venison steaks. This recipe is fairly spicy. If you prefer a very mild pepper flavor, drain the cooled peppercorns in a fine-mesh strainer in step 1, toss them with 5 tablespoons of fresh oil, add the salt, and proceed. We like these steaks cooked to medium-rare, but if you prefer them more or less done, see our guidelines on page 154. When making the sauce, make sure that the ghee is still hot (about 180 degrees) so that the egg yolks cook sufficiently.

STEAKS

- ¼ **cup black peppercorns, cracked**
- 6 **tablespoons extra-virgin olive oil**
- 1 **tablespoon kosher salt**
- 4 **(8-ounce) center-cut venison loin steaks, trimmed**

BÉARNAISE SAUCE

- ½ **cup white wine vinegar**
- 2 **sprigs fresh tarragon, plus 1½ tablespoons minced**
- 1 **shallot, sliced thin**
- 2 **large egg yolks**
- 1½ **teaspoons lemon juice**
  Kosher salt and pepper
- 10 **tablespoons ghee, melted and still hot**

1. FOR THE STEAKS Cook peppercorns and 5 tablespoons oil in 12-inch skillet over low heat until fragrant, 2 to 4 minutes; transfer to bowl, stir in salt, and let cool to room temperature.

2. Coat steaks with peppercorn mixture, pressing gently to adhere. Pat steaks to uniform 1½ inches thick and tie with kitchen twine around equator; let sit at room temperature for 1 hour.

3. Meanwhile, adjust oven rack to middle position, place baking sheet on oven rack, and heat oven to 450 degrees. When oven reaches 450 degrees, heat remaining 1 tablespoon oil in now-empty skillet over medium-high heat until just smoking. Place steaks in skillet and cook until well browned and crusty, about 3 minutes per side.

4. Transfer steaks to hot sheet in oven and roast until meat registers 120 to 125 degrees (for medium-rare), 5 to 7 minutes. Transfer steaks to platter and discard twine; let rest while making sauce.

5. FOR THE BÉARNAISE SAUCE Wipe skillet clean with paper towels. Bring vinegar, tarragon sprigs, and shallot to simmer in skillet over medium heat and cook until vinegar is reduced to about 2 tablespoons, 5 to 7 minutes. Discard shallot and tarragon sprigs.

6. Process egg yolks, lemon juice, ¼ teaspoon salt, and vinegar mixture in blender until frothy, about 10 seconds. With blender running, slowly drizzle in hot melted ghee until fully emulsified, about 1½ minutes. Adjust sauce consistency with hot water as needed, 1 teaspoon at a time, until sauce slowly drips from spoon. Stir in minced tarragon and season with salt and pepper to taste. Serve.

Shredded Beef Tacos with Cabbage Slaw

Serves 4 to 6

☑ **WHY THIS RECIPE WORKS** Robust, flavorful shredded beef tacos are a Mexican food favorite. But to make a paleo version, we would have to eliminate the canned tomatoes, store-bought broth, and beer used in the sauce, and ensure that our beef was flavorful enough to work without any cheese, sour cream, or other nonpaleo taco toppings. We started with collagen-rich chuck-eye roast and braised it gently in a covered Dutch oven. To achieve plenty of flavorful browning without having to sear the meat, we raised the beef out of the braising liquid by resting it on onion rounds. Next, we built a bold braising liquid with tomato paste, ancho chiles, and plenty of spices. The potently flavored liquid infused the beef with big flavor, and it pulled double duty as a base for our sauce—once the beef had finished cooking, we pureed the cooking liquid into a sauce with a smooth, luxurious consistency. A bright, tangy, and lightly spicy cabbage slaw provided a nice counterbalance to the rich meat.

2	cups water, plus extra as needed
1¼	cups cider vinegar
4	teaspoons dried oregano
	Kosher salt and pepper
4	cups shredded green cabbage
2	large carrots, peeled and shredded
1	jalapeño chile, stemmed, seeded, and minced
4	dried ancho chiles, stemmed, seeded, and torn into ½-inch pieces (1 cup)
3	tablespoons tomato paste
6	garlic cloves, lightly crushed and peeled
1	tablespoon ground cumin
¾	teaspoon ground cinnamon
½	teaspoon ground cloves
3	bay leaves
1	large onion, sliced into ½-inch-thick rounds
2	pounds boneless beef chuck-eye roast, pulled apart at seams, trimmed, and cut into 2-inch pieces
1	cup chopped fresh cilantro
12	(6-inch) Paleo Wraps, warmed (page 24)
	Lime wedges

1. Whisk ½ cup water, ¾ cup vinegar, 1 teaspoon oregano, and 1 tablespoon salt together in large bowl until salt is dissolved. Add cabbage, carrot, and jalapeño and toss to combine. Cover and refrigerate until ready to serve. (Slaw can be refrigerated for up to 24 hours.)

2. Adjust oven rack to lower-middle position and heat oven to 325 degrees. Combine anchos, tomato paste, garlic, cumin, cinnamon, cloves, bay leaves, 1 tablespoon salt, ½ teaspoon pepper, remaining 1½ cups water, remaining ½ cup vinegar, and remaining 1 tablespoon oregano in Dutch oven. Arrange onion rounds in single layer on bottom of pot. Place beef on top of onion rounds in single layer.

3. Fit large piece of aluminum foil over pot, pressing to seal, then cover tightly with lid. Transfer pot to oven and cook until meat is well browned and tender, 2½ to 3 hours.

4. Using slotted spoon, transfer beef to large bowl and cover. Being careful of hot pot handles, strain cooking liquid through fine-mesh strainer into 2-cup liquid measuring cup (do not wash pot). Discard onion rounds and bay leaves, then transfer remaining solids to blender. Using wide, shallow spoon, skim excess fat from surface of liquid. Add water as needed to equal 1 cup. Add liquid to blender with solids and process until smooth, about 2 minutes; transfer to now-empty pot.

5. Using 2 forks, shred beef into bite-size pieces, discarding excess fat. Bring sauce to simmer over medium heat. Stir in shredded beef and season with salt to taste. Drain slaw and stir in cilantro. Serve shredded beef with warm wraps, slaw, and lime wedges.

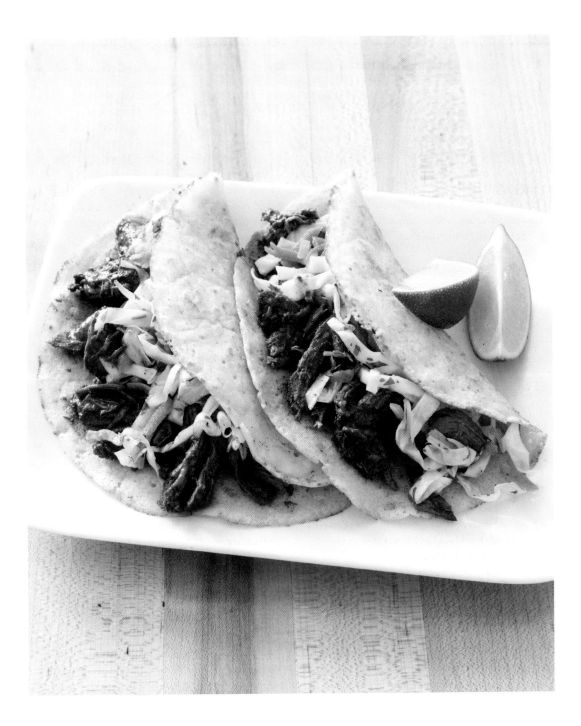

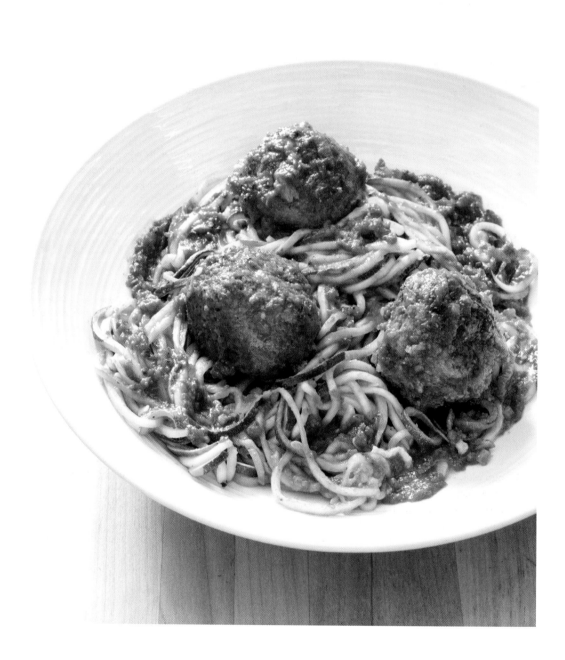

Zucchini "Spaghetti" and Meatballs

Serves 4

✓ **WHY THIS RECIPE WORKS** Recipes for spaghetti and meatballs are fraught with nonpaleo ingredients: pasta, canned tomato sauce, bread, milk, and cheese. To devise a paleo-friendly version of this dish, we needed to successfully replace the wheat pasta, bind the meatballs, and make a hearty sauce out of fresh tomatoes. First, we tackled the meatballs. In the test kitchen, we often use a panade in meatball and meatloaf recipes to help the ground meat stay moist and hold its shape. A panade is a mixture of starch and liquid—most commonly white bread and whole milk, two nonstarters on the paleo diet. We tried making meatballs without a panade, but as expected, they turned out tough and rubbery. We tested our way through a number of binding and tenderizing options, including almond flour, coconut flour, gelatin, and boiled, pureed cashews. Coconut flour and gelatin left our meatballs spongy, but the cashew puree worked perfectly—its neutral flavor wasn't noticeable, and it helped the meatballs stay together and kept the meat tender. Cooking the aromatics all at once and dividing them between the meatballs and the sauce saved time and ensured that the finished dish was consistently seasoned. We found that using ripe, flavorful tomatoes was essential to the sauce's success; we processed the tomatoes in the food processor to achieve a near-smooth consistency. To fortify our sauce, we used the fat left in the skillet from our meatballs to brown the aromatics and some tomato paste, which gave our sauce good body and depth. We then braised the meatballs in the sauce, allowing the sauce to pick up more meaty flavor. With our sauce and meatballs done, all we needed was to find the perfect substitute for spaghetti. We tested a variety of vegetables, but tasters liked spiralized zucchini for its ability to be twirled around a fork like real spaghetti. Roasting the noodles rid them of excess moisture and ensured that our sauce didn't become watered down. If possible, use smaller, in-season zucchini, which have thinner skins and less seeds. For more information on spiralizing, see page 14. This recipe calls for a 12-inch nonstick skillet; however, a well-seasoned cast-iron skillet can be used instead.

¼ cup raw cashews

3 tablespoons extra-virgin olive oil

2 onions, chopped fine

6 garlic cloves, minced

1 tablespoon dried oregano

¼ teaspoon red pepper flakes

¼ cup plus 2 tablespoons chopped fresh basil

1 large egg
Kosher salt and pepper

1 pound 85 percent lean ground beef

2 pounds tomatoes, cored and chopped

¼ cup tomato paste

3 pounds zucchini or yellow summer squash, trimmed

1. Bring 4 cups water to boil in medium saucepan over medium-high heat. Add cashews and cook until softened, about 15 minutes. Drain and rinse well.

2. Heat 1 tablespoon oil in 12-inch nonstick skillet over medium heat until shimmering. Add onions and cook until softened and lightly browned, 8 to 10 minutes. Stir in garlic, oregano, and pepper flakes and cook until fragrant, about 30 seconds. Transfer half of onion mixture to bowl and set aside.

3. Process remaining onion mixture, boiled cashews, ¼ cup basil, egg, and 1½ teaspoons salt in food processor to fine paste, about 1 minute, scraping down sides of bowl as needed; transfer to large bowl. Add ground beef and knead with your hands until well combined. Pinch off and roll mixture into 1½-inch meatballs (you should have 12 meatballs).

4. Process tomatoes in clean, dry workbowl until smooth, about 30 seconds. Heat 1 tablespoon oil in now-empty skillet over medium heat until just smoking. Brown meatballs on all sides, about 10 minutes; transfer to plate.

5. Add reserved onion mixture and tomato paste to fat left in skillet and cook over medium heat until tomato paste begins to brown, about 1 minute. Stir in processed tomatoes, bring to simmer, and cook until sauce is thickened, about 20 minutes.

6. Return browned meatballs and any accumulated juices to skillet. Reduce heat to medium-low, cover, and simmer gently until meatballs are cooked through, about 10 minutes. Adjust sauce consistency with hot water as needed. Stir in remaining 2 tablespoons basil and season with salt and pepper to taste. (Sauce and meatballs can be refrigerated for up to 3 days or frozen for up to 1 month; gently reheat before serving.)

7. Meanwhile, adjust oven rack to middle position and heat oven to 375 degrees. Using spiralizer, cut zucchini into ⅛-inch-thick noodles, then cut noodles into 12-inch lengths. Toss zucchini with 1 teaspoon salt, ½ teaspoon pepper, and remaining 1 tablespoon oil on rimmed baking sheet and roast until tender, 20 to 25 minutes. Transfer zucchini to colander and shake to remove any excess liquid. Transfer zucchini to large serving bowl, add several spoonfuls of sauce (without meatballs), and gently toss to combine. Serve zucchini with remaining sauce and meatballs.

VARIATION
Butternut Squash "Spaghetti" and Meatballs

This recipe uses only the solid necks of the squash. Reserve the bulbs for another use. Cooked squash noodles will be delicate and may break when transferring to serving platter.

Using sharp vegetable peeler or chef's knife, remove skin and fibrous threads from 2 (3-pound) butternut squashes. Trim off top of squash and cut squash in half where narrow neck and wide curved base meet; reserve squash bases for another use. Using spiralizer, cut squash necks into ⅛-inch-thick noodles, then cut noodles into 12-inch lengths (you should have 14 cups). Substitute squash noodles for zucchini noodles in step 7, covering tightly with aluminum foil for first 15 minutes of roasting; do not drain in colander. Gently transfer squash to serving platter and top with meatballs and several spoonfuls of sauce (do not toss). Serve with remaining sauce.

TEST KITCHEN TIP **MAKING PALEO MEATBALLS**

For tender paleo meatballs, we bind them with boiled, pureed cashews instead of bread crumbs and milk.

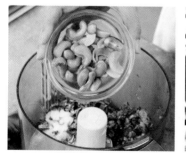 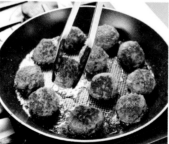 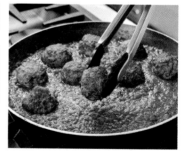

1. Cook cashews in boiling water until softened. Process cooked cashews with sautéed aromatics, basil, egg, and salt to fine paste. This paste incorporates easily into ground meat.

2. Add ground beef to cashew paste and knead until combined. Pinch off and roll mixture into 1½-inch meatballs, then brown meatballs to enhance meaty, savory flavor.

3. Once tomato sauce has thickened, return browned meatballs to sauce and continue to simmer. This allows meatballs to gently cook through and contribute meaty flavor to sauce.

Shepherd's Pie

Serves 4 to 6

✓ **WHY THIS RECIPE WORKS** Old-fashioned shepherd's pie traditionally consists of a meat-and-gravy base topped with fluffy mashed potatoes. But the flour-thickened gravy and the potato topping mean that most recipes aren't paleo. We set out to make a paleo-friendly version that was as hearty as the original, and, to streamline the often arduous cooking process, we decided to make our pie in a skillet. Ground beef made an easy, meaty base for our pie; it cooked in less than half the time required by bigger chunks and needed no butchering. Because searing ground meat turns it pebbly, we ensured that the meat stayed tender by skipping the browning and simmering the meat right in the gravy. But in most recipes, browning does more than just parcook the meat—it also provides savory depth. We found that we could achieve the flavor we were after by browning onions, mushrooms, and tomato paste instead, creating a rich fond. We deglazed the pan with beef broth for even more savory flavor. But without the flour, the sauce was thin—not the satisfying, luxurious gravy we expect in shepherd's pie. We tried thickening it with arrowroot and tapioca flours, but they turned the gravy gloppy. We decided instead to stir some of the pureed vegetable topping into the filling to thicken it naturally—but first, we needed to figure out what the topping would be. We tested a variety of vegetables; tasters found the distinct flavor of sweet potatoes too overwhelming, while celery root turned a little too gluey. Neutral-tasting cauliflower worked perfectly: We browned it briefly to bring out some savory notes, then steamed it and processed it to a smooth consistency. Just half a cup of the puree thickened the filling beautifully. We stirred a beaten egg into the remaining puree to give it some heft and to help it hold up on top of the pie. Don't use ground beef that's less than 90 percent lean or the dish will be greasy. We prefer to use homemade beef broth; however, you can substitute your favorite store-bought broth. You will need a 10-inch broiler-safe skillet for this recipe.

3	tablespoons ghee
1	head cauliflower (2½ pounds), cored and cut into ½-inch pieces (8 cups)
	Kosher salt and pepper
1	large egg, lightly beaten
3	tablespoons minced fresh chives
4	ounces cremini mushrooms, trimmed and chopped
1	onion, chopped fine
2	tablespoons tomato paste
¼	ounce dried porcini mushrooms, rinsed and minced
2	garlic cloves, minced
1	teaspoon minced fresh thyme or ¼ teaspoon dried
1¼	cups Paleo Beef Broth (page 17)
2	carrots, peeled and chopped
1½	pounds 90 percent lean ground beef

1. Heat 2 tablespoons ghee in large saucepan over medium-low heat until shimmering. Add cauliflower and cook, stirring occasionally, until softened and beginning to brown, about 10 minutes. Stir in ½ cup water and 1 teaspoon salt, cover, and cook until cauliflower falls apart easily when poked with fork, about 10 minutes. Off heat, remove lid and allow steam to escape for 2 minutes.

2. Process cauliflower in food processor until smooth, about 45 seconds. Measure out and reserve ½ cup processed cauliflower for filling. Transfer remaining cauliflower to large bowl and stir in beaten egg and chives; set aside.

3. Heat remaining 1 tablespoon ghee in 10-inch broiler-safe skillet over medium heat until shimmering. Add cremini mushrooms, onion, 1 teaspoon salt, and ¼ teaspoon pepper and cook until softened and lightly browned, 8 to 10 minutes. Stir in tomato paste, porcini mushrooms, garlic, and thyme and cook until fragrant, about 1 minute. Stir in broth and carrots, scraping up any browned bits.

4. Reduce heat to medium-low, add ground beef in 2-inch chunks, and bring to gentle simmer. Cover and cook until beef is cooked through, 10 to 12 minutes, stirring and breaking up meat chunks with 2 forks halfway through cooking. Off heat, stir in reserved processed cauliflower and season with salt and pepper to taste.

5. Adjust oven rack 5 inches from broiler element and heat broiler. Transfer cauliflower/chive mixture to 1-gallon zipper-lock bag and snip off 1 corner to create 1-inch opening. Pipe mixture in even layer over filling, making sure to cover entire surface. Smooth mixture with back of spoon, then use tines of fork to make ridges over surface. Place skillet on rimmed baking sheet and broil until topping is golden brown and crusty and filling is bubbly, 10 to 15 minutes. Let cool for 10 minutes before serving.

TEST KITCHEN TIP **MAKING SHEPHERD'S PIE TOPPING**

Since potatoes are not included in the paleo diet, we make a smooth, creamy, and flavorful Shepherd's Pie topping using cauliflower.

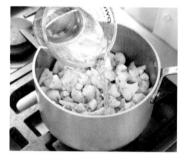

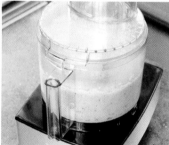

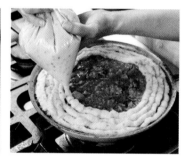

1. Lightly brown cauliflower in ghee to bring out its nutty flavor, then stir in water and let steam. Off heat, remove lid and allow steam to escape so cauliflower puree does not become watered down.

2. Puree cauliflower in food processor until smooth. Set aside ½ cup for filling; transfer remaining puree to bowl and stir in beaten egg to give puree more structure.

3. Transfer cauliflower mixture to 1-gallon zipper-lock bag and snip off 1 corner. Pipe mixture over filling in even layer. Smooth with back of spoon, then make decorative ridges with fork before broiling.

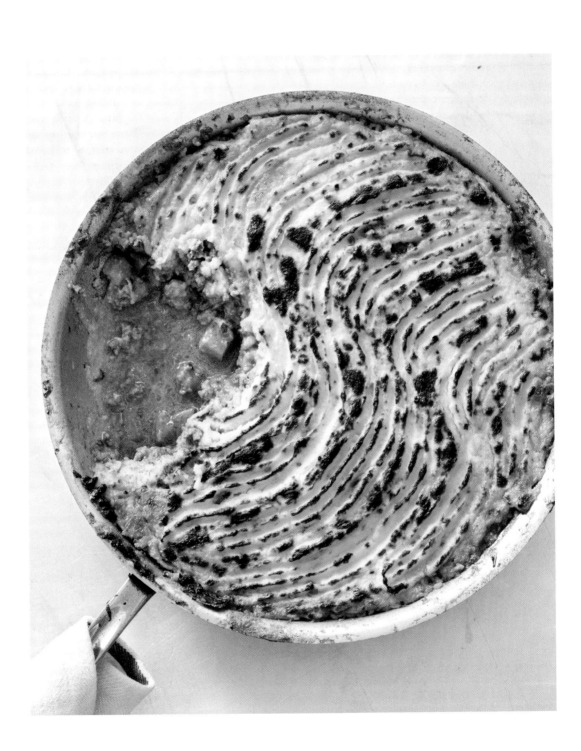

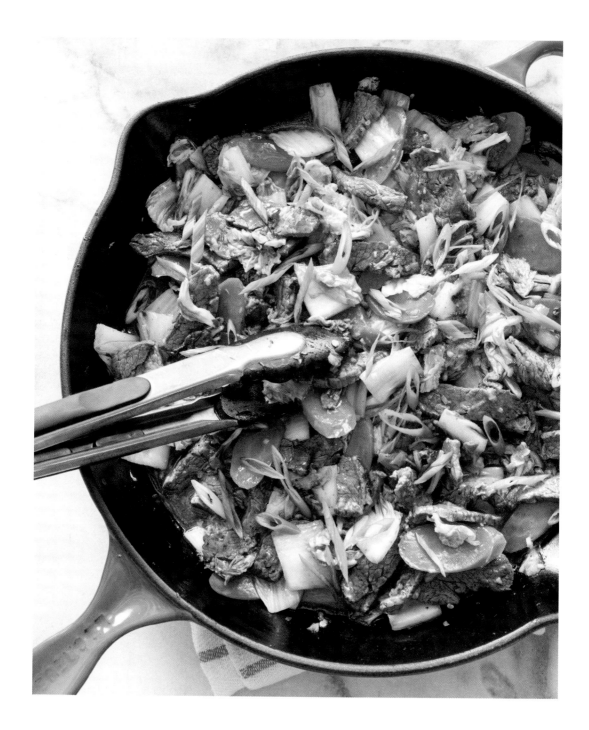

Spicy Korean-Style Stir-Fried Beef

Serves 4

✓ **WHY THIS RECIPE WORKS** We set out to create a simple beef stir-fry inspired by the flavors of kimchi, a traditional Korean dish of spicy, fermented vegetables. Store-bought kimchi often contains preservatives that aren't paleo, so we re-created the flavor using a few potent ingredients: fish sauce, coconut aminos (a common paleo replacement for soy sauce), lime juice, scallions, garlic, ginger, and a generous amount of red pepper flakes. Cabbage and carrots, which are typical ingredients in kimchi, made a perfect slate for the intense flavors. With our flavor profile down, we turned to the beef. Flank steak is the classic choice for beef stir-fry because it's quick-cooking and has great meaty depth. We cut the meat against the grain into thin strips to ensure that it would be tender and easy to eat. We found that freezing the beef for at least 15 minutes made it easier to cut into wide, flat slices that would cook quickly and brown nicely. To encourage deep, flavorful browning, we cooked the steak over high heat in two batches. This recipe calls for a 12-inch nonstick skillet; however, a well-seasoned cast-iron skillet can be used instead. For more information on coconut aminos, see page 11. Serve with Cauliflower Rice (page 288).

SAUCE

- ¼ **cup coconut aminos**
- 2 **tablespoons lime juice**
- 2 **teaspoons fish sauce**
- 1½ **teaspoons tapioca flour**

STIR-FRY

- 2 **teaspoons lime juice**
- 1 **teaspoon coconut aminos**
- 1 **pound flank steak, trimmed and sliced thin against grain into 2-inch-long pieces**
- 5 **scallions, white parts minced, green parts sliced thin on bias**
- 4 **garlic cloves, minced**
- 1 **tablespoon grated fresh ginger**
- 1½ **teaspoons red pepper flakes**
- 3 **tablespoons coconut oil, melted**
- 3 **carrots, peeled and sliced ¼ inch thick on bias**
- 1 **small head napa cabbage (1½ pounds), cored and cut into 1-inch pieces**

1. FOR THE SAUCE Whisk all ingredients together in bowl.

2. FOR THE STIR-FRY Whisk lime juice and coconut aminos together in medium bowl, then stir in beef and let marinate for 10 minutes. In separate bowl, combine scallion whites, garlic, ginger, pepper flakes, and 1 tablespoon melted oil.

3. Heat 2 teaspoons melted oil in 12-inch nonstick skillet over high heat until just smoking. Add half of beef, break up any clumps, and cook, without stirring, for 1 minute. Stir beef and continue to cook until browned, about 1 minute; transfer to clean bowl. Repeat with 2 teaspoons melted oil and remaining beef; transfer to bowl.

4. Heat remaining 2 teaspoons melted oil in now-empty skillet over medium-high heat until shimmering. Add carrots and cook until softened, about 5 minutes. Add cabbage and cook, stirring occasionally, until spotty brown and crisp-tender, about 3 minutes.

5. Push vegetables to sides of skillet. Add scallion mixture to center and cook, mashing mixture into skillet, until fragrant, about 1 minute. Stir mixture into vegetables.

6. Stir cooked beef and any accumulated juices into vegetables. Whisk sauce to recombine, then add to skillet. Cook, stirring constantly, until sauce is thickened, about 1 minute. Transfer to serving platter and sprinkle with scallion greens. Serve.

French Pot Roast with Mustard-Parsley Sauce

Serves 6 to 8

✔ **WHY THIS RECIPE WORKS** The elegant French pot roast known as *pot-au-feu* delivers more complex flavor than the average American pot roast but is just as comforting and rich. Traditional pot-au-feu recipes utilize multiple cuts of boneless and bone-in beef that can be hard to find, so we simplified and streamlined by using a boneless chuck-eye roast, which was easy to carve and serve, and beef bones, which imparted deep, meaty flavor. The oven's gentle, ambient heat made cooking simple and hands-off. To make it paleo, we left out the traditional potatoes and freshened up the pot with whole spears of asparagus. To brighten up the finished dish, we used the marrow from the bones in a piquant finishing sauce of minced herbs, vinegar, mustard, and cornichons. Marrow bones (also sold as soup bones) can often be found in the freezer section of the grocery store; if using frozen bones, be sure to thaw them completely. If your bones do not yield 2 tablespoons of marrow, supplement with the fat skimmed from the broth in step 4.

⅔ cup minced fresh parsley
¼ cup minced fresh chives
¼ cup Dijon mustard
3 tablespoons white wine vinegar
10 cornichons, minced
Kosher salt and pepper
1 (3½- to 4-pound) boneless beef chuck-eye roast, pulled into 2 pieces at natural seam and trimmed of large pieces of fat
1½ pounds marrow bones
1 onion, quartered
1 celery rib, sliced thin
3 bay leaves
1 teaspoon black peppercorns
4 cups cold tap water, plus extra as needed
1 pound turnips, peeled and cut into 1-inch pieces
6 carrots, peeled, halved crosswise, thick ends quartered lengthwise, thin ends halved lengthwise
1 pound asparagus, trimmed

1. Adjust oven rack to lower-middle position and heat oven to 300 degrees. Combine parsley, chives, mustard, vinegar, cornichons, and 1½ teaspoons pepper in bowl; cover and set aside.

2. Season roasts with salt and tie each into loaf shape using 3 pieces of kitchen twine. Place beef, bones, onion, celery, bay leaves, and peppercorns in Dutch oven. Add water (water should come halfway up roasts) and bring to simmer over high heat. Partially cover pot, transfer to oven, and cook until sharp knife slips easily in and out of meat, 3¼ to 3¾ hours.

3. Remove pot from oven and turn oven off. Transfer beef to serving platter, cover with aluminum foil, and place in turned-off oven.

4. Being careful of hot pot handles, transfer bones to cutting board and use end of spoon to extract 2 tablespoons marrow; discard bones. Mince marrow into paste and add to parsley sauce. Using wide, shallow spoon, skim excess fat from surface of broth. Strain broth through fine-mesh strainer into 8-cup liquid measuring cup; discard solids. Add extra water to broth as needed to make 6 cups.

5. Return broth to now-empty pot. Add turnips and carrots, bring to simmer over medium heat, and cook for 10 minutes. Stir in asparagus and cook until vegetables are tender, 3 to 5 minutes.

6. Using slotted spoon, transfer vegetables to serving bowl. Toss with 3 tablespoons parsley sauce and season with salt and pepper to taste. Season broth with salt to taste.

7. Transfer roasts to carving board, remove twine, and slice into ½-inch-thick slices. Arrange meat on serving platter, drizzle with ¼ cup broth, and dollop with half of sauce. Serve beef and vegetables, passing remaining broth and sauce separately.

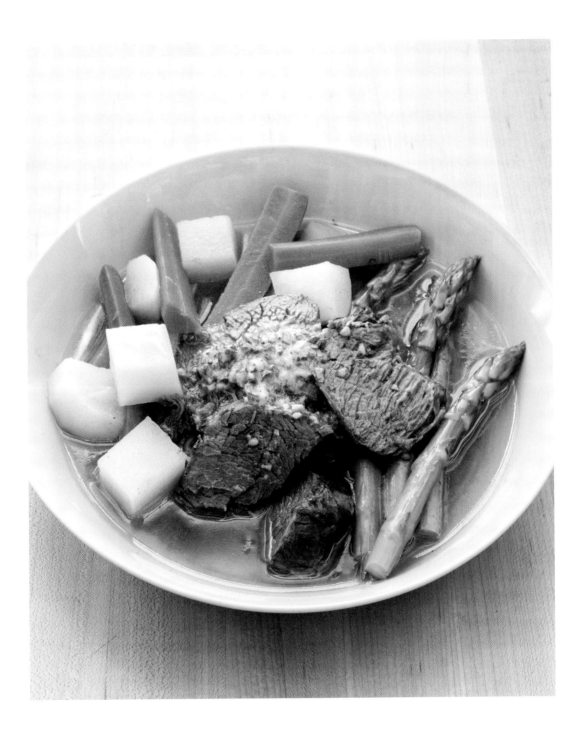

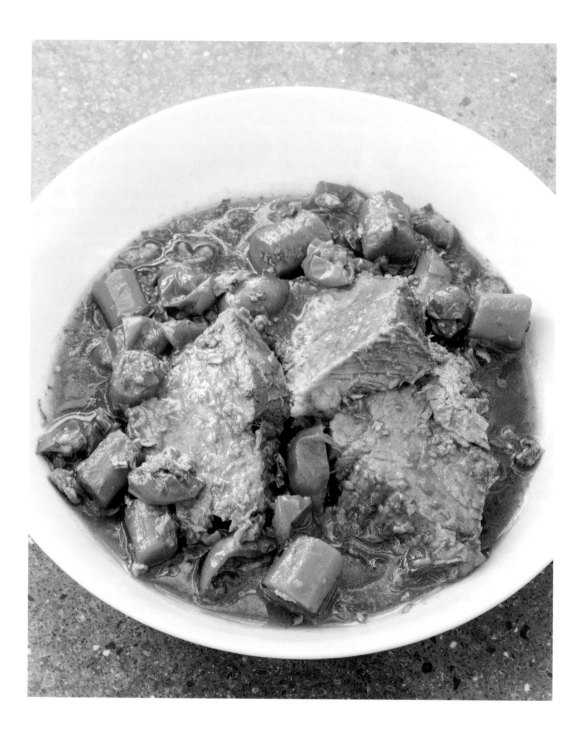

Slow-Cooker Italian-Style Pot Roast

Serves 6 to 8

✓ **WHY THIS RECIPE WORKS** For a tender pot roast recipe with an Italian spin, we started with boneless chuck-eye roast—our favorite cut for pot roast because it's well marbled with fat and connective tissue. The slow cooker, with its even and moist heat, is the perfect environment for braising a pot roast until fork-tender, but many slow-cooker recipes call for canned tomatoes as the base of the braise. We found that halved cherry tomatoes cooked perfectly along with the roast, breaking down to create a flavorful, fresh-tasting tomato sauce. We reinforced the Italian flavors in the pot roast with the addition of garlic, oregano, red pepper flakes, and dried porcini mushrooms. Since store-bought broth was off the table, we gave our pot roast a boost of meaty flavor by getting out a skillet: We sautéed bacon, browned the aromatics in the rendered bacon fat, and deglazed the pan to capture all the flavorful browned bits. A sprinkling of fresh basil before serving highlighted the fresh, bold flavors of our sauce. Many markets sell chuck-eye roast with elastic netting, which should be removed. Re-tie the roast using kitchen twine. You will need an oval 5½- to 7-quart slow cooker for this recipe.

8 slices bacon, chopped
2 onions, chopped
4 carrots, peeled and sliced 1 inch thick
   Kosher salt and pepper
3 tablespoons tomato paste
6 garlic cloves, minced
2 tablespoons minced fresh oregano
   or 2 teaspoons dried
½ ounce dried porcini mushrooms,
   rinsed and minced
½ teaspoon red pepper flakes
½ cup water
1 pound cherry tomatoes, halved
2 bay leaves
1 (3½- to 4-pound) boneless beef chuck-eye
   roast, trimmed and tied at 1-inch intervals
¼ cup chopped fresh basil

1. Cook bacon in 12-inch skillet over medium heat until crisp, 5 to 7 minutes. Using slotted spoon, transfer bacon to paper towel–lined plate; set aside.

2. Pour off all but 2 tablespoons fat from skillet. Add onions, carrots, and 1 teaspoon salt and cook over medium heat until softened and lightly browned, 8 to 10 minutes. Stir in tomato paste, garlic, oregano, mushrooms, and pepper flakes

and cook until fragrant, about 1 minute. Stir in water, scraping up any browned bits; transfer to slow cooker.

3. Stir tomatoes and bay leaves into slow cooker. Season roast with salt and pepper and nestle into slow cooker. Cover and cook until sharp knife slips easily in and out of meat, 9 to 10 hours on low or 6 to 7 hours on high.

4. Transfer roast to carving board, tent loosely with aluminum foil, and let rest for 20 minutes.

5. Meanwhile, discard bay leaves. Using large, shallow spoon, skim excess fat from surface of sauce. Stir in crisp bacon and basil and season with salt and pepper to taste. Remove twine from roast, slice against grain into ½-inch-thick slices, and arrange on serving platter. Spoon 1 cup sauce over meat and serve with remaining sauce.

TEST KITCHEN TIP **TYING POT ROAST**

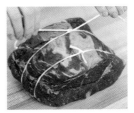

Chuck-eye roasts can be oddly shaped; to ensure roast cooks evenly, tie with kitchen twine at 1-inch intervals.

Pomegranate-Braised Beef Short Ribs

Serves 6

✅ **WHY THIS RECIPE WORKS** Rich, beefy short ribs turn fall-apart tender when braised, but most recipes rely on copious amounts of red wine or beer in the braising liquid. We wanted an equally flavorful and robust dish made with paleo ingredients. Instead of red wine, we decided on a fresh, modern spin, starting with a combination of unsweetened pomegranate juice, orange zest and juice, thyme, and garlic. Adding a carrot to the braising liquid provided complementary sweetness to balance the tart pomegranate juice. Bacon provided savory, meaty depth. We chose bone-in short ribs because the bones contain marrow, which contributed flavor and body to our braise. Most recipes call for browning the short ribs on the stovetop in batches, but we wanted a simpler option. We found we could brown all of the ribs at once in a roasting pan in the oven. This had the added benefit of rendering some fat from the ribs. Deglazing the roasting pan with the pomegranate juice ensured that we captured all of the flavorful browned bits from the pan. To prevent the sauce from being greasy, we defatted the liquid before blending the liquid and solids together into a smooth, velvety sauce for our succulent ribs. This recipe will also work with flanken-style short ribs (if using, flip ribs halfway through roasting in step 2). Any brand of 100 percent unsweetened pomegranate juice will work; avoid sweetened juice or juice blends. Serve with Celery Root Puree (page 291).

6 pounds bone-in English-style short ribs, trimmed
  Kosher salt and pepper
3 cups unsweetened pomegranate juice
2 slices bacon, chopped fine
1 onion, chopped fine
1 carrot, chopped
6 garlic cloves, minced
1 tablespoon minced fresh thyme or 1 teaspoon dried
1 cup water
4 (2-inch) strips orange zest plus ½ cup juice
3 bay leaves
2 tablespoons chopped fresh parsley

1. Adjust oven rack to lower-middle position and heat oven to 450 degrees. Pat short ribs dry with paper towels and season with salt and pepper. Arrange ribs bone side down in single layer in large roasting pan and roast until meat begins to brown, about 45 minutes.

2. Discard any accumulated juices in pan, if necessary, and continue to roast until meat is well browned, 15 to 20 minutes. Transfer ribs to plate; set aside.

3. Reduce oven temperature to 300 degrees. Stir pomegranate juice into roasting pan, scraping up any browned bits; set aside.

4. Cook bacon in Dutch oven over medium-high heat until crisp, about 5 minutes. Add onion and carrot and cook until softened, about 5 minutes. Stir in garlic and thyme and cook until fragrant, about 30 seconds. Stir in juice from roasting pan, water, orange zest and juice, bay leaves, 2 teaspoons salt, and ½ teaspoon pepper and bring to simmer. Nestle browned ribs into pot, completely submerging meat in liquid. Cover, transfer to oven, and cook until ribs are tender, about 2½ hours.

5. Transfer ribs to serving platter and tent loosely with aluminum foil. Discard loose bones and bay leaves. Using wide, shallow spoon, skim excess fat from surface of braising liquid. Being careful of hot pot handles, transfer braising liquid to blender in batches. Process braising liquid until smooth, about 30 seconds. Return sauce and ribs to now-empty pot, bring to gentle simmer over medium heat, and cook until ribs are heated through, about 5 minutes. Season with salt and pepper to taste. Return ribs to serving platter and sprinkle with parsley. Serve, passing remaining sauce separately.

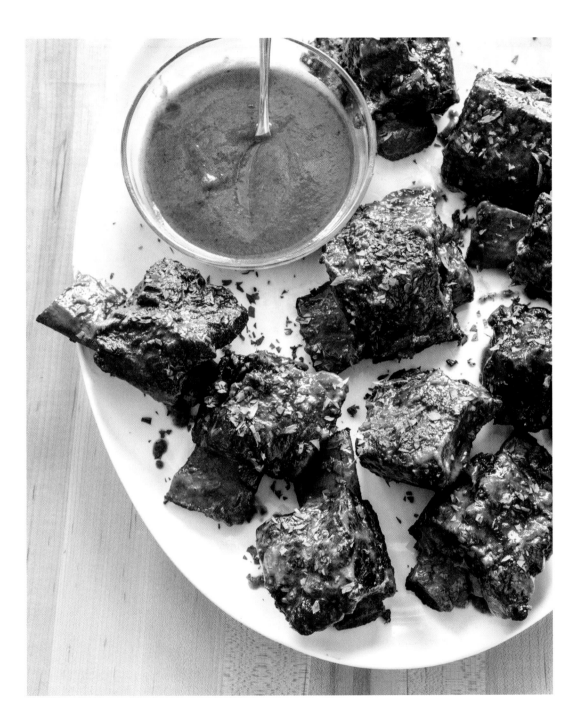

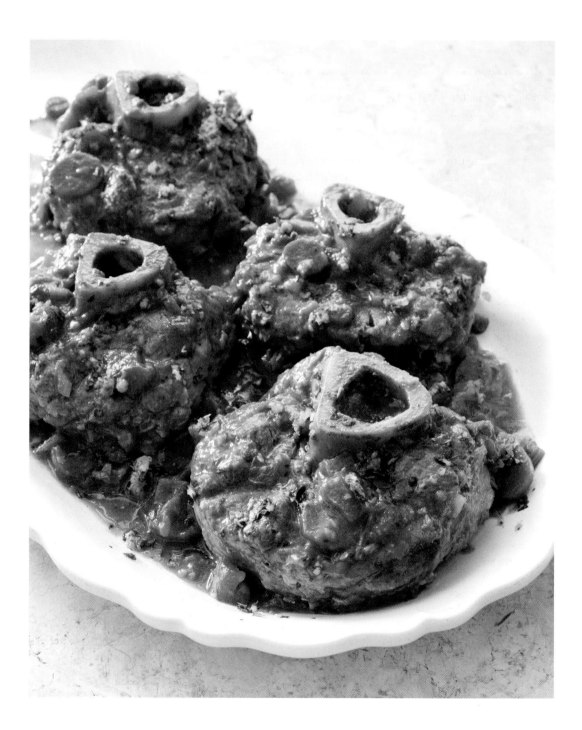

Osso Buco

Serves 6

✔ **WHY THIS RECIPE WORKS** This well-known Italian classic is made from simple ingredients, but the rich, flavorful braising liquid typically depends on wine and canned tomatoes. To provide a savory backbone for the veal using paleo ingredients, we started with the stock. Veal stock is traditional, but few cooks have homemade veal stock on hand. We found that chicken broth along with garlic, onions, carrots, and celery made a sturdy yet subtle flavor base for our braising liquid. A combination of tomato paste and fresh tomatoes worked perfectly in place of canned, and they added enough acidity and brightness that tasters didn't miss the wine. At the end of cooking, we processed the marrow from the veal shanks with the braising liquid to give it a lush, thick consistency. Gremolata—a mixture of minced garlic, parsley, and lemon zest—is a classic component of osso bucco. We stirred half of the gremolata right into the braise, and also used it to garnish each serving for a final hit of fresh flavor. We prefer to use homemade chicken broth; however, you can substitute your favorite store-bought broth. Serve with Celery Root Puree (page 291).

¼	cup minced fresh parsley
9	garlic cloves, minced
2	teaspoons grated lemon zest
6	(8- to 10-ounce) veal shanks, 1½ inches thick, trimmed and tied around equator
	Kosher salt and pepper
6	tablespoons extra-virgin olive oil
2	onions, chopped
2	carrots, peeled and sliced ¼ inch thick
2	celery ribs, cut into ½-inch pieces
3	tablespoons tomato paste
¼	ounce dried porcini mushrooms, rinsed and minced
¼	teaspoon red pepper flakes
3	cups Paleo Chicken Broth (page 16)
2	tomatoes, cored and chopped
2	bay leaves
1	sprig fresh thyme

1. Adjust oven rack to lower-middle position and heat oven to 325 degrees. Combine parsley, one-third of garlic, and lemon zest in bowl; set aside.

2. Pat shanks dry with paper towels and season with salt and pepper. Heat 2 tablespoons oil in Dutch oven over medium-high heat until just smoking. Brown half of shanks on all sides, 8 to 10 minutes; transfer to large bowl. Repeat with 2 tablespoons oil and remaining shanks; transfer to bowl.

3. Add remaining 2 tablespoons oil to fat left in pot and heat over medium heat until shimmering. Add onions, carrots, celery, and 1 teaspoon salt and cook until softened and lightly browned, 8 to 10 minutes. Stir in tomato paste, mushrooms, pepper flakes, and remaining garlic and cook until fragrant, about 1 minute. Stir in broth, tomatoes, bay leaves, and thyme sprig, scraping up any browned bits, and bring to simmer.

4. Nestle browned shanks into pot along with any accumulated juices. Cover, transfer to oven, and cook until veal is tender and sharp knife slips easily in and out of meat, but meat is not falling off bone, about 2½ hours.

5. Transfer shanks to platter and discard twine. Extract marrow from bones using end of spoon and reserve. Tent shanks loosely with aluminum foil.

6. Being careful of hot pot handles, discard bay leaves and thyme sprig. Process reserved marrow and 1½ cups braising liquid in blender until smooth, about 30 seconds. Stir marrow mixture and half of parsley mixture into remaining braising liquid and season with salt and pepper to taste. Place shanks in individual serving bowls, ladle braising liquid over top, and sprinkle with remaining parsley mixture. Serve.

Orange Chipotle–Glazed Pork Chops

Serves 4

☑ **WHY THIS RECIPE WORKS** Quick-cooking boneless pork chops make a great weeknight meal, and a tangy-sweet glaze is an easy way to boost the flavor of this mild cut. To prevent our skillet-browned chops from curling as they cooked, we made a few slashes through the fat and silverskin. We didn't want to spend extra time brining or marinating our chops, so we seared them over medium-high heat and then gently simmered them in a simple glaze made from orange juice, coconut sugar, lime zest and juice, and chipotle chile powder, which infused the chops with flavor and kept them from drying out. Once the chops were done, we let them rest while we reduced the glaze until it was thick and glossy, but not overly syrupy. We added the juices from the rested meat to give the glaze a savory backbone. Be careful not to overreduce the glaze in step 4. If the glaze thickens to the correct consistency before the chops reach 145 degrees, add a few tablespoons of water to the skillet. Serve with Slow-Cooker Mashed Sweet Potatoes (page 300), pictured.

⅔ **cup orange juice**

1½ **tablespoons coconut sugar**

½ **teaspoon grated lime zest plus 1 teaspoon juice**

½ **teaspoon chipotle chile powder**

4 **(8-ounce) boneless pork chops, ¾ to 1 inch thick, trimmed Kosher salt and pepper**

1 **tablespoon extra-virgin olive oil**

1. Combine orange juice, sugar, lime zest and juice, and chile powder in bowl.

2. Cut 2 slits, about 2 inches apart, through outer layer of fat and silverskin on each chop. Pat chops dry with paper towels and season with salt and pepper. Heat oil in 12-inch skillet over medium-high heat until just smoking. Place chops in skillet and cook until well browned on first side, about 5 minutes.

3. Flip chops and add glaze. Reduce heat to medium-low and cook until pork registers 145 degrees, 5 to 8 minutes.

4. Transfer chops to serving platter and tent loosely with aluminum foil. Increase heat to medium and simmer glaze until thick and syrupy, 2 to 6 minutes, adding any accumulated pork juices. Pour glaze over chops and serve.

VARIATION

Maple-Glazed Pork Chops

Substitute following mixture for orange glaze: ½ cup maple syrup, ¼ cup cider vinegar, 2 teaspoons Dijon mustard, and 2 teaspoons minced fresh thyme. Simmer glaze as directed.

TEST KITCHEN TIP

PREVENTING CURLED PORK CHOPS

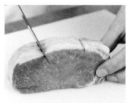

To prevent pork chops from curling and encourage even browning, cut 2 slits, 2 inches apart, through outer layer of fat and silverskin of each chop.

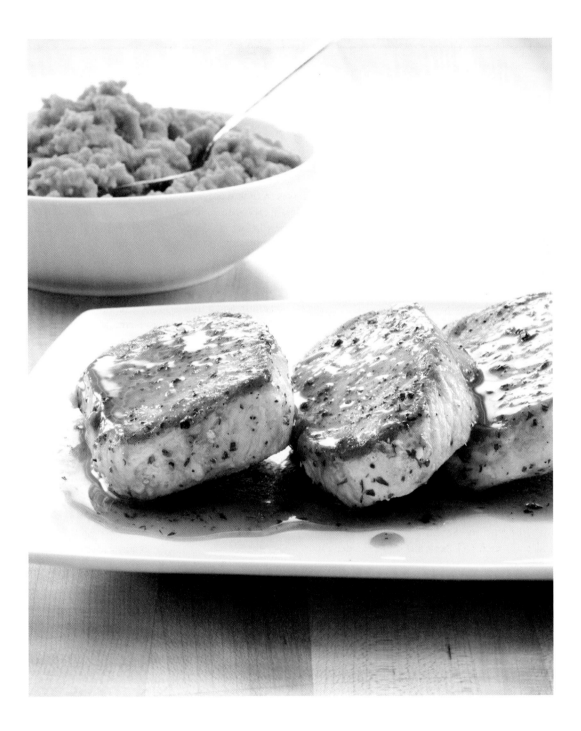

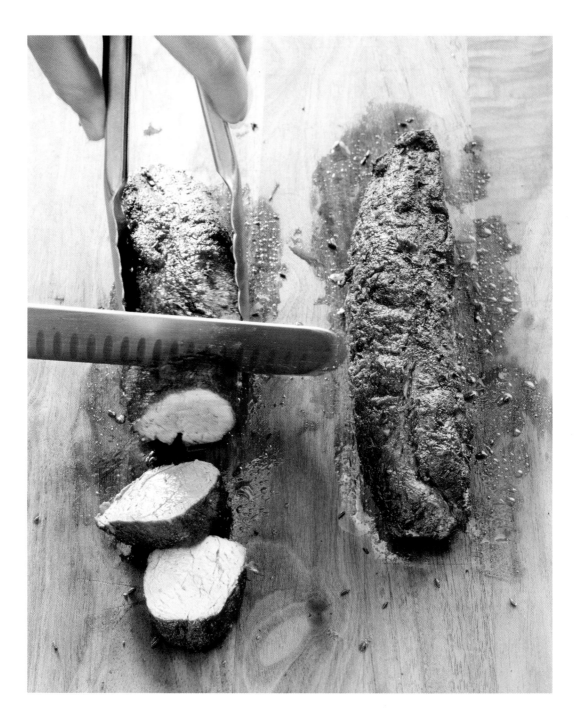

Spiced Pork Tenderloins

Serves 4

✓ **WHY THIS RECIPE WORKS** Quick-cooking pork tenderloins, with their buttery, fine-grained texture and mild flavor, make the perfect backdrop for a variety of seasonings. But cooking this lean cut can be a challenge—too often, the meat turns out dry and overcooked. We wanted a recipe that would produce flavorful and juicy pork tenderloins every time. After attempting to cook the tenderloins in the oven at a wide range of temperatures, we discovered that the best approach was to start them on the stovetop (for a good sear) and then finish them in the oven (for gentle, even cooking). A spice rub was a great way to add flavor, and we created a simple one by combining aromatic caraway seeds, allspice, coriander, and nutmeg. To ensure that the tenderloins don't curl during cooking, remove the silverskin from the meat.

- 2 teaspoons kosher salt
- 1 teaspoon caraway seeds
- ½ teaspoon pepper
- ½ teaspoon ground allspice
- ½ teaspoon ground coriander
- ¼ teaspoon ground nutmeg
- 2 (12- to 16-ounce) pork tenderloins, trimmed
- 2 tablespoons extra-virgin olive oil

1. Adjust oven rack to lower-middle position and heat oven to 450 degrees. Combine salt, caraway seeds, pepper, allspice, coriander, and nutmeg in bowl. Pat tenderloins dry with paper towels and rub with spice mixture.

2. Heat oil in 12-inch ovensafe skillet over medium-high heat until just smoking. Brown pork on all sides, about 10 minutes. Transfer skillet to oven and roast until pork registers 145 degrees, 10 to 15 minutes, flipping meat halfway through roasting.

3. Transfer pork to carving board, tent loosely with aluminum foil, and let rest for 5 to 10 minutes. Slice pork into ½-inch-thick slices and serve.

TEST KITCHEN TIP **REMOVING PORK SILVERSKIN**

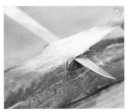

To ensure even browning on tenderloin, slip knife under silverskin, angle knife upward, and use gentle back-and-forth motion to remove silverskin.

Grilled Stuffed Pork Tenderloins

Serves 4 to 6

✓ **WHY THIS RECIPE WORKS** For a paleo-friendly stuffed pork tenderloin recipe, we created a bold, breadless stuffing with potent ingredients like olives, anchovies, and sun-dried tomatoes. For brightness and balance, we added fresh baby spinach leaves. To encourage deep browning, we rubbed the outside of the pork with a small amount of maple sugar. Cooking our tenderloin over indirect heat on the grill allowed the stuffing to heat through before the delicate meat overcooked. For more information on maple sugar, see page 10.

½ cup pitted kalamata olives

½ cup oil-packed sun-dried tomatoes, rinsed and chopped

4 anchovy fillets, rinsed

2 garlic cloves, minced

1 teaspoon minced fresh thyme

1 teaspoon grated lemon zest

2 (1¼- to 1½-pound) pork tenderloins, trimmed

Kosher salt and pepper

2 teaspoons maple sugar

1 ounce (1 cup) baby spinach

2 tablespoons extra-virgin olive oil

1. Pulse olives, tomatoes, anchovies, garlic, thyme, and lemon zest in food processor until coarsely chopped, 5 to 10 pulses.

2. Cut each tenderloin in half horizontally, stopping ½ inch from edge so halves remain attached. Open up tenderloins, cover with plastic wrap, and pound to even ¼-inch thickness. Trim any ragged edges to create rough rectangle about 10 inches by 6 inches. Sprinkle interior of each tenderloin with ⅛ teaspoon salt and ⅛ teaspoon pepper.

3. Combine sugar, 1 teaspoon salt, and ½ teaspoon pepper in bowl. With long side of 1 tenderloin facing you, spread half of olive mixture over bottom half of pork followed by ½ cup of spinach. Roll tenderloin away from you into tight cylinder, taking care not to squeeze stuffing out ends. Position tenderloin seam side down, evenly space 5 pieces kitchen twine underneath, and tie. Repeat with remaining tenderloin, olive mixture, and spinach. Coat tenderloins with oil, then rub evenly with sugar mixture.

4A. FOR A CHARCOAL GRILL Open bottom vent completely. Light large chimney starter filled with charcoal briquettes (6 quarts). When top coals are partially covered with ash, pour evenly over half of grill. Set cooking grate in place, cover, and open lid vent completely. Heat grill until hot, about 5 minutes.

4B. FOR A GAS GRILL Turn all burners to high, cover, and heat grill until hot, about 15 minutes. Leave primary burner on high and turn off other burner(s).

5. Clean and oil cooking grate. Place pork on cooler side of grill, cover, and cook until meat registers 145 degrees, 25 to 30 minutes, rotating pork halfway through cooking. Transfer pork to carving board, tent loosely with aluminum foil, and let rest for 5 to 10 minutes. Remove twine and slice pork into ½-inch-thick slices. Serve.

TEST KITCHEN TIP

MAKING STUFFED PORK TENDERLOINS

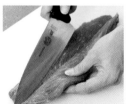

1. Cut tenderloins in half horizontally, stopping ½ inch from edge. Open tenderloins, cover with plastic wrap, and pound to ¼-inch thickness.

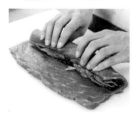

2. With long side of 1 tenderloin facing you, spread half of olive mixture and ½ cup spinach over bottom half of pork. Roll into tight cylinder.

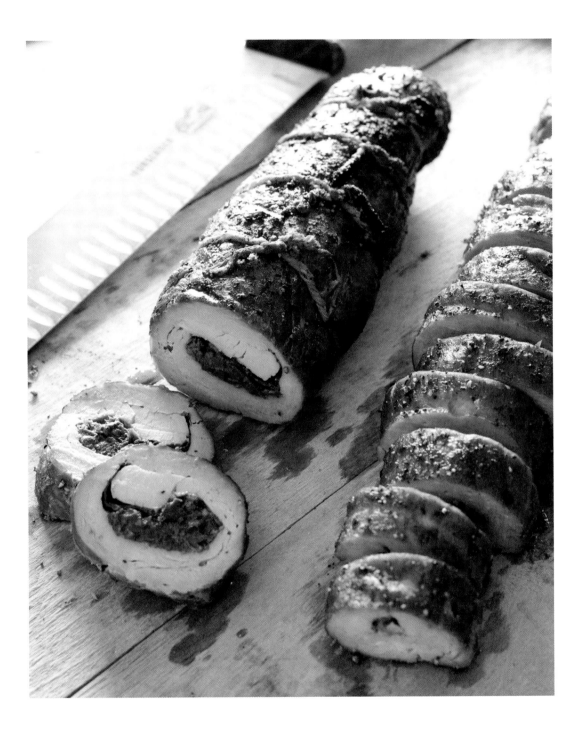

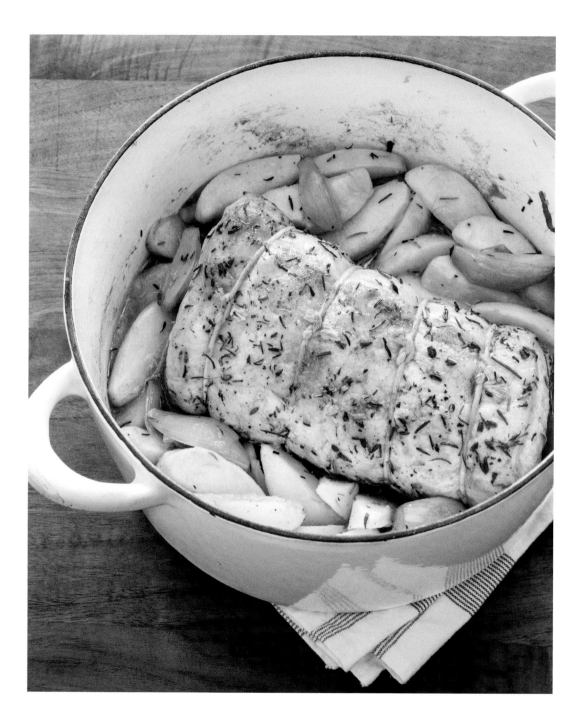

One-Pot Pork Roast with Apples and Shallots

Serves 4 to 6

✓ **WHY THIS RECIPE WORKS** This remarkably flavorful dish relies on just a few well-chosen ingredients to deliver an impressive meal. We browned our boneless pork loin roast on the stovetop, then let it cook through slowly in a 250-degree oven. Herbes de Provence—a fragrant mixture of dried herbs that typically includes basil, fennel seed, lavender, marjoram, rosemary, sage, summer savory, and thyme—provided lots of aromatic flavor and meant that we didn't have to buy eight different dried herbs. As the herbs simmered in the savory pork juices, their flavor bloomed and intensified. Since apples are a traditional pairing with pork, we decided to incorporate them into our dish. But we knew the apples would release a considerable amount of liquid, which could dull the flavor of the meat. To combat this, we removed the pork from the pot after we browned it and parcooked the apples separately to allow some of their juices to evaporate. We then added the pork back to the pot and let everything finish in the oven. At the end, we had a rustic, chunky applesauce to accompany our tender, juicy pork roast. This recipe works best with a pork roast that is about 7 to 8 inches long and 4 to 5 inches wide. If your roast has a thick layer of fat on top, trim the fat until it measures about ¼ inch thick. You can find herbes de Provence in the spice aisle of most supermarkets; however, 1 teaspoon each dried thyme, dried rosemary, and dried marjoram can be substituted.

1 **(2½- to 3-pound) boneless pork loin roast, trimmed and tied at 1½-inch intervals**
4 **teaspoons herbes de Provence**
   Kosher salt and pepper
3 **tablespoons extra-virgin olive oil**
12 **shallots, peeled and quartered**
1½ **pounds Golden Delicious apples, peeled, cored, and cut into ½-inch-thick wedges**
1 **tablespoon lemon juice**

1. Adjust oven rack to lowest position and heat oven to 250 degrees. Pat pork dry with paper towels, sprinkle with herbes de Provence, and season with salt and pepper. Heat 2 tablespoons oil in Dutch oven over medium-high heat until just smoking. Brown pork on all sides, 7 to 10 minutes; transfer to plate.

2. Add remaining 1 tablespoon oil to fat left in pot and heat over medium heat until shimmering. Add shallots and cook until softened, about 3 minutes. Stir in apples and cook until shallots and apples are lightly browned, 5 to 7 minutes. Off heat, nestle pork into pot fat side up along with any accumulated juices.

3. Fit large piece of aluminum foil over pot, pressing to seal, then cover tightly with lid. Transfer pot to oven and cook until pork registers 140 degrees, 35 to 55 minutes.

4. Transfer pork to carving board, tent loosely with foil, and let rest for 20 minutes.

5. Meanwhile, being careful of hot pot handles, stir lemon juice into shallot mixture and season with salt and pepper to taste; cover to keep warm. Slice pork thin and transfer to serving platter. Spoon shallot mixture over pork and serve.

TEST KITCHEN TIP **TYING A ROAST**

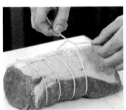

To ensure roast browns evenly, wrap piece of kitchen twine snugly around roast and fasten with double knot. Repeat every 1½ inches down length of roast.

Slow-Roasted Pork with Red Pepper Chutney

Serves 8 to 12

☑ **WHY THIS RECIPE WORKS** A pork shoulder roast is an ultraversatile cut: It's inexpensive, loaded with flavorful intramuscular fat, and crowned with a thick fat cap that renders to a beautifully bronzed, bacon-like crust. But to achieve that coveted crust, we needed a caramelizing agent, which usually comes in the form of granulated sugar. For a less processed and more flavorful approach, we turned to maple sugar. We rubbed the roast's exterior with a mixture of maple sugar and salt and then let it rest overnight to thoroughly season the meat. We cooked the pork slowly, and found that cooking it to 190 degrees (well past the typical doneness temperature of 140 degrees) allowed the intramuscular fat to melt and the fat cap to fully render and crisp, resulting in rich, tender meat. Pork butt roast is often labeled Boston shoulder, Boston butt, or pork butt in the supermarket. Note that the pork must be refrigerated for at least 12 hours before cooking. Add more water to the roasting pan as necessary during the last hours of cooking to prevent the fond from burning. For more information on maple sugar, see page 10.

1   (6- to 8-pound) bone-in pork butt roast
    Kosher salt and pepper
¼   cup maple sugar
1   tablespoon extra-virgin olive oil
1   red onion, chopped fine
4   red bell peppers, stemmed, seeded,
    and chopped fine
1   cup white wine vinegar
¼   cup honey
2   garlic cloves, peeled and smashed
1   (1-inch) piece ginger, peeled, sliced into
    thin coins, and smashed
1   teaspoon yellow mustard seeds
½   teaspoon red pepper flakes

1. Using sharp knife, cut slits, spaced 1 inch apart, in crosshatch pattern in fat cap of roast, being careful to cut down to but not into meat. Combine ⅓ cup salt and sugar in bowl and rub mixture over entire roast and into slits. Wrap roast tightly in double layer of plastic wrap, place on rimmed baking sheet, and refrigerate for at least 12 hours or up to 24 hours.

2. Adjust oven rack to lowest position and heat oven to 325 degrees. Unwrap roast and brush any excess salt mixture from surface. Season roast with pepper. Set greased V-rack in large roasting pan and place roast on rack. Add 4 cups water to roasting pan.

3. Cook roast, basting twice during cooking, until pork is extremely tender and meat near (but not touching) bone registers 190 degrees, 5 to 6 hours. Transfer roast to carving board, tent loosely with aluminum foil, and let rest for 1 hour.

4. Meanwhile, heat oil in medium saucepan over medium heat until shimmering. Add onion and cook until softened, about 5 minutes. Stir in bell peppers, vinegar, honey, garlic, ginger, mustard seeds, pepper flakes, and 1 teaspoon salt. Bring to simmer and cook until thickened, about 40 minutes. Off heat, discard garlic and ginger and let sauce cool slightly.

5. Using sharp paring knife, cut around inverted T-shaped bone until it can be pulled free from roast (use clean dish towel to grasp bone). Using serrated knife, slice roast thin. Serve, passing sauce separately.

TEST KITCHEN TIP **SCORING PORK SHOULDER**

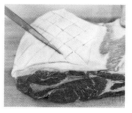

To help fat render, use sharp knife to cut slits, spaced 1 inch apart, in crosshatch pattern in fat cap of roast. Be careful to cut down to but not into meat.

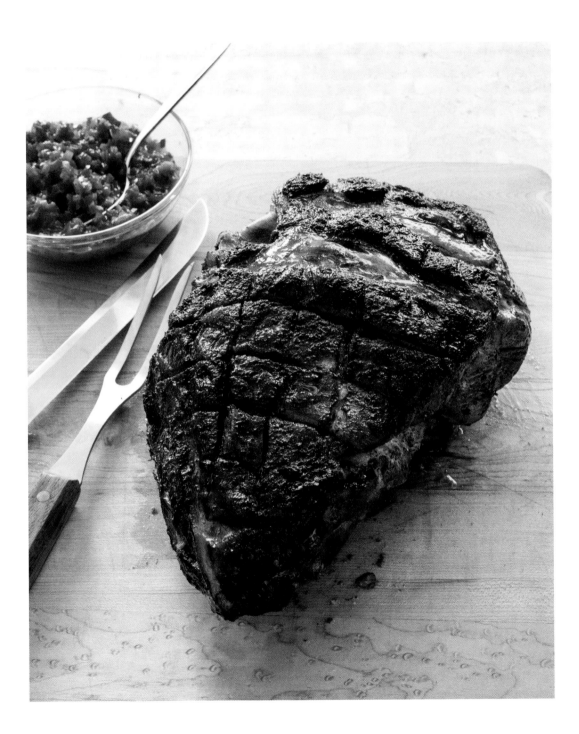

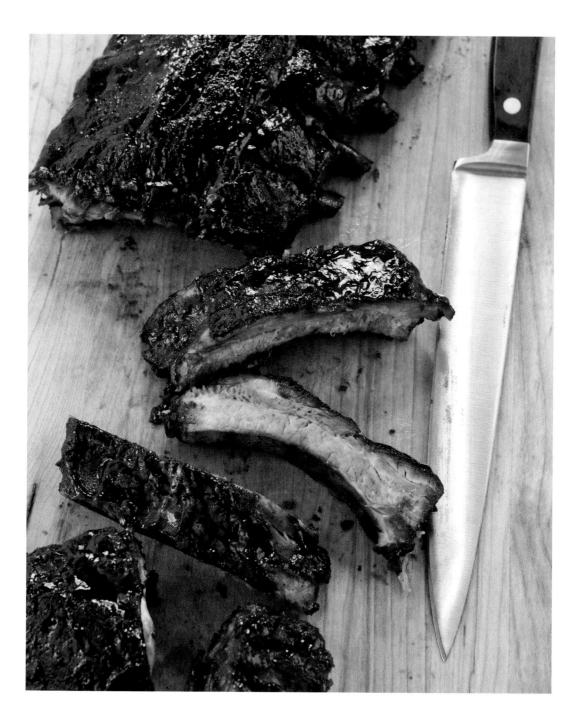

Slow-Cooker "Barbecued" Spareribs

Serves 4 to 6

✔ **WHY THIS RECIPE WORKS** Saucy, fall-off-the-bone-tender ribs are undeniably appealing, but they present a challenge in the paleo kitchen: Store-bought barbecue sauce (and most recipes for homemade sauces) contain hefty amounts of sugar and other nonpaleo ingredients. We set out to make an easy paleo-friendly sauce, and we decided to make this a year-round recipe by moving the cooking from the grill to the slow cooker. We started by rubbing two racks of ribs with a potent dry rub of smoked paprika, cayenne, salt, and pepper, which infused both the ribs and the sauce with flavor. For our sauce, we built an aromatic base with onion, tomato paste, and garlic. Mustard and cider vinegar offered tang, while maple syrup provided subtle sweetness. Reducing the sauce on the stovetop after cooking gave it just the right consistency. Once the ribs were fully tender, we transferred them from the slow cooker to the oven and broiled them to develop caramelized, lightly charred exteriors. Avoid buying racks of ribs labeled only "spareribs"; their large size and irregular shape make them unwieldy in a slow cooker. St. Louis–style spareribs are smaller and more uniform in size, making them ideal for the slow cooker. You will need an oval 6½- to 7-quart slow cooker for this recipe.

1	onion, chopped fine
3	tablespoons tomato paste
4	garlic cloves, minced
1	tablespoon extra-virgin olive oil
½	cup water
3	tablespoons maple syrup
2	tablespoons Dijon mustard
2	tablespoons cider vinegar
3	tablespoons smoked paprika
¼	teaspoon cayenne pepper
	Kosher salt and pepper
2	(2½- to 3-pound) racks St. Louis–style spareribs, trimmed

1. Microwave onion, tomato paste, garlic, and oil in bowl, stirring occasionally, until onion is softened, about 5 minutes; transfer to slow cooker. Whisk in water, maple syrup, mustard, and 1 tablespoon vinegar.

2. Combine paprika, cayenne, 1½ tablespoons salt, and 1 tablespoon pepper in bowl and rub mixture evenly over ribs. Arrange ribs upright in slow cooker with meaty sides facing outward. Cover and cook until ribs are tender, 5 to 6 hours on low.

3. Adjust oven rack 10 inches from broiler element and heat broiler. Set greased wire rack in aluminum foil–lined rimmed baking sheet. Transfer ribs meaty side up to prepared rack.

4. Using wide, shallow spoon, skim excess fat from surface of cooking liquid. Process defatted liquid in blender until smooth, about 30 seconds. Transfer liquid to small saucepan, bring to simmer over medium heat, and cook, stirring occasionally, until thickened and reduced to 1½ cups, about 5 minutes. Off heat, stir in remaining 1 tablespoon vinegar and season with salt and pepper to taste.

5. Brush ribs with some of sauce, then broil until browned and sticky, about 10 minutes, flipping and brushing with additional sauce every few minutes. Transfer ribs to carving board and let rest for 10 minutes. Slice ribs between bones and serve with remaining sauce.

TEST KITCHEN TIP
ARRANGING RIBS IN A SLOW COOKER

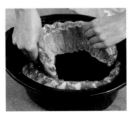

To ensure that ribs cook evenly, stand racks up along perimeter of slow cooker with wide end down and meatier side of ribs facing wall of slow-cooker insert.

Stir-Fried Sesame Pork and Eggplant

Serves 4

✓ **WHY THIS RECIPE WORKS** This aromatic stir-fry combines tender, caramelized slices of pork and vegetables in a smooth, piquant sauce. We used a paleo-friendly tapioca flour mixture to protect the meat from the heat and keep it juicy, and we created a flavorful base for our sauce using coconut aminos (instead of soy sauce), fish sauce, and toasted sesame oil. The combination of supple eggplant, aromatic red onion, and fresh basil leaves gave our stir-fry layers of texture and flavor. To ensure that every element was done perfectly, we cooked the pork, eggplant, and onion separately, and carefully timed the return of each one to the pan to avoid overcooking. We prefer to use homemade chicken broth; however, you can substitute your favorite store-bought broth. This recipe calls for a 12-inch nonstick skillet; however, a well-seasoned cast-iron skillet can be used instead. To make the pork easier to slice, freeze it for 15 minutes. For more information on coconut aminos, see page 11. Serve with Cauliflower Rice (page 288).

SAUCE

- ½ cup Paleo Chicken Broth (page 16)
- 6 tablespoons coconut aminos
- 3 tablespoons toasted sesame oil
- 2 tablespoons fish sauce
- 1½ teaspoons tapioca flour

STIR-FRY

- 2 tablespoons plus 1 teaspoon toasted sesame oil
- 2 teaspoons coconut aminos
- 1½ teaspoons tapioca flour
- 1 (1-pound) pork tenderloin, trimmed, halved lengthwise, and sliced ¼ inch thick
- 2 tablespoons grated fresh ginger
- 5 garlic cloves, minced
- 2 scallions, minced
- 2 tablespoons coconut oil
- 1 pound eggplant, peeled and cut into ¾-inch pieces
- 1 small red onion, halved and sliced ½ inch thick
- 1 cup coarsely chopped fresh basil
- 2 teaspoons sesame seeds, toasted

1. FOR THE SAUCE Whisk all ingredients together in bowl.

2. FOR THE STIR-FRY Whisk 2 tablespoons sesame oil, coconut aminos, and flour together in medium bowl until smooth, then stir in pork. In separate bowl, combine ginger, garlic, scallions, and remaining 1 teaspoon sesame oil.

3. Heat 1 teaspoon coconut oil in 12-inch nonstick skillet over high heat until just smoking. Add half of pork, break up any clumps, and cook, without stirring, for 1 minute. Stir pork and continue to cook until lightly browned, about 30 seconds; transfer to clean bowl. Repeat with 1 teaspoon coconut oil and remaining pork; transfer to bowl.

4. Heat 2 teaspoons coconut oil in now-empty skillet over medium-high heat until just smoking. Add eggplant and cook until softened and lightly browned, about 3 minutes; transfer to separate bowl. Add remaining 2 teaspoons coconut oil and onion to now-empty skillet and cook until softened and lightly browned, about 3 minutes. Return eggplant to skillet, reduce heat to medium, and cook until vegetables are tender, about 2 minutes.

5. Push vegetables to sides of skillet. Add ginger mixture and cook, mashing mixture into skillet, until fragrant, about 1 minute. Stir mixture into vegetables.

6. Whisk sauce to recombine, then add to skillet. Cook, stirring constantly, until sauce is thickened, about 2 minutes. Stir in cooked pork and any accumulated juices. Off heat, stir in basil. Transfer to serving platter and sprinkle with sesame seeds. Serve.

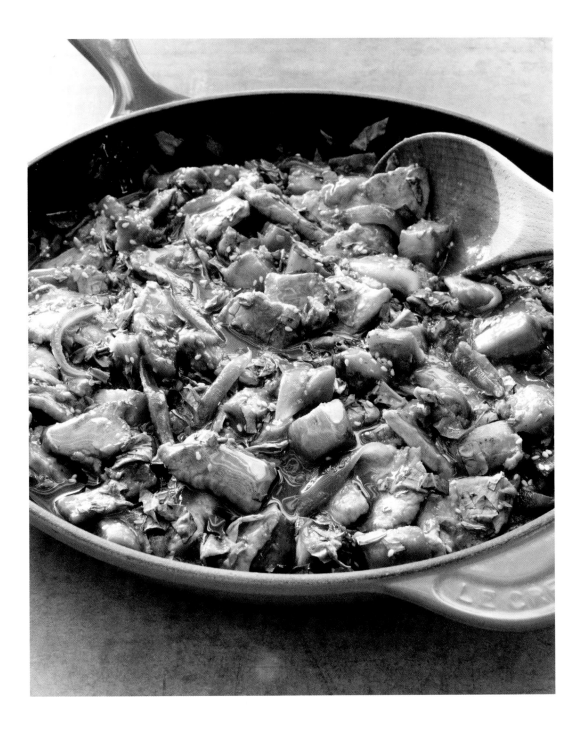

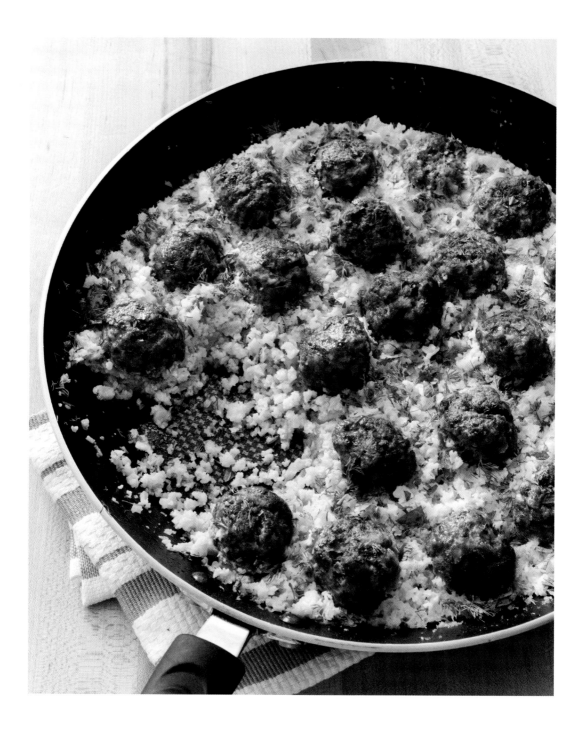

Greek Lamb Meatballs with Cauliflower Rice

Serves 4

✓ **WHY THIS RECIPE WORKS** Meatballs are a surefire crowd pleaser, so we decided to develop a recipe with a Greek spin, using ground lamb seasoned with mint and dill. To make them paleo, we replaced the typical panade—a paste made from bread and milk that's used to keep ground meat moist—with boiled and pureed cashews. The mild-tasting cashew paste helped to bind the meatballs and keep them tender without interfering with the meatballs' flavor. We made our lamb meatballs a little smaller than traditional Italian-style meatballs, and browned them well to enhance their savory flavor and render away some of their fat. Since these meatballs were so flavorful on their own, we decided not to douse them in sauce. Instead, we wanted to let them shine by serving them on a bed of cauliflower rice. To give the dish a unified flavor profile, we sautéed the cauliflower in some of the fat rendered from the meatballs, and seasoned the rice with more mint and dill. A splash of lemon juice and some zest added brightness and acidity to the cauliflower rice, which perfectly balanced the richness of the meatballs. We prefer to use homemade chicken broth; however, you can substitute your favorite store-bought broth. This recipe calls for a 12-inch nonstick skillet; however, a well-seasoned cast-iron skillet can be used instead. You can substitute 85 percent lean ground beef for the lamb. For more information on making cauliflower rice, see step photo on page 288.

½ cup raw cashews

1 head cauliflower (2 pounds), cored and cut into 1-inch florets (6 cups)

1½ pounds ground lamb

1 small red onion, chopped fine

2 tablespoons chopped fresh mint

2 tablespoons chopped fresh dill

2 garlic cloves, minced

Kosher salt and pepper

1 teaspoon extra-virgin olive oil

½ cup Paleo Chicken Broth (page 16)

1 teaspoon grated lemon zest plus 2 tablespoons juice, plus lemon wedges for serving

1. Bring 4 cups water to boil in medium saucepan over medium-high heat. Add cashews and cook until softened, about 15 minutes. Drain and rinse well. Meanwhile, working in 2 batches, pulse cauliflower in food processor until finely ground into ¼- to ⅛-inch pieces, 6 to 8 pulses, scraping down sides of bowl as needed; set aside.

2. Process boiled cashews in now-empty food processor until smooth, about 1 minute, scraping down sides of bowl as needed; transfer to large bowl. Add ground lamb, onion, 1 tablespoon mint, 1 tablespoon dill, garlic, 2 teaspoons salt, and ½ teaspoon pepper and knead with your hands until well combined. Pinch off and roll mixture into 1½-inch meatballs (you should have 24 meatballs).

3. Heat oil in 12-inch nonstick skillet over medium heat until just smoking. Brown meatballs on all sides, about 10 minutes; transfer to plate.

4. Pour off all but 2 tablespoons fat from skillet and return to medium heat until shimmering. Add processed cauliflower, broth, lemon zest and juice, and 1 teaspoon salt. Nestle browned meatballs into skillet along with any accumulated juices. Reduce heat to medium-low, cover, and cook until cauliflower is tender and meatballs are cooked through, 12 to 15 minutes.

5. Uncover and continue to cook until cauliflower rice is almost completely dry, about 3 minutes. Off heat, sprinkle with remaining 1 tablespoon mint and remaining 1 tablespoon dill and season with salt and pepper to taste. Serve with lemon wedges.

Grilled Lamb Chops with Asparagus

Serves 4

✓ **WHY THIS RECIPE WORKS** Lamb shoulder chops are significantly less expensive than rib or loin chops, and their flavor is much more complex due to their delicate networks of fat and collagen-rich connective tissue—an appealing option, we thought, for a quick, economical, anytime-meal from the grill. What we found, however, is that producing a grilled shoulder chop with a beautifully browned exterior and a moist and tender interior can be a challenge. Because the chops are relatively thin, we had trouble achieving good color on the outside of our chops before they overcooked. We also found that the texture of our cooked chops was uneven—meatier parts might be tender while other parts stayed chewy and tough. We knew from past recipes that a quick soak in a baking soda brine can help speed up the browning process and also tenderize meat, but when we tried it with our shoulder chops, we detected an unappealing aftertaste. We needed a gentler approach, so we tried a simple marinade of oil, garlic, salt, oregano, and just a small amount of baking soda. In under 10 minutes on a hot grill, our chops were perfectly browned, succulent, and full of flavor. We paired them with grilled asparagus (which cooked while our chops were resting) and a bright, refreshing vinaigrette. We like these chops cooked to medium-rare, but if you prefer them more or less done, see our guidelines on page 154.

¾   cup extra-virgin olive oil

6   tablespoons red wine vinegar

¼   cup chopped fresh mint

1   shallot, minced

2   teaspoons Dijon mustard
     Kosher salt and pepper

2   garlic cloves, minced

2   teaspoons minced fresh oregano

1   teaspoon baking soda

4   (8- to 12-ounce) lamb shoulder chops (blade or round bone), ¾ to 1 inch thick, trimmed

1½   pounds thick asparagus, trimmed

1. Whisk ½ cup oil, vinegar, mint, shallot, mustard, 1 teaspoon salt, and ¼ teaspoon pepper together in bowl; set aside for serving.

2. Whisk remaining ¼ cup oil, garlic, oregano, baking soda, 1 teaspoon salt, and ½ teaspoon pepper together in bowl. Combine oil mixture and chops in 1-gallon zipper-lock bag and toss to coat; press out as much air as possible and seal bag. Refrigerate for 30 minutes or up to 1 hour, flipping bag halfway through marinating. Remove lamb from marinade and let excess marinade drip off but do not pat dry.

3A. FOR A CHARCOAL GRILL Open bottom vent completely. Light large chimney starter filled with charcoal briquettes (6 quarts). When top coals are partially covered with ash, pour evenly over grill. Set cooking grate in place, cover, and open lid vent completely. Heat grill until hot, about 5 minutes.

3B. FOR A GAS GRILL Turn all burners to high, cover, and heat grill until hot, about 15 minutes. Leave all burners on high.

4. Clean and oil cooking grate. Place chops on grill. Cook until well browned and meat registers 120 to 125 degrees (for medium-rare), 2 to 4 minutes per side. Transfer chops to serving platter, tent loosely with aluminum foil, and let rest while cooking asparagus.

5. As lamb finishes cooking, place asparagus on grill and cook, turning as needed, until crisp-tender and lightly browned, about 5 minutes; transfer to platter. Drizzle vinaigrette over lamb and asparagus and serve.

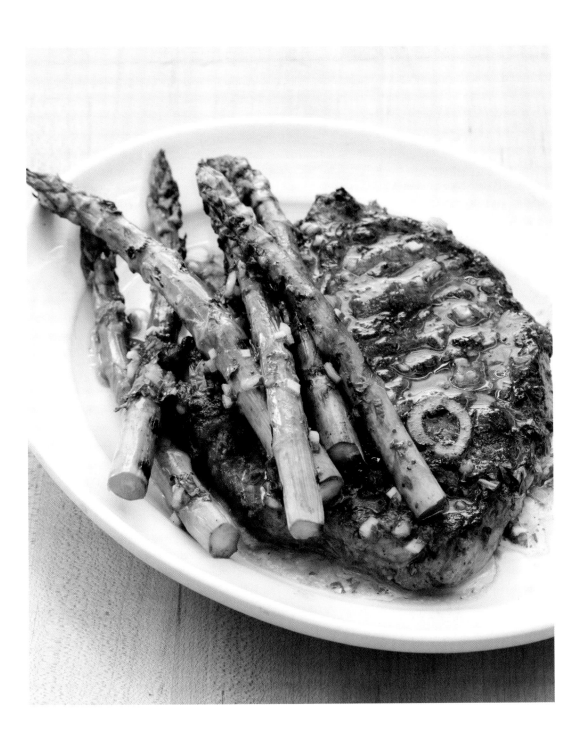

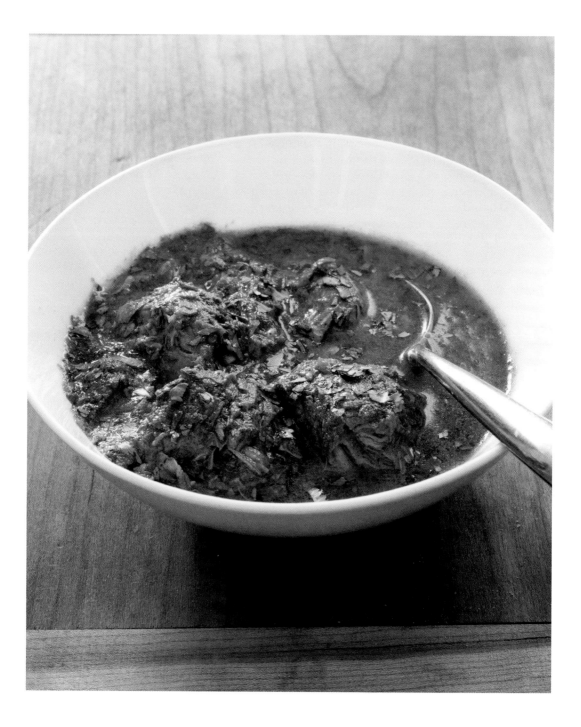

Slow-Cooker Indian-Style Lamb Curry

Serves 6 to 8

✓ **WHY THIS RECIPE WORKS** Every paleo cook should have an arsenal of incredibly flavorful, cook-all-day meals from the slow cooker, so we turned to a classic Indian curry known as Rogan Josh for inspiration. This stew-like dish is typically made by cutting lamb shoulder into small pieces and braising them in a sauce redolent with warm spices, mild Kashmiri chiles, and aromatics. We started with the lamb. A boneless lamb shoulder was easy to work with, and we found that cutting the meat into small pieces to cook was unnecessary; we simply cut the roast into four pieces and then shredded it into bite-size pieces after cooking. To re-create the traditional flavor of the sauce, we started with paprika, a good substitute for hard-to-find Kashmiri chiles. Onion, garlic, and ginger gave the sauce an aromatic backbone, and whole cumin seeds, coriander seeds, cloves, cardamom pods, and a cinnamon stick rounded out the flavor. But tasters weren't fond of crunching down on whole cloves or cardamom pods in the finished dish, since the flavors overwhelmed their palates. Switching to ground versions easily solved this problem. Tomato paste enhanced the color and body of the sauce. A relatively small amount of water was all we needed, since the meat released so much liquid as it cooked. After many hours in the slow cooker, the lamb was tender and bathed in a fragrant, warm-spiced sauce. A dollop of yogurt might typically be added to the dish before serving, but tasters found that a sprinkling of cilantro added enough bright freshness that the dairy wasn't missed. You will need a 4- to 7-quart slow cooker for this recipe. For a spicier curry, use the larger amount of cayenne.

1	**(4- to 5-pound) boneless lamb shoulder, trimmed and quartered**
	Kosher salt and pepper
3	**tablespoons ghee**
2	**onions, chopped fine**
¼	**cup tomato paste**
8	**garlic cloves, minced**
2	**tablespoons paprika**
1½	**tablespoons cumin seeds**
1	**tablespoon grated fresh ginger**
2	**teaspoons coriander seeds**
¾	**teaspoon ground cardamom**
¼–½	**teaspoon cayenne pepper**
⅛	**teaspoon ground cloves**
1	**cinnamon stick**
1½	**cups water, plus extra as needed**
½	**cup chopped fresh cilantro**

1. Pat lamb dry with paper towels and season with salt and pepper. Heat 1 tablespoon ghee in 12-inch skillet over medium-high heat until just smoking. Brown half of lamb, about 5 minutes per side; transfer to slow cooker. Repeat with remaining lamb.

2. Heat remaining 2 tablespoons ghee in now-empty skillet over medium heat until shimmering. Add onions and cook until softened and lightly browned, 8 to 10 minutes. Stir in tomato paste, garlic, paprika, cumin seeds, ginger, coriander seeds, cardamom, cayenne, cloves, cinnamon stick, and 1 teaspoon salt. Cook until fragrant and tomato paste begins to brown, about 5 minutes. Stir in water, scraping up any browned bits; transfer to slow cooker. Cover and cook until lamb is tender, 9 to 11 hours on low or 5 to 7 hours on high.

3. Transfer lamb to cutting board, let cool slightly, then pull into large pieces using 2 spoons; discard any excess fat. Discard cinnamon stick. Using wide, shallow spoon, skim excess fat from surface of stew.

4. Gently stir lamb into stew and let sit until heated through, about 5 minutes. Adjust stew consistency with extra hot water as needed. Stir in cilantro and season with salt and pepper to taste. Serve.

Roast Butterflied Leg of Lamb

Serves 8

✅ **WHY THIS RECIPE WORKS** Lamb has a rich flavor and a meaty texture that can be as supple as that of tenderloin. We wanted a foolproof recipe for a perfect leg of lamb. To get a good ratio of crispy crust to evenly cooked meat we decided to use a butterflied leg of lamb rather than a tied roast. This cut had several benefits: a uniform thickness for even cooking; easy access to big pockets of chewy intramuscular fat and connective tissue (making removal of these portions easy); and the ability to be seasoned thoroughly and efficiently. Rubbing a generous amount of salt into the leg produced well-seasoned, juicy, and tender meat, and created a relatively dry surface that browned and crisped well during roasting. Scoring the fat cap in a crosshatch pattern ensured that the salt penetrated the meat thoroughly. After slowly roasting our lamb at 250 degrees, we finished it under the broiler to achieve a burnished, crisp crust. A spice rub scorched under the intense heat of the broiler, so we flavored the meat with a spice-infused oil, which later doubled as a base for a quick serving sauce. We prefer the subtler flavor and larger size of lamb labeled "domestic" or "American" for this recipe. We like this lamb cooked to medium-rare, but if you prefer it more or less done, see our guidelines on page 154.

1   **(4-pound) boneless leg of lamb**
    Kosher salt and pepper
⅓   **cup extra-virgin olive oil**
4   **shallots (3 sliced thin, 1 minced)**
4   **garlic cloves, peeled and smashed**
1   **(1-inch) piece ginger, peeled, sliced into ½-inch-thick rounds, and smashed**
1   **tablespoon coriander seeds**
1   **tablespoon cumin seeds**
1   **tablespoon mustard seeds**
3   **bay leaves**
2   **(2-inch) strips lemon zest plus 2 tablespoons juice**
⅓   **cup chopped fresh mint**
⅓   **cup chopped fresh cilantro**

1. Place lamb on cutting board with fat cap facing down. Using sharp knife, trim any pockets of fat and connective tissue from underside of lamb. Flip lamb over, trim fat cap to between ⅛ and ¼ inch thick, and pound roast to even 1-inch thickness. Cut slits, spaced ½ inch apart, in crosshatch pattern in fat cap, being careful to cut down to but not into meat. Rub 4 teaspoons salt over entire roast and into slits. Let sit, uncovered, at room temperature for 1 hour.

2. Meanwhile, adjust 1 oven rack to lower-middle position and second rack 4 to 5 inches from broiler element and heat oven to 250 degrees. Combine oil, sliced shallots, garlic, ginger, coriander seeds, cumin seeds, mustard seeds, bay leaves, and lemon zest on rimmed baking sheet and bake on lower rack until spices are softened and fragrant and shallots and garlic turn golden, about 1 hour. Remove sheet from oven and discard bay leaves.

3. Pat lamb dry with paper towels and transfer fat side up to sheet (directly on top of spices). Roast on lower rack until lamb registers 120 degrees, about 30 minutes. Remove sheet from oven and heat broiler. Broil lamb on upper rack until surface is well browned and charred in spots and lamb registers 125 degrees (for medium-rare), 3 to 5 minutes.

4. Remove sheet from oven and, using 2 pairs of tongs, transfer lamb to carving board (some spices will cling to bottom of roast). Tent lamb loosely with aluminum foil and let rest for 20 minutes.

5. Meanwhile, carefully pour pan juices through fine-mesh strainer into medium bowl, pressing on solids to extract as much liquid as possible; discard solids. Stir in mint, cilantro, minced shallot, and lemon juice. Add any accumulated lamb juices to sauce and season with salt and pepper to taste.

6. With long side facing you, slice lamb with grain into 3 equal pieces. Turn each piece and slice against grain into ¼-inch-thick slices. Serve with sauce. (Briefly warm sauce in microwave if it has cooled and thickened.)

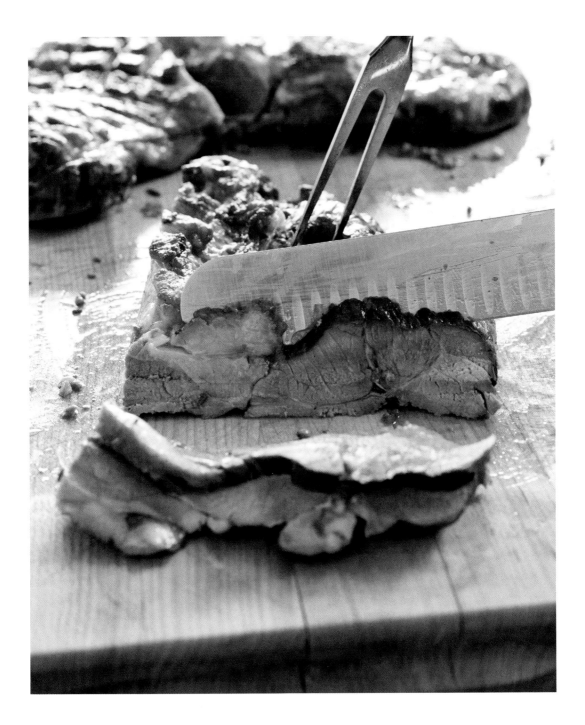

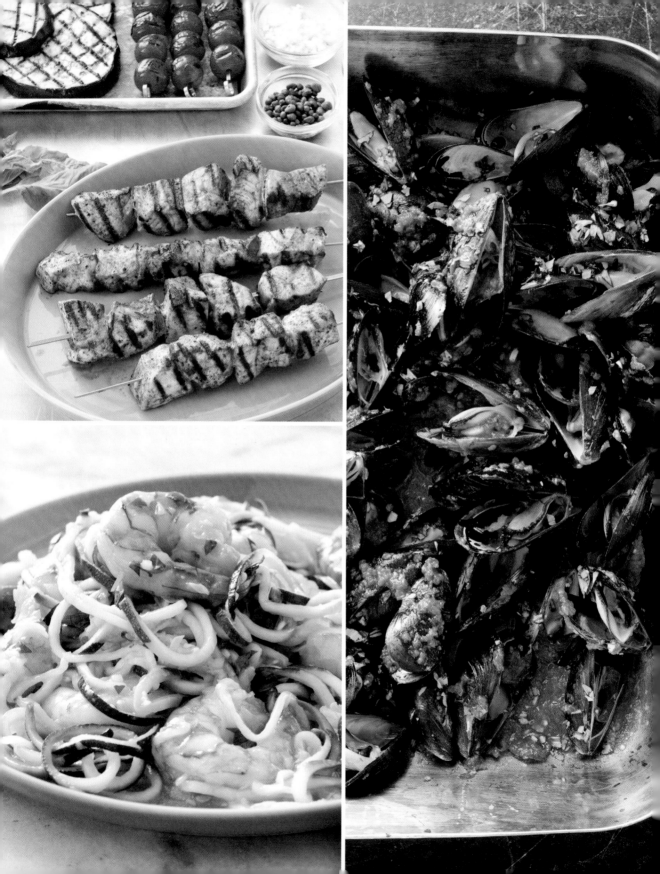

SEAFOOD
CHAPTER 5

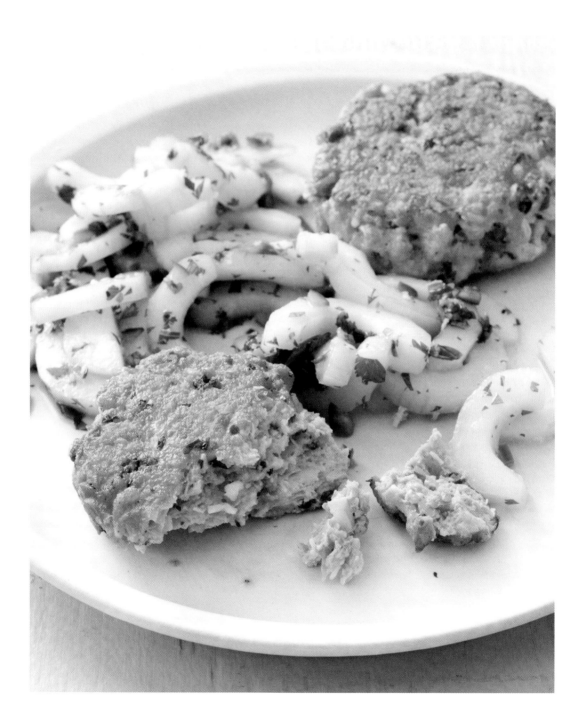

Salmon Cakes with Spicy Cucumber Salad

Serves 4

✓ **WHY THIS RECIPE WORKS** Crispy on the outside and rich and tender inside, salmon cakes are a perfect way to prepare fresh salmon. But all too often they're held together with store-bought mayonnaise and bread crumbs, neither of which are paleo-friendly. We were after salmon cakes with a fresh flavor profile along with a bold, interesting accompaniment. We opted to use a mixture of coconut oil and an egg yolk to replace the mayonnaise. A bit of shredded coconut was a great replacement for the bread crumbs; it helped to absorb any excess moisture and bind the salmon. For cakes that held together but weren't pasty, we pulsed 1-inch pieces of fresh salmon in the food processor. To boost the flavor of our cakes, we chose some Asian-inspired ingredient additions that would go nicely with the mild coconut flavor in the cakes. Scallion, ginger, cayenne pepper, cilantro, and lime juice worked perfectly. A refreshing salad of crunchy cucumbers, fresh cilantro, thinly sliced scallions, and minced serrano chiles, tossed in a honey-sesame dressing, made a perfect counterpoint to the rich cakes. If buying a skin-on salmon fillet, purchase 1⅓ pounds of fish in order to yield 1¼ pounds after the skin is removed. This recipe calls for a 12-inch nonstick skillet; however, a well-seasoned cast-iron skillet can be used instead. When processing the salmon it is OK to have some pieces that are larger than ¼ inch. It is important to avoid overprocessing the fish.

2 cucumbers, peeled, halved lengthwise, seeded, and cut into ¼-inch-thick slices
¼ cup minced fresh cilantro
2 serrano chiles, stemmed, seeded, and minced
2 scallions, white parts minced, green parts sliced thin on bias
3 tablespoons lime juice (2 limes), plus extra for seasoning
1 tablespoon honey
2 teaspoons toasted sesame oil
2 teaspoons grated fresh ginger
 Kosher salt and pepper
6 tablespoons coconut oil, melted
3 tablespoons unsweetened shredded coconut, toasted
1 large egg yolk
 Pinch cayenne pepper
1¼ pounds skinless wild-caught salmon, cut into 1-inch pieces

1. Combine cucumbers, 2 tablespoons cilantro, serranos, scallion greens, 2 tablespoons lime juice, honey, sesame oil, 1 teaspoon ginger, and 1 teaspoon salt in serving bowl. Season with salt, pepper, and extra lime juice to taste; set aside for serving.

2. Adjust oven rack to middle position and heat oven to 200 degrees. Set wire rack in rimmed baking sheet. Combine 2 tablespoons melted coconut oil, coconut, egg yolk, cayenne, scallion whites, 1¼ teaspoons salt, ¼ teaspoon pepper, remaining 2 tablespoons cilantro, remaining 1 tablespoon lime juice, and remaining 1 teaspoon ginger in large bowl. Working in 3 batches, pulse salmon in food processor until coarsely chopped into ¼-inch pieces, about 2 pulses; transfer to bowl with coconut mixture. Gently mix until uniformly combined.

3. Transfer salmon mixture to parchment paper–lined rimmed baking sheet, divide into 8 lightly packed balls, then gently flatten into ¾-inch-thick patties.

4. Heat 2 tablespoons melted coconut oil in 12-inch nonstick skillet over medium-high heat until just smoking. Place 4 cakes in skillet and cook until golden brown, about 2 minutes per side. Drain cakes briefly on paper towel–lined plate, then transfer to prepared rack and keep warm in oven. Repeat with remaining 2 tablespoons melted coconut oil and remaining 4 cakes. Serve with salad.

Crab Cakes

Serves 4

✓ **WHY THIS RECIPE WORKS** We wanted a recipe for sweet and plump crab cakes with big seafood flavor, but since bread crumbs and store-bought mayonnaise are usually used as binders, we had to reimagine our approach. First we made a batch of mayo from scratch and folded in lump crabmeat along with a bit of sautéed celery, onion, and garlic, but because our homemade mayo had no stabilizers, our crab cakes fell apart while they cooked. Looking for a paleo-friendly alternative, we turned to toasted coconut and an egg, which had helped us to bind together our salmon cakes (see page 205). But after sliding our cakes into a hot pan we found that the coconut caused them to fall apart even more. We wondered why our salmon cakes had held together well and the crab cakes fell apart. Our science editor explained that the raw proteins in the salmon help to bind the cakes; since crabmeat is sold already cooked, it doesn't have the same sticking power. To add raw seafood proteins to our mix, we decided to use shrimp. We made a quick shrimp puree in a food processor to see if it would hold our cakes together. The shrimp puree bound the crab perfectly; after searing we were left with beautiful golden-brown cakes with plenty of sweet seafood flavor. A squeeze of fresh lemon over the finished crab cakes was a welcome addition. Be sure to purchase fresh or pasteurized crabmeat (usually sold next to the fresh seafood) rather than canned crabmeat (packed in tuna fish–like cans) found in the supermarket aisles. This recipe calls for a 12-inch nonstick skillet; however, a well-seasoned cast-iron skillet can be used instead.

2   **celery ribs, chopped**
½   **cup chopped onion**
1   **garlic clove, peeled and smashed**
5   **tablespoons extra-virgin olive oil**
     Kosher salt and pepper
5   **ounces shrimp, peeled, deveined, and tails removed**
2   **tablespoons water**
2   **teaspoons Dijon mustard**
1   **teaspoon lemon juice**
½   **teaspoon hot sauce**
½   **teaspoon Old Bay seasoning**
1   **pound lump crabmeat, picked over for shells**
     Lemon wedges

1. Adjust oven rack to middle position and heat oven to 200 degrees. Set wire rack in rimmed baking sheet. Pulse celery, onion, and garlic in food processor until finely chopped, 5 to 8 pulses, scraping down sides of bowl as needed. Heat 1 tablespoon oil in 12-inch nonstick skillet over medium heat. Add processed vegetables, ½ teaspoon salt, and ⅛ teaspoon pepper and cook until softened and dry, 4 to 6 minutes; transfer to large bowl and let cool to room temperature.

2. Pulse shrimp in now-empty food processor until finely ground, 12 to 15 pulses, scraping down sides of bowl as needed. Add water and pulse to combine, 2 to 4 pulses. Stir shrimp paste, mustard, lemon juice, hot sauce, and Old Bay into cooled vegetable mixture. Gently fold in crabmeat with rubber spatula until uniformly combined.

3. Transfer crab mixture to parchment paper–lined rimmed baking sheet, divide into 8 lightly packed balls, then gently flatten into ½-inch-thick patties. Cover and refrigerate for 30 minutes.

4. Wipe skillet clean with paper towels. Add 2 tablespoons oil and heat over medium heat until shimmering. Place 4 cakes in skillet and cook until golden brown, 3 to 4 minutes per side. Drain cakes briefly on paper towel–lined plate, then transfer to prepared rack and keep warm in oven. Repeat with remaining 2 tablespoons oil and remaining 4 cakes. Serve with lemon wedges.

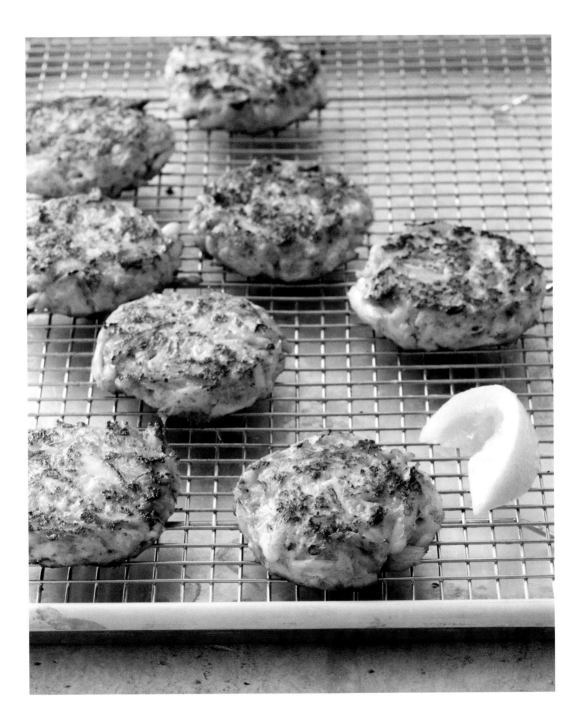

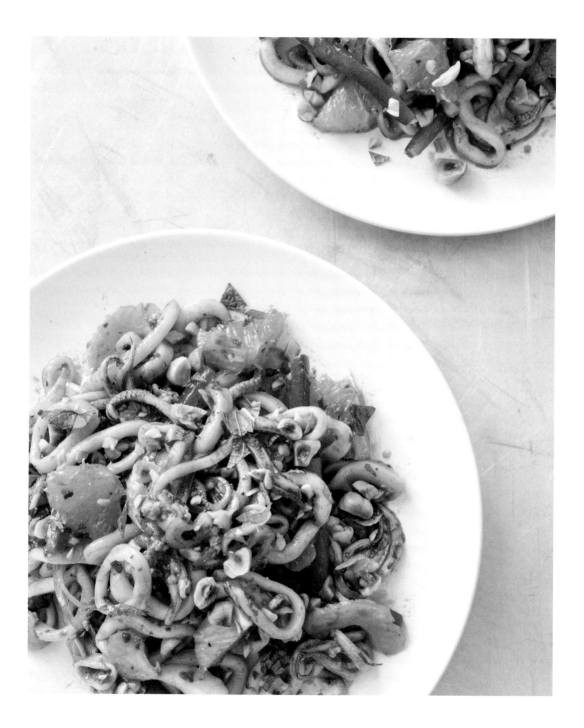

Chile-Marinated Calamari Salad with Oranges

Serves 4 to 6

✔ **WHY THIS RECIPE WORKS** Calamari is a super-lean, mild-tasting protein that takes well to a wide range of flavors. We wanted to use this often-overlooked seafood as a base for a bold, aromatic salad. Since squid cooks quickly, we made it a goal to keep the recipe as streamlined and simple as possible. First, we needed to settle on a cooking method for the squid. After trying grilling, broiling, and sautéing, all of which resulted in overcooked, chewy squid, we settled on blanching the squid in boiling water. To ensure that both the bodies and the tentacles were perfectly cooked, we added the tentacles to the pot 30 seconds before adding the bodies. After blanching, we transferred the squid to an ice bath to halt the cooking. While tasters preferred the blanched calamari to other methods we had tried, it was still too chewy and the method had no margin for error. Our science editor mentioned that alkaline solutions are often used to keep proteins tender. We wondered if baking soda, which is alkaline, would improve the texture of our calamari. We made a quick brine from water and baking soda and soaked the squid briefly before cooking. This batch cooked up perfectly tender, even after cooking for a full 90 seconds. Since calamari can be relatively mild, we decided to dress it with a piquant mixture of tangy red wine vinegar and spicy harissa chile paste. We tossed the squid with our dressing before stirring in pieces of orange, bell pepper, and celery. Marinating the salad in the fridge allowed the flavors to meld. Hazelnuts, stirred in just before serving, gave the salad some welcome crunch. Harissa, a chile paste, can be found in the international aisle of most supermarkets, usually with the Middle Eastern or Indian ingredients. For the best flavor and texture we recommend allowing the salad to marinate for the full 24 hours before serving.

2 tablespoons baking soda
    Kosher salt and pepper
2 pounds squid, bodies sliced crosswise
    into ¼-inch-thick rings, tentacles halved
2 oranges
¼ cup extra-virgin olive oil
3 tablespoons red wine vinegar
2½ tablespoons harissa
2 garlic cloves, minced
1 teaspoon Dijon mustard
1 red bell pepper, stemmed, seeded, and cut
    into 2-inch-long matchsticks
2 celery ribs, sliced thin on bias
1 shallot, sliced thin
⅓ cup hazelnuts, toasted, skinned,
    and chopped
3 tablespoons chopped fresh mint

1. Dissolve baking soda and 2 tablespoons salt in 3 cups cold water in large container. Submerge squid in brine, cover, and refrigerate for 15 minutes.

2. Bring 8 cups water to boil in large saucepan over medium-high heat. Remove squid from brine and separate bodies from tentacles. Fill large bowl with ice water. Add tentacles and 2 tablespoons salt to boiling water and cook for 30 seconds. Add bodies and cook until bodies are firm and opaque throughout, about 90 seconds. Drain squid, transfer to ice water, and let sit until chilled, about 5 minutes.

3. Cut away peel and pith from oranges. Quarter oranges, then slice crosswise into ½-inch-thick pieces. Whisk oil, vinegar, harissa, garlic, mustard, 1½ teaspoons salt, and ½ teaspoon pepper together in large bowl. Drain squid well and transfer to bowl with dressing. Add oranges, bell pepper, celery, and shallot and toss to coat. Cover and refrigerate for at least 1 hour or up to 24 hours. Stir in hazelnuts and mint and season with salt and pepper to taste. Serve.

Shrimp Ceviche

Serves 4

👉 **WHY THIS RECIPE WORKS** This simple and refreshing seafood dish is equally at home when served as an appetizer or on a bed of greens for a light meal. Rather than using heat to cook the seafood, ceviche relies on acidic juices, such as lime or lemon juice, to do the "cooking." Although there are many takes on the dish around the world, one of our favorites is a Mexican version made with shrimp. We tested several combinations of acidic liquids, even white wine vinegar and cider vinegar, and settled on equal parts lime and lemon juice for the most well-rounded, balanced flavor. To bring the lime flavor to the fore, we also added a bit of lime zest. We sliced each shrimp in half lengthwise, which helped all of the pieces to cook evenly and gave our ceviche a pleasant chunky texture. We rounded out the fresh flavor of the shrimp with a few seasoning ingredients: jalapeño, garlic, scallions, and cilantro. We also liked the addition of tomato, which provided a welcome color and texture contrast to the shrimp. A bit of extra-virgin olive oil stirred in before serving helped meld the flavors and add some depth.

1   tomato, cored, seeded, and chopped fine
½   cup lemon juice (3 lemons)
1   jalapeño chile, stemmed, seeded, and minced
1   teaspoon grated lime zest plus ½ cup juice (4 limes)
1   garlic clove, minced
    Kosher salt and pepper
1   pound extra-large shrimp (21 to 25 per pound), peeled, deveined, tails removed, and halved lengthwise
¼   cup extra-virgin olive oil
4   scallions, sliced thin
3   tablespoons minced fresh cilantro
½   teaspoon honey

1. Combine tomato, lemon juice, jalapeño, lime zest and juice, garlic, and ½ teaspoon salt in medium bowl. Pat shrimp dry with paper towels, then stir into tomato mixture. Cover and refrigerate until shrimp are firm and opaque throughout, 45 minutes to 1 hour, stirring halfway through refrigerating.

2. Drain shrimp mixture in colander, leaving shrimp slightly wet, and transfer to serving bowl. Stir in oil, scallions, cilantro, and honey. Season with salt and pepper to taste. Serve.

TEST KITCHEN TIP **DEVEINING SHRIMP**

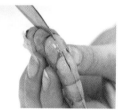

1. Use paring knife to make shallow cut along back of shrimp to expose vein.

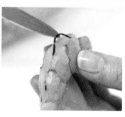

2. Use tip of knife to lift out vein. Discard vein by wiping blade on paper towel.

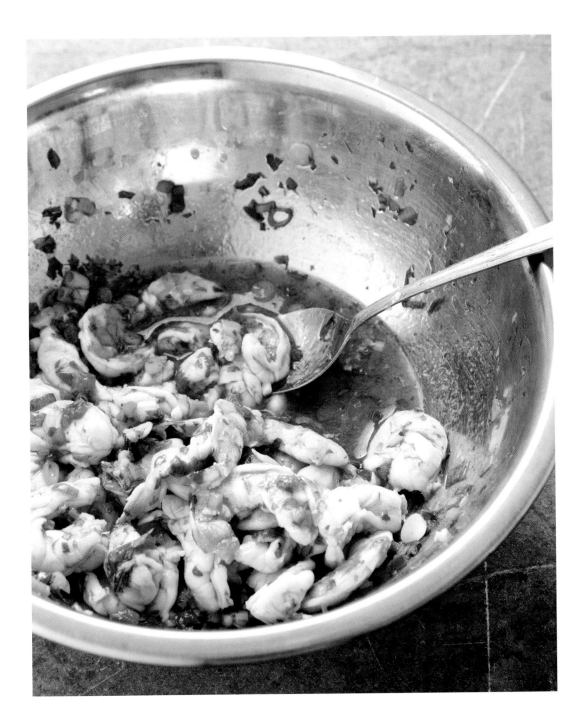

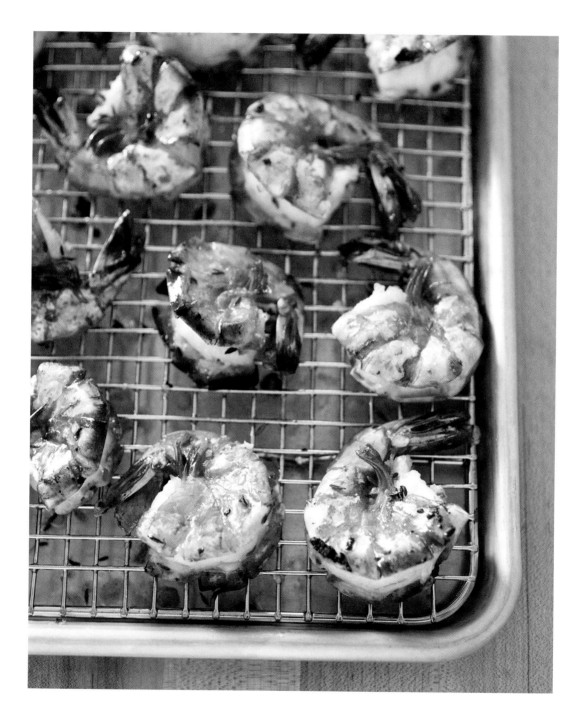

Garlicky Roasted Shrimp with Anise

Serves 4 to 6

✓ **WHY THIS RECIPE WORKS** These aromatic, intensely flavored jumbo shrimp are a cinch to prepare, making them great for a weeknight meal or for entertaining. To keep our shrimp tender under the high heat of the broiler (which helped give them their deep roasted flavor), we brined them briefly in a simple solution of kosher salt and water to season and plump them up. We then tossed them in a potent mix of aromatics—including a hefty amount of minced garlic, red pepper flakes, and anise seeds, which impart a uniquely sweet perfume— taking care to gently coat each shrimp with the mixture. A combination of olive oil and ghee provided a rich, buttery flavor. To ensure that they didn't become tough as they cooked, we left their shells on. When we broiled them in a single layer on a wire rack (to enable quick, even cooking), the shells browned in the heat of the oven, giving the delicate meat beneath a potent, umami-rich flavor. Don't be tempted to use smaller shrimp with this cooking technique; they will be overseasoned and prone to overcooking.

⅓ cup kosher salt

2 pounds shell-on jumbo shrimp (16 to 20 per pound)

3 tablespoons ghee, melted

3 tablespoons extra-virgin olive oil

6 garlic cloves, minced

1 teaspoon anise seeds

½ teaspoon red pepper flakes

¼ teaspoon pepper

2 tablespoons minced fresh parsley

Lemon wedges

1. Dissolve salt in 4 cups cold water in large container. Using kitchen shears or sharp paring knife, cut through shell of shrimp and devein but do not remove shell. Using paring knife, continue to cut shrimp ½ inch deep, taking care not to cut in half completely. Submerge shrimp in brine, cover, and refrigerate for 15 minutes.

2. Adjust oven rack 4 inches from broiler element and heat broiler. (If necessary, set upside-down rimmed baking sheet on oven rack to get closer to broiler element.) Combine melted ghee, oil, garlic, anise seeds, pepper flakes, and pepper in large bowl. Remove shrimp from brine and pat dry with paper towels. Add shrimp and parsley to ghee mixture and toss well, making sure ghee mixture gets into interior of shrimp. Arrange shrimp in single layer on wire rack set in rimmed baking sheet.

3. Broil shrimp until opaque and shells are beginning to brown, 2 to 4 minutes, rotating sheet halfway through broiling. Flip shrimp and continue to broil until second side is opaque and shells are beginning to brown, 2 to 4 minutes, rotating sheet halfway through broiling. Transfer shrimp to serving platter and serve immediately with lemon wedges.

VARIATION

Garlicky Roasted Shrimp with Cumin, Ginger, and Sesame

Omit ghee, anise seeds, pepper, and lemon wedges. Increase oil to 6 tablespoons and decrease garlic to 2 cloves. Add 2 teaspoons toasted sesame oil, 1½ teaspoons grated fresh ginger, and 1 teaspoon cumin seeds to oil mixture in step 2. Substitute 2 thinly sliced scallion greens for parsley.

TEST KITCHEN TIP **BUTTERFLYING SHRIMP**

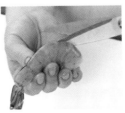

To ensure thorough seasoning, use kitchen shears or paring knife to cut through shell; do not remove it. Remove vein. Continue to cut shrimp ½ inch deep.

Shrimp Scampi

Serves 4

WHY THIS RECIPE WORKS For a paleo version of classic Italian shrimp scampi, we needed to find a creative substitution for the wheat-based pasta while retaining all of the rich garlic and seafood flavors of the original. First, we tested a number of different vegetables to take the place of the pasta. The naturally short strands of roasted and scraped spaghetti squash left tasters desiring something more akin to real pasta. While tasters enjoyed the texture of spiralized butternut squash noodles, we found that the squash's sweetness overwhelmed the flavor of the shrimp. Tasters preferred long strands of spiralized zucchini; the mild flavor allowed the shrimp and garlic to be the stars of the dish, and the texture closely resembled that of real pasta. Once we settled on the noodles, we set out to perfect the sauce. First we infused our cooking oil with minced garlic and a pinch of red pepper flakes. We deglazed the pan with clam juice to reinforce the seafood flavor before stirring in chopped parsley. The sauce tasted great, but stirring in the zucchini resulted in a thin and watery sauce as the zucchini released its moisture. By roasting the spiralized zucchini separately, we were able to drive off most of the excess liquid. We also added the garlic-marinated shrimp to the zucchini during the last few minutes of roasting to quickly cook the shrimp through. While roasting rid the zucchini of a good deal of moisture, combining it with the sauce still resulted in a watery mess. Adding arrowroot flour to the sauce before combining it with the noodles created a thicker mixture that coated the noodles and shrimp perfectly. A tablespoon of ghee and a teaspoon of lemon juice gave our scampi its classic, buttery-rich finish. If possible, use smaller, in-season zucchini, which have thinner skins and fewer seeds. For more information on spiralizing, see page 14.

- 9 garlic cloves, minced
- ¼ cup extra-virgin olive oil
- Kosher salt and pepper
- 1 pound large shrimp (26 to 30 per pound), peeled, deveined, and tails removed
- 3 pounds zucchini, trimmed
- ¼ teaspoon red pepper flakes
- ¾ cup bottled clam juice
- 2½ teaspoons arrowroot flour
- ½ cup chopped fresh parsley
- 1 tablespoon ghee
- 1 teaspoon lemon juice, plus lemon wedges for serving

1. Adjust oven rack to middle position and heat oven to 375 degrees. Combine 2 teaspoons garlic, 1 tablespoon oil, and ½ teaspoon salt in bowl. Add shrimp and toss to coat.

2. Using spiralizer, cut zucchini into ⅛-inch-thick noodles, then cut noodles into 12-inch lengths. Toss zucchini noodles with 1 tablespoon oil and 1 teaspoon salt on rimmed baking sheet and roast until zucchini is softened, about 15 minutes.

3. Scatter shrimp over zucchini and bake until zucchini is tender and shrimp are opaque throughout, about 8 minutes. Transfer zucchini and shrimp to colander and shake to remove any excess liquid; transfer to large serving bowl.

4. Cook remaining 2 tablespoons oil, remaining garlic, and pepper flakes in medium saucepan over low heat, stirring constantly, until garlic is sticky and golden brown, about 4 minutes. Whisk clam juice and flour together, then whisk into skillet and cook until sauce is very thick, about 3 minutes. Off heat, whisk in parsley, ghee, and lemon juice. Add sauce to bowl with zucchini and shrimp and gently toss to combine. Season with salt and pepper to taste. Serve with lemon wedges.

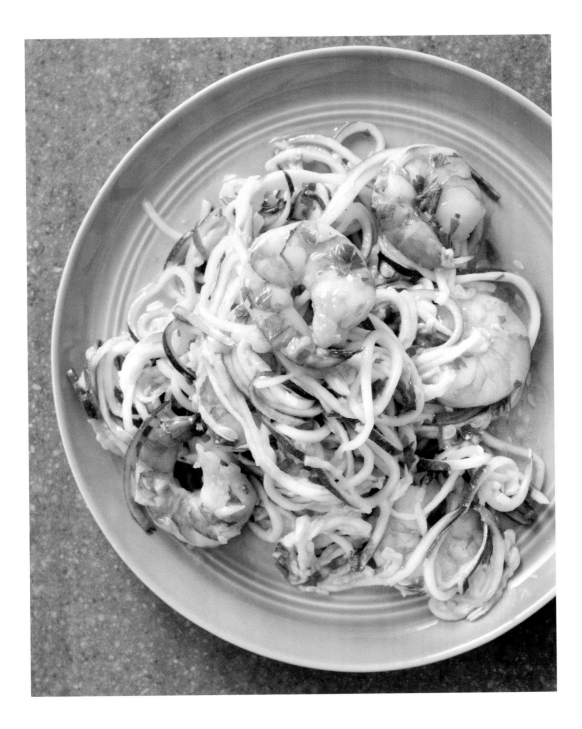

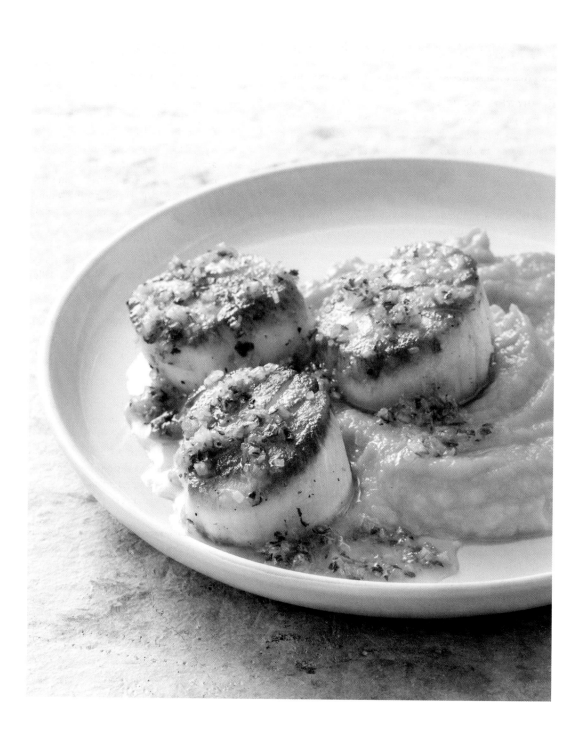

Seared Scallops with Butternut Squash Puree

Serves 4

✓ **WHY THIS RECIPE WORKS** For an elegant meal that was remarkably easy to prepare, we combined perfectly seared, succulent sea scallops with a velvety butternut squash puree. Steaming the squash in the microwave enabled us to significantly reduce the meal's overall preparation time. The puree needed only a tablespoon of ghee and a touch of cayenne to bring its flavor into focus. For maximum caramelization on our scallops, we rested them on dish towels to remove excess moisture, and we pan-seared them in two batches to avoid crowding (and steaming) in the pan. A simple yet fragrant pan sauce of ghee, shallots, fresh sage, and briny juices from the scallops tied the dish together. Be sure to purchase "dry" scallops, which don't have chemical additives. Dry scallops will look ivory or pinkish; "wet" scallops are bright white. This recipe calls for a 12-inch nonstick skillet; however, a well-seasoned cast-iron skillet can be used instead.

1½ **pounds large sea scallops, tendons removed**

2 **pounds butternut squash, peeled, seeded, and cut into 1-inch pieces (7 cups)**

½ **cup ghee**

1 **tablespoon water**

Salt and pepper

⅛ **teaspoon cayenne pepper**

1 **shallot, minced**

2 **teaspoons minced fresh sage**

1 **tablespoon lemon juice**

1. Place scallops on rimmed baking sheet lined with clean dish towel. Place second dish towel on top of scallops and press gently on towel to blot liquid. Let scallops sit at room temperature for 10 minutes.

2. Microwave squash in covered bowl, stirring occasionally, until tender, 12 to 14 minutes; drain well. Process squash, 1 tablespoon ghee, water, 1 teaspoon salt, and cayenne in food processor until smooth, about 30 seconds, scraping down sides of bowl as needed; transfer to serving bowl and cover to keep warm.

3. Season scallops with salt and pepper. Heat 2 tablespoons ghee in 12-inch nonstick skillet over high heat until just smoking. Add half of scallops in single layer, flat side down, and cook, without moving, until well browned, 1½ to 2 minutes.

4. Flip scallops and continue to cook, using large spoon to baste scallops with melted ghee (tilt skillet so ghee runs to 1 side), until sides of scallops are firm and centers are opaque, 30 to 90 seconds (remove smaller scallops as they finish cooking). Transfer scallops to large plate and tent loosely with aluminum foil. Wipe skillet clean with paper towels and repeat with 2 tablespoons ghee and remaining scallops; transfer to plate.

5. Wipe skillet clean with paper towels. Heat remaining 3 tablespoons ghee in skillet over medium heat until shimmering. Add shallot and sage and cook until fragrant, about 1 minute. Stir in lemon juice and any accumulated scallop juices and cook for 30 seconds. Season with salt and pepper to taste. Pour sauce over scallops and serve with squash.

TEST KITCHEN TIP **PREPPING SCALLOPS**

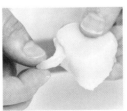

Use your fingers to peel away small, crescent-shaped muscle that is sometimes attached to scallops, as this tendon becomes tough when cooked.

Grilled Bacon-Wrapped Scallops with Celery and Apple Salad

Serves 4

✓ **WHY THIS RECIPE WORKS** Salty, smoky bacon is the perfect foil for sweet, briny scallops, but this combo presents a challenging cooking problem. Delicate scallops are best when seared quickly over high heat. Bacon, on the other hand, needs low and slow heat to render its fat before becoming crisp. We knew we would have to give our bacon a head start so that it could become crispy before our scallops were overdone. Rendering bacon on the grill can cause flare-ups, so we microwaved the bacon on a plate between layers of paper towels to absorb excess grease. Weighing the bacon down with a second plate prevented it from curling. We tossed the scallops with olive oil to encourage browning and prevent them from sticking to the grill grate. Using one piece of bacon to bundle two scallops gave us a perfect bacon-to-scallop ratio. A two-level grill fire, which has a hotter and cooler side, allowed us to gently crisp the two bacon sides of the skewers and then quickly finish cooking the scallops over high heat. A hearty salad of crunchy apples and celery provided a fresh complement to the dish. Be sure to purchase "dry" scallops, which don't have chemical additives. Dry scallops will look ivory or pinkish; "wet" scallops are bright white. You will need four 12-inch metal skewers for this recipe.

5 tablespoons extra-virgin olive oil
3 tablespoons cider vinegar
4 teaspoons Dijon mustard
1 tablespoon honey
1 Granny Smith apple, cored and cut into 2-inch-long matchsticks
6 celery ribs, sliced thin on bias
¼ cup fresh parsley leaves
1 shallot, sliced thin
   Kosher salt and pepper
12 slices bacon
24 large sea scallops, tendons removed

1. Whisk 3 tablespoons oil, vinegar, mustard, and honey together in large bowl. Add apple, celery, parsley, and shallot and toss to combine. Season with salt and pepper to taste. Set aside for serving.

2. Place triple layer of paper towels on large plate and arrange 6 slices bacon in single layer on towels. Top with 3 more paper towels, remaining 6 slices bacon, and second plate. Microwave until bacon is slightly shriveled but still pliable, about 4 minutes.

3. Toss scallops with remaining 2 tablespoons oil, 1 teaspoon salt, and ⅛ teaspoon pepper. Press 2 scallops together, side to side, and wrap sides of bundle with 1 slice bacon. Thread onto 12-inch metal skewer through bacon. Repeat with remaining scallops and bacon, threading 3 bundles onto each of 4 skewers.

4A. FOR A CHARCOAL GRILL Open bottom vent completely. Light large chimney starter filled with charcoal briquettes (6 quarts). When top coals are partially covered with ash, pour two-thirds evenly over half of grill, then pour remaining coals over other half of grill. Set cooking grate in place, cover, and open lid vent completely. Heat grill until hot, about 5 minutes.

4B. FOR A GAS GRILL Turn all burners to high, cover, and heat grill until hot, about 15 minutes. Leave primary burner on high and turn other burner(s) to medium.

5. Clean and oil cooking grate. Place skewers, bacon side down, on cooler side of grill. Cook (covered if using gas) until bacon is crisp on first side, about 4 minutes. Flip skewers onto other bacon side and cook until crisp, about 4 minutes. Flip skewers so one flat side of scallops is facing down and move to hotter side of grill. Grill until sides of scallops are firm and centers are opaque, about 4 minutes. Serve with salad.

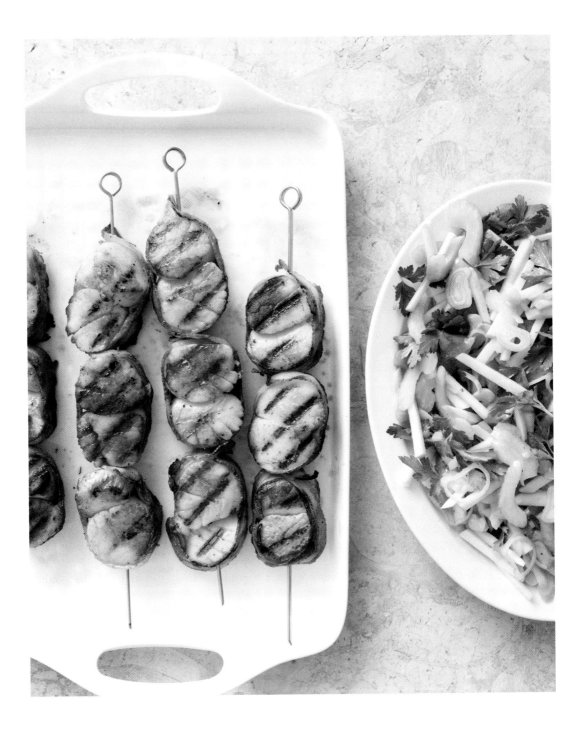

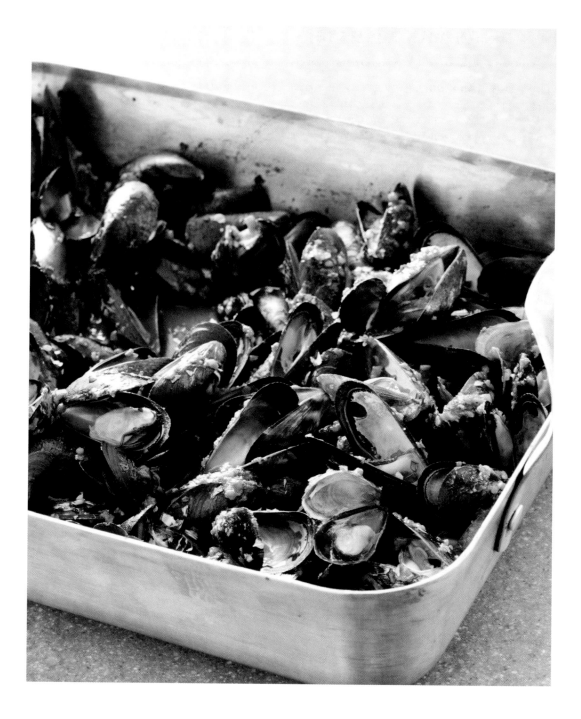

Oven-Steamed Mussels with Coconut Curry

Serves 4

✓ **WHY THIS RECIPE WORKS** Mussels are often braised in white wine and then finished with butter; we set out to put a paleo spin on this easy-to-prepare shellfish. To bring out the sweet, mineral quality of the mussels, we decided to create a coconut curry braising liquid. Since canned coconut milk often contains preservatives, we skipped it and made a quick coconut base for our mussels by sautéing shallots, curry paste, jalapeño, garlic, and ginger before stirring in water and shredded coconut. Simmering the sauce for a few minutes allowed the flavors to meld and softened the coconut, making it easy to puree the mixture into a smooth sauce. Adding a bit of arrowroot ensured that the sauce coated the mussels, and a dash of fish sauce rounded out the flavor. Braising the mussels in the oven ensured that they cooked evenly. Before cooking, discard any mussels with an unpleasant odor or with a cracked shell or a shell that won't close. Serve with lime wedges.

COCONUT CURRY

2	tablespoons coconut oil
3	shallots, minced
3	tablespoons Thai green curry paste
1	jalapeño chile, stemmed, seeded, and minced
6	garlic cloves, minced
1	tablespoon grated fresh ginger
3	cups water
2	cups unsweetened shredded coconut
2	tablespoons plus 2 teaspoons arrowroot flour
1	tablespoon fish sauce

MUSSELS

4	pounds mussels, scrubbed and debearded
3	tablespoons chopped fresh cilantro

1. FOR THE COCONUT CURRY Heat oil in medium saucepan over medium heat until shimmering. Add shallots and cook until softened, about 3 minutes. Stir in curry paste, jalapeño, garlic, and ginger and cook until fragrant, about 30 seconds. Stir in water and coconut, bring to simmer, and cook until coconut is softened, about 5 minutes.

2. Process coconut mixture in blender until coconut is finely ground, about 2 minutes. Strain mixture through fine-mesh strainer set over bowl, pressing on solids to extract as much liquid as possible;

discard spent pulp. Whisk flour and fish sauce into coconut broth. (Coconut curry can be refrigerated for up to 3 days.)

3. FOR THE MUSSELS Adjust oven rack to lowest position and heat oven to 500 degrees. Bring coconut curry to simmer in large roasting pan over medium heat and cook until thickened, about 1 minute. Stir in mussels, cover pan tightly with aluminum foil, and transfer to oven. Cook until mussels have opened, 16 to 20 minutes. Discard any unopened mussels. Stir in cilantro and serve.

VARIATION

Oven-Steamed Mussels Marinara

We prefer to use our Paleo Tomato Sauce (page 21) here; however, you can substitute your favorite store-bought sauce.

Substitute 4 cups tomato sauce for coconut curry and skip steps 1 and 2. Substitute 3 tablespoons chopped fresh basil for cilantro and stir 2 tablespoons extra-virgin olive oil into mussels before serving.

TEST KITCHEN TIP **DEBEARDING MUSSELS**

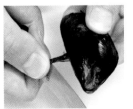

Grasp beard between your thumb and flat side of paring knife and tug gently to remove.

Smoky Braised Clams with Kale

Serves 4

✓ **WHY THIS RECIPE WORKS** For a one-pot paleo meal with big flavor, we turned to briny-sweet littleneck clams, which are simple to prepare and cook quickly. To create a potently flavored bath to steam the clams, we added smoky bacon, juicy tomatoes, and plenty of spices. For a heartier final dish, we also added kale. The large pieces of kale broke down during cooking, becoming soft and absorbing some of the flavorful liquid from the pot. Starting with a Dutch oven large enough to eventually hold the clams, we rendered our bacon until it was browned and crisp. We reserved the crunchy bits of bacon for serving and used the remaining fat to soften the onion. Then we stirred in tomato paste for depth, garlic for its pungency, oregano for its peppery bite, smoked paprika for its unique flavor, and cayenne for heat. After blooming our spices, we added the tomatoes and kale to the pot so they could begin to break down; we also added half a cup of water to ensure there would be plenty of liquid to steam our clams. Once the kale was tender we cranked the heat to high and stirred in 4 pounds of littleneck clams, covered the pot, and allowed them to cook undisturbed for a few minutes. We gave the pot a stir and kept cooking a few minutes more while we waited for the clams to open. To add some finishing touches, we added parsley for a bit of freshness, sherry vinegar to cut through the pungent spices, and olive oil for a rich fruitiness. Before cooking, discard any clams with an unpleasant odor or with a cracked shell or a shell that won't close.

6   slices thick-cut bacon, cut into 1-inch pieces
1   onion, chopped fine
2   tablespoons tomato paste
5   garlic cloves, sliced thin
1   tablespoon minced fresh oregano
     or 1 teaspoon dried
1   teaspoon smoked paprika
¼   teaspoon cayenne pepper
1½   pounds tomatoes, cored and cut
     into 1-inch pieces
1   pound kale, stemmed and cut
     into 1-inch pieces
½   cup water
4   pounds littleneck clams, scrubbed
2   tablespoons minced fresh parsley
1   tablespoon sherry vinegar
1   tablespoon extra-virgin olive oil

1. Cook bacon in Dutch oven over medium heat until crisp, 8 to 10 minutes. Using slotted spoon, transfer bacon to paper towel–lined plate.

2. Pour off all but 2 tablespoons fat from pot. Add onion and cook over medium heat until softened, about 5 minutes. Stir in tomato paste, garlic, oregano, paprika, and cayenne and cook until fragrant, about 30 seconds. Stir in tomatoes, kale, and water, cover, and cook, stirring occasionally, until kale is tender, about 15 minutes.

3. Increase heat to high. Stir in clams, cover, and cook for 3 minutes. Stir clams thoroughly, cover, and continue to cook until clams have opened, 2 to 4 minutes. Discard any unopened clams. Stir in crisp bacon, parsley, vinegar, and oil. Serve.

TEST KITCHEN TIP **SCRUBBING CLAMS**

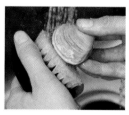

Before cooking clams, use soft brush to scrape away any bits of sand trapped in shell.

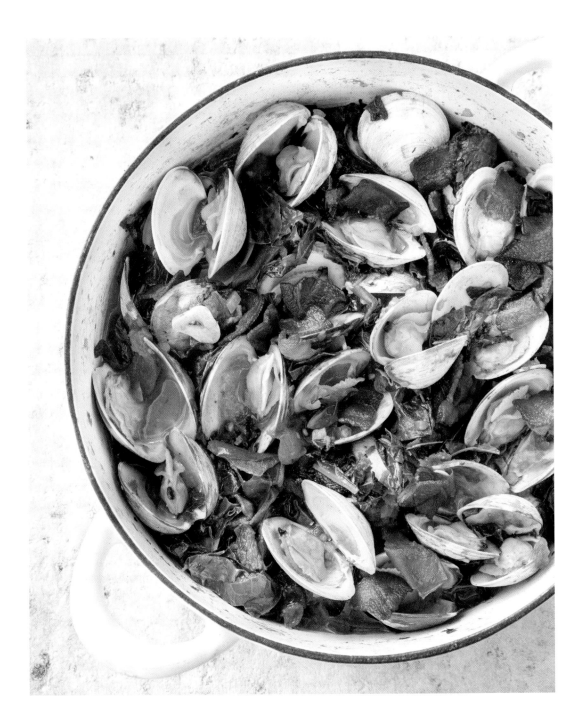

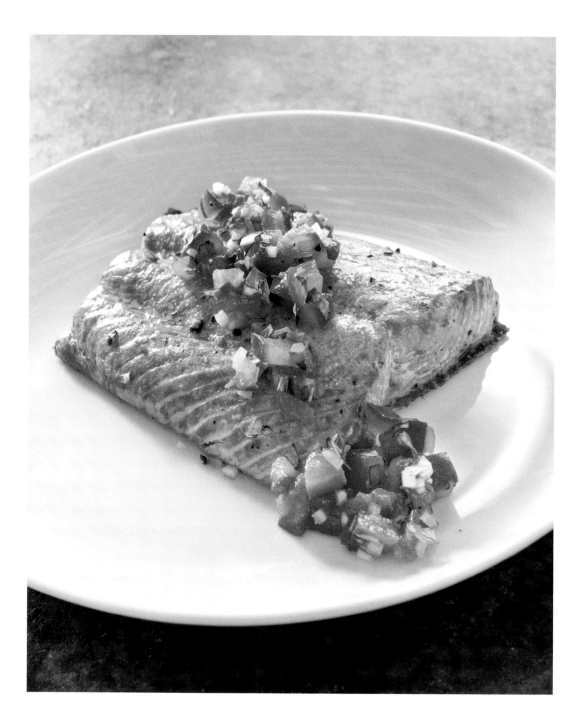

Oven-Roasted Salmon with Tomato Relish

Serves 4

✓ **WHY THIS RECIPE WORKS** Fresh, wild-caught salmon is a staple of the paleo diet, but cooking it can be intimidating for even the most seasoned home cook. Oven roasting is a great hands-off approach, but often the price is an overcooked interior. To ensure that our fillets were perfectly cooked all the way through, we developed a hybrid roasting method, preheating the oven and baking sheet to 500 degrees and then turning down the heat just before placing the fish in the oven. The initial blast of high heat firmed the exterior of the fish; cutting a few small slashes in the skin rendered some excess fat. The fish cooked gently and stayed moist as the temperature slowly dropped. We paired our roasted salmon with a quickly marinated salad of fresh tomatoes, sweet basil, pungent shallots, and peppery olive oil. Mixing the vegetables with the dressing before cooking our salmon gave the shallots time to mellow and allowed all of the flavors to meld. The brightly flavored salad acted as a vibrant counterpoint to the rich salmon. If your knife is not sharp enough to cut through the skin easily, try a serrated knife. It is important to keep the skin on during cooking; remove it afterward if you choose not to serve it.

2   **tomatoes, cored, seeded, and cut into ¼-inch pieces**

1   **small shallot, minced**

2   **tablespoons chopped fresh basil**

5   **teaspoons extra-virgin olive oil**

1   **teaspoon red wine vinegar**
    Kosher salt and pepper

4   **(6- to 8-ounce) skin-on wild-caught salmon fillets, 1 inch thick**

1. Adjust oven rack to lowest position, place rimmed baking sheet on rack, and heat oven to 500 degrees. Combine tomatoes, shallot, basil, 1 tablespoon oil, and vinegar in bowl. Season with salt and pepper to taste; set aside for serving.

2. Make 4 or 5 shallow slashes, about 1 inch apart, on skin side of each fillet, being careful not to cut into flesh. Pat salmon dry with paper towels, rub with remaining 2 teaspoons oil, and season with salt and pepper.

3. Reduce oven temperature to 275 degrees. Carefully place salmon skin side down on hot sheet and roast until center is still translucent when checked with tip of paring knife and registers 125 degrees (for medium rare), 6 to 9 minutes. Serve salmon with relish.

VARIATION

Oven Roasted Salmon with Grapefruit-Basil Relish

Substitute following mixture for tomato relish: Cut away peel and pith from 2 grapefruits. Holding fruit over bowl (to collect juice), use paring knife to slice between membranes to release segments; cut segments into ½-inch pieces. Combine grapefruit and juice, 1 minced shallot, 2 tablespoons chopped fresh basil, and 2 teaspoons extra-virgin olive oil. Season with salt and pepper to taste.

TEST KITCHEN TIP

SCORING SALMON FOR ROASTING

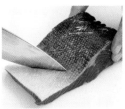

To help fat render, use sharp knife to cut 4 or 5 shallow slashes, about 1 inch apart, through skin on each fillet. Be careful not to cut into flesh.

Cod Baked in Foil with Leeks and Carrots

Serves 4

✓ **WHY THIS RECIPE WORKS** Cooking mild fish like cod *en papillote*—in which individual portions are steamed quickly and gently within tightly sealed parchment parcels—is a simple way to enhance its delicate flavor. While most recipes call for a small amount of wine to impart a heady fragrance, we wanted to find a paleo-friendly alternative, so we created a flavor-packed paste of ghee, fresh herbs, and lemon zest to gently bathe the cod as it steamed. Leeks and carrots, cut into matchsticks, provided subtle sweetness. To simplify the preparation, we found that foil was easier to work with than parchment paper, since it stayed sealed without much effort. Placing the fish on top of the vegetables prevented the fillets from drying out by ensuring that the delicate fish wasn't in direct contact with the hot baking sheet. We baked the parcels on the oven's lower-middle rack to concentrate the exuded liquid and deepen the flavor. Finally, we sprinkled the finished dish with a bright mixture of parsley, lemon zest, and garlic. Haddock, red snapper, halibut, and sea bass will also work well in this recipe as long as the fillets are 1 to 1¼ inches thick. Open each packet promptly after baking to prevent overcooking.

1   pound leeks, white and light green parts only, halved lengthwise, cut into 2-inch-long matchsticks, and washed thoroughly

2   carrots, peeled and cut into 2-inch-long matchsticks

     Kosher salt and pepper

¼   cup ghee, softened

2   garlic cloves, minced

1½   teaspoons grated lemon zest, plus lemon wedges for serving

1   teaspoon minced fresh thyme

2   tablespoons minced fresh parsley

¼   cup water

4   (6- to 8-ounce) skinless cod fillets, 1 to 1¼ inches thick

1. Adjust oven rack to lower-middle position and heat oven to 450 degrees. Combine leeks and carrots in bowl and season with salt and pepper. In separate bowl, combine ghee, half of garlic, ½ teaspoon lemon zest, thyme, ½ teaspoon salt, and ⅛ teaspoon pepper. In third bowl, combine parsley, remaining garlic, and remaining 1 teaspoon zest; set aside for serving.

2. Cut eight 12-inch-square sheets of aluminum foil and arrange 4 sheets flat on counter. Divide vegetable mixture among foil sheets, mounding it in center, and sprinkle with water. Season cod with salt and pepper and place on top of vegetables. Spread ghee mixture evenly over cod.

3. Place second square of foil on top of cod. Press edges of foil together and fold over several times until packet is well sealed and measures about 7 inches. Place packets on rimmed baking sheet, overlapping as needed, and bake for 15 minutes.

4. Carefully open foil, allowing steam to escape away from you. Using thin metal spatula, gently slide cod and vegetables and any accumulated juices onto plates. Sprinkle with parsley mixture and serve with lemon wedges.

TEST KITCHEN TIP **ASSEMBLING FOIL PACKETS**

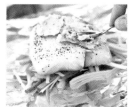

1. To protect cod from drying out, place vegetables in center of foil sheets; place fillets on top. Spread ghee mixture evenly over cod.

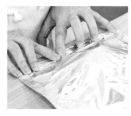

2. Place second square of foil on top of fish. Press edges of foil together and fold over several times until packet is well sealed.

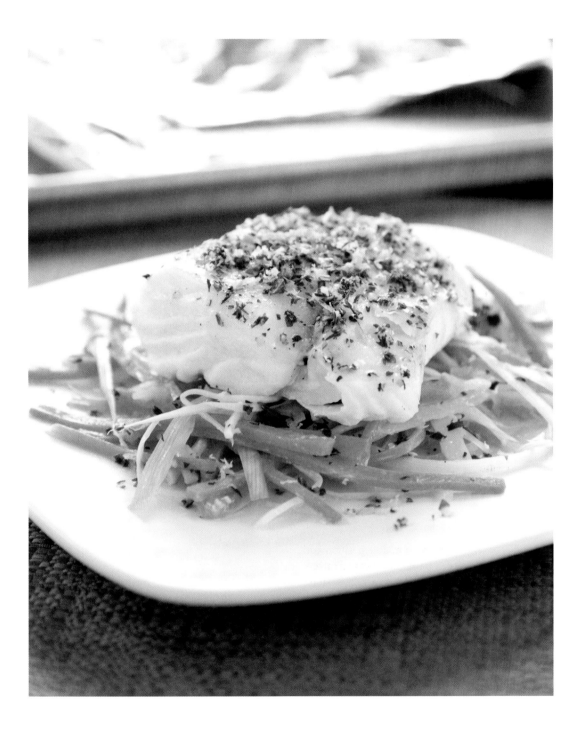

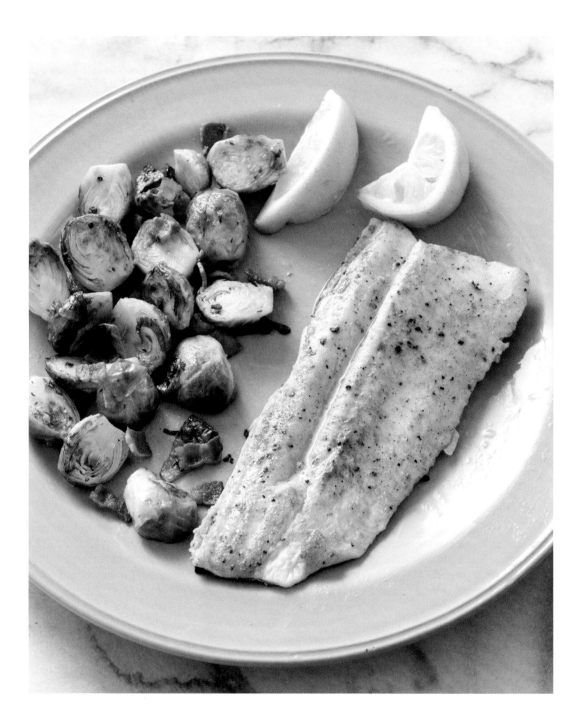

Seared Trout with Brussels Sprouts and Bacon

Serves 4

✓ **WHY THIS RECIPE WORKS** We loved the idea of a quick and paleo-friendly fish dinner, complete with a vegetable side, which could go from stovetop to table in under 45 minutes. Pairing crispy bacon and caramelized Brussels sprouts with trout seemed to fit the bill, but the long roasting time typically required for Brussels sprouts made them appear to be a nonstarter for our quick weeknight dinner. We worked around this by jump-starting the sprouts in the microwave with a tablespoon of water, steaming them until almost tender in just 6 minutes. While the sprouts were in the microwave, we took the opportunity to crisp some bacon on the stovetop. To boost the flavor of our microwaved Brussels sprouts, we sautéed them in the rendered bacon fat; in just a few minutes they had crisp, browned edges and big bacon flavor. We kept the sprouts warm in a low oven while we quickly sautéed our trout in batches. Nixing the flour or cornstarch often used to dredge the thin fish, we turned to a spice mixture of coriander and dry mustard powder to help with browning and give our trout a crisp crust. Lemon wedges provided a bright counterpoint to the fish and rich Brussels sprouts. This recipe calls for a 12-inch nonstick skillet; however, a well-seasoned cast-iron skillet can be used instead.

1½ pounds Brussels sprouts, trimmed and halved
Kosher salt and pepper
4 slices bacon, cut into ½-inch pieces
1 shallot, sliced thin
2 garlic cloves, minced
½ teaspoon minced fresh thyme
1 teaspoon ground coriander
½ teaspoon dry mustard
4 (6-ounce) skin-on trout fillets
¼ cup ghee
Lemon wedges

1. Adjust oven rack to middle position and heat oven to 200 degrees. Microwave Brussels sprouts, 1 tablespoon water, 1½ teaspoons salt, and ¼ teaspoon pepper in covered bowl, stirring occasionally, until Brussels sprouts are just tender, about 6 minutes; drain well.

2. Cook bacon in 12-inch nonstick skillet over medium-high heat until crisp, about 5 minutes. Using slotted spoon, transfer bacon to paper towel–lined plate; set aside for serving.

3. Add shallot to fat left in skillet and cook over medium-high heat until softened, about 1 minute. Stir in garlic and thyme and cook until fragrant, about 30 seconds. Add drained Brussels sprouts and cook until spotty brown, about 3 minutes. Stir in crisp bacon, then transfer to ovensafe serving platter and keep warm in oven.

4. Wipe skillet clean with paper towels. Combine coriander, mustard, 2 teaspoons salt, and ½ teaspoon pepper in bowl. Pat trout dry with paper towels and season with spice mixture. Heat 2 tablespoons ghee in now-empty skillet over medium-high heat until shimmering. Place 2 fillets flesh side down in skillet and cook until browned on first side, about 3 minutes. Carefully flip fillets and cook until browned on second side and trout flakes apart when gently prodded with paring knife, about 3 minutes; transfer to platter in oven. Repeat with remaining 2 tablespoons ghee and remaining 2 fillets. Serve with lemon wedges.

Whole Roasted Snapper with Citrus Vinaigrette

Serves 4

✓ **WHY THIS RECIPE WORKS** Roasting a whole fish delivers a richer, deeper flavor than cooking boneless fillets; sweet, mild red snapper is perfectly suited for this technique. Roasting the fish on a large rimmed baking sheet allowed for plenty of air circulation, which gave the snapper an evenly firm, flaky texture. A relatively brief stint in a hot oven helped the fish to stay moist. We made shallow diagonal slashes in the skin to ensure even cooking and seasoning; the slashes also allowed us to gauge the doneness of the fish more easily. We rubbed the fish with a quick, intensely flavorful citrus salt; letting the rubbed fish sit for a few minutes infused the fish with flavor. A quick vinaigrette made with citrus juice, extra-virgin olive oil, fresh cilantro, shallot, and red pepper flakes gave our aromatic fish a vibrant punch of flavor. Bass is a good substitute for the snapper.

½ cup plus 2 tablespoons extra-virgin olive oil

2 teaspoons grated lime zest plus ¼ cup juice (2 limes)

2 teaspoons grated orange zest plus ¼ cup juice

⅓ cup minced fresh cilantro

1 shallot, minced

¼ teaspoon red pepper flakes
  Kosher salt and pepper

2 (1½- to 2-pound) whole red snappers, scaled, gutted, and fins snipped off with scissors

1. Adjust oven rack to middle position and heat oven to 500 degrees. Line rimmed baking sheet with parchment paper and grease parchment. Whisk ½ cup oil, lime juice, orange juice, cilantro, shallot, and pepper flakes together in bowl. Season with salt and pepper to taste; set aside for serving.

2. In separate bowl, combine lime zest, orange zest, 1 tablespoon salt, and ½ teaspoon pepper. Rinse each snapper under cold running water and pat inside and outside dry with paper towels. Make 3 or 4 shallow slashes, about 2 inches apart, along both sides of fish. Open cavity of each snapper and sprinkle 1 teaspoon salt mixture over flesh. Brush 1 tablespoon oil over outside of each snapper and season with remaining salt mixture; transfer to prepared sheet and let sit for 10 minutes.

3. Roast until fish flakes apart when gently prodded with paring knife and registers 140 degrees, 15 to 20 minutes. Using 2 thin metal spatulas, transfer snappers to carving board and let rest for 5 to 10 minutes.

4. To serve, use sharp knife to make vertical cut just behind head from top to belly, then make another cut along top of snapper from head to tail. Use metal spatula to lift meat away from bones in single piece, starting at head end and running spatula over bones to lift out fillet. Repeat on second side of fish, discarding head and skeleton. Whisk dressing to recombine and serve with snapper.

TEST KITCHEN TIP

SERVING WHOLE ROASTED FISH

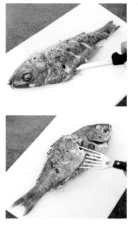

1. To create attractive whole fillet, make vertical cut just behind head from top to belly, then cut along back of fish from head to tail.

2. Starting at head and working toward tail, use metal spatula to lift meat away from bones. Repeat on second side.

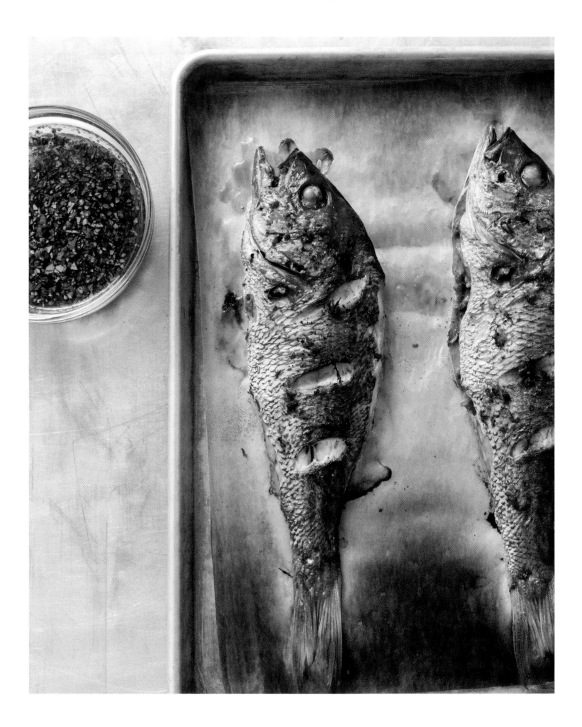

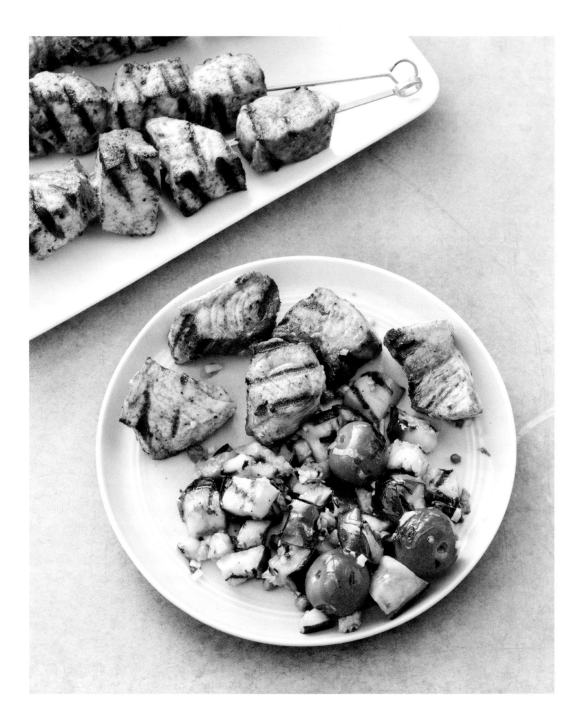

Grilled Swordfish Skewers with Charred Eggplant and Tomato Salad

Serves 4

👨‍🍳 **WHY THIS RECIPE WORKS** This naturally paleo recipe highlights the pure flavor and meaty texture of swordfish by grilling it with a simple spice rub. To maintain the clean flavor profile of the dish, we opted to pair the fish with fresh summer produce. Cutting the fish into 1¼-inch pieces and stringing the pieces onto skewers made the swordfish easier to grill and serve. For some aromatic flavor, we coated the fish with a simple mixture of ground coriander, paprika, salt, and pepper. While the grill was hot, we took the opportunity to make a salad to serve with our fish. We grilled eggplant rounds that we salted to pull out their excess moisture; we also added a handful of tomato skewers to the grill when we grilled our fish. Once everything was cooked, we combined our vegetables and seasoned them with a mixture of oil, shallot, basil, capers, and red wine vinegar for a pop of freshness. Mahi-mahi or halibut are good substitutes for the swordfish. You will need seven 12-inch metal skewers for this recipe.

2	pounds eggplant, sliced into ½-inch-thick rounds
	Kosher salt and pepper
5	tablespoons extra-virgin olive oil
12	ounces cherry tomatoes
1	teaspoon ground coriander
1	teaspoon paprika
1½	pounds skinless swordfish steaks, 1¼ inches thick, cut into 1¼-inch pieces
1	small shallot, minced
2	tablespoons chopped fresh basil
2	tablespoons capers, rinsed
2	tablespoons red wine vinegar

1. Toss eggplant with 1½ teaspoons salt and let drain in colander until it releases about 2 tablespoons liquid, 30 to 40 minutes; wipe excess salt from eggplant. Line baking sheet with triple layer of paper towels, spread eggplant over top, and cover with more paper towels. Press firmly on eggplant to remove as much liquid as possible. Brush both sides of eggplant with 1 tablespoon oil and season with pepper.

2. Toss tomatoes with 1 tablespoon oil, then thread onto three 12-inch metal skewers. Combine 2 tablespoons oil, coriander, paprika, ½ teaspoon salt, and ½ teaspoon pepper in large bowl. Pat swordfish dry with paper towels, add to spice mixture, and gently toss to coat. Thread swordfish tightly onto four 12-inch metal skewers.

3A. FOR CHARCOAL GRILL Open bottom vent completely. Light large chimney starter filled with charcoal briquettes (6 quarts). When top coals are partially covered with ash, pour evenly over grill. Set cooking grate in place, cover, and open lid vent completely. Heat grill until hot, about 5 minutes.

3B. FOR GAS GRILL Turn all burners to high, cover, and heat grill until hot, about 15 minutes. Turn all burners to medium-high.

4. Clean and oil cooking grate. Grill eggplant, turning as needed, until tender and spotty brown, 5 to 10 minutes; transfer to cutting board.

5. Clean cooking grate, then repeatedly brush grate with well-oiled paper towels until black and glossy, 5 to 10 times. Place swordfish and tomato skewers on grill. Cook (covered if using gas), turning as needed, until swordfish flakes apart when gently prodded with paring knife and registers 140 degrees and tomato skins begin to blister, 5 to 10 minutes; transfer to serving platter.

6. Chop eggplant coarse and transfer to bowl. Using fork, remove tomatoes from skewers and transfer to bowl with eggplant. Add shallot, basil, capers, vinegar, and remaining 1 tablespoon oil and toss to combine. Season with salt and pepper to taste. Serve.

Grilled Fish Tacos with Pineapple Salsa

Serves 4 to 6

✓ **WHY THIS RECIPE WORKS** Classic fish tacos consist of tender white fish encased in a crispy fried beer-batter coating, drizzled with cooling Mexican *crema* or sour cream, and served in warm corn tortillas. But with beer, flour, dairy, and corn off the table, we wanted to figure out a paleo-friendly way to enjoy fresh and flavorful fish tacos. With our homemade Paleo Wraps in hand (a great substitute for corn tortillas), we set out to find the best fish for the job. We knew we wanted to grill the fish; it would give our tacos a great smoky flavor. We tested a variety of types of fish, easily ruling out delicate white-fleshed fish like cod since it fell apart on the grill. Although salmon grilled up nicely, its strong flavor was overpowering. We landed on swordfish, which was easy to find and didn't break apart when flipped on the grill. Plus, the thick pieces could stand up to the heat of the grill long enough to pick up plenty of flavorful char before the interior cooked through. Cutting the fish into 1-inch-wide strips meant that the fish could go from grill to taco with minimal additional prep. To infuse the fish with flavor, we looked to some classic Mexican spices. Since a plain spice rub tended to burn in the heat of the grill, we made an oil-based paste that we could rub onto the fish. We added ancho and chipotle chile powders, oregano, and ground coriander, and bloomed their flavors by warming them in the oil. Tomato paste provided a savory-sweet punch, and a combination of lime and orange juices gave the paste some complex tang. With our fish settled, we turned to creating some complementary accompaniments to finish off our tacos. We decided to make a fresh pineapple salsa, which would play off of the spicy, earthy flavors in the fish. We grilled the pineapple and a jalapeño along with the fish to give our salsa some smoky depth. Red bell pepper provided crunch, while minced cilantro offered a pop of clean, fresh flavor. Mahi-mahi or halibut are good substitutes for the swordfish. The recipe for the pineapple salsa makes more than is needed for the tacos; leftovers can be refrigerated for up to two days. Serve with shredded lettuce, diced avocado, and lime wedges.

3 tablespoons extra-virgin olive oil

1 tablespoon ancho chile powder

2 teaspoons chipotle chile powder

2 garlic cloves, minced

1 teaspoon dried oregano

1 teaspoon ground coriander
    Kosher salt

2 tablespoons tomato paste

½ cup orange juice

6 tablespoons lime juice (3 limes)

1½ pounds skinless swordfish steaks, 1 inch thick, cut lengthwise into 1-inch-thick strips

1 pineapple, peeled, quartered lengthwise, cored, and each quarter halved lengthwise

1 jalapeño chile

1 red bell pepper, stemmed, seeded, and cut into ¼-inch pieces

2 tablespoons minced fresh cilantro

12 (6-inch) Paleo Wraps, warmed (page 24)

1. Heat 2 tablespoons oil, ancho chile powder, and chipotle chile powder in 8-inch skillet over medium heat, stirring constantly, until fragrant and some bubbles form, 2 to 3 minutes. Add garlic, oregano, coriander, and 2 teaspoons salt and continue to cook until fragrant, about 30 seconds. Add tomato paste and, using spatula, mash tomato paste with spice mixture until combined, about 20 seconds. Stir in

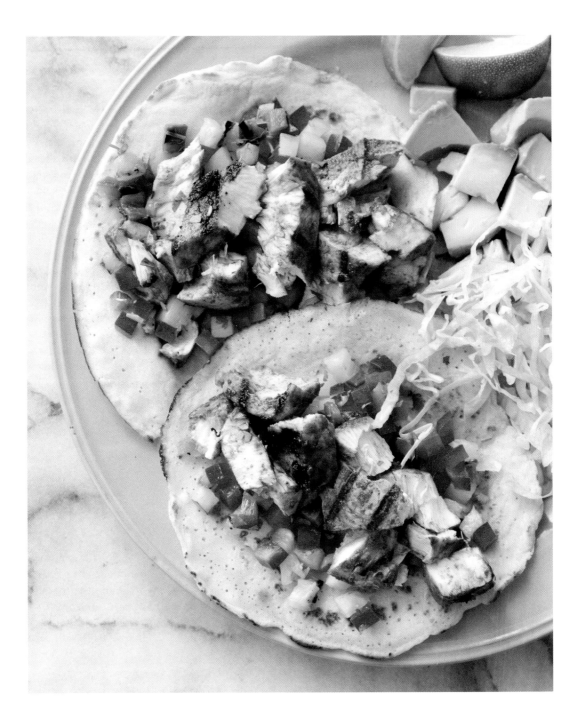

orange juice and 2 tablespoons lime juice. Cook, stirring constantly, until thoroughly mixed and reduced slightly, about 2 minutes. Transfer chile mixture to large bowl and let cool to room temperature.

2. Add swordfish to chile mixture and gently toss to coat. Cover and refrigerate for at least 30 minutes or up to 2 hours. Brush pineapple and jalapeño with remaining 1 tablespoon oil.

3A. FOR CHARCOAL GRILL Open bottom vent completely. Light large chimney starter mounded with charcoal briquettes (7 quarts). When top coals are partially covered with ash, pour evenly over grill. Set cooking grate in place, cover, and open lid vent completely. Heat grill until hot, about 5 minutes.

3B. FOR GAS GRILL Turn all burners to high, cover, and heat grill until hot, about 15 minutes. Turn all burners to medium-high.

4. Clean cooking grate, then repeatedly brush grate with well-oiled paper towels until black and glossy, 5 to 10 times. Place swordfish, pineapple, and jalapeño on grill. Cover and cook until swordfish, pineapple, and jalapeño have begun to brown, 3 to 5 minutes. Using thin metal spatula, turn swordfish, pineapple, and jalapeño. Cover and cook until pineapple and jalapeño are well browned and swordfish flakes apart when gently prodded with paring knife and registers 140 degrees, 3 to 5 minutes; transfer to serving platter and tent loosely with aluminum foil.

5. Chop pineapple and jalapeño fine and combine with bell pepper, cilantro, and remaining ¼ cup lime juice in bowl. Season with salt to taste. Using 2 forks, pull fish apart into large flakes and serve with pineapple salsa and warm wraps.

TEST KITCHEN TIP **MAKING GRILLED FISH TACOS**

Marinating our fish in a chile-citrus marinade allows us to skip nonpaleo beer-battering and frying. Grilling both the fish and some of the salsa ingredients gives our tacos great depth of flavor.

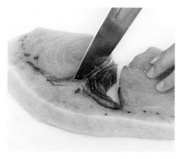 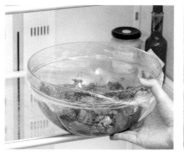 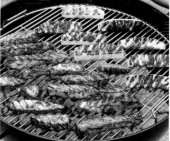

1. Using sharp knife, trim dark lines from flesh. Cut flesh into 1-inch-thick strips to make assembling tacos simple.

2. Toss swordfish with cooled chile marinade and refrigerate for at least 30 minutes to infuse it with deep flavor.

3. Place fish, pineapple, and jalapeño on grill over hot fire to ensure plenty of flavorful char before fish pieces overcook.

Spanish Shellfish Stew

Serves 4 to 6

☑ **WHY THIS RECIPE WORKS** This deeply flavorful shellfish stew is based on *zarzuela*, a popular dish from Spain's Mediterranean coast. But classic versions contain several ingredients that we wanted to avoid, such as canned tomatoes and bread (which gives the stew body). We found that the key to preparing a great zarzuela was to carefully coax the best flavor possible from each of its simple ingredients—adding each at the right moment, at the right temperature, and for the right amount of time helped to build layer upon layer of delicate aromas and ultimately produce a complex and satisfying dish. We began by making a powerful, umami-rich broth by toasting the shells from our shrimp and then allowing them to steep, covered, as we prepared the rest of the dish. Next, we made a *sofrito*—the foundation of countless dishes across Spain—by slowly cooking some finely chopped onion and pepper in olive oil over low heat. This concentrated their flavors and created a hearty, savory base. We intensified the sofrito with garlic, tomato paste, a pinch of saffron, and smoked paprika, which gave the stew a complex, aromatic backbone. To build up our stew's characteristic tomatoey richness, we needed to make the most of fresh tomatoes. After briefly processing them with the sofrito, we allowed the mixture to simmer gently until the flavors became deep and robust. We stirred in our potent seafood broth and then carefully timed the additions of our clams, mussels, scallops, and shrimp, enabling them to cook to perfection as they released their sweet, briny liquid into the stew. Finally, following Spanish tradition, we incorporated a *picada*, a flavorful blend of fresh parsley, toasted almonds, garlic, and olive oil; we left out the bread found in most traditional recipes. Added off the heat, the picada gave our finished stew a vibrant boost. Do not buy peeled shrimp; you will need the shrimp shells to make the broth. Be sure to purchase "dry" scallops, which don't have chemical additives. Dry scallops will look ivory or pinkish; "wet" scallops are bright white. Before cooking, discard any clams or mussels with an unpleasant odor or with a cracked shell or a shell that won't close.

5	tablespoons extra-virgin olive oil
8	ounces medium-large shrimp (31 to 40 per pound), peeled, deveined, and tails removed, shells reserved
2	cups water
2	bay leaves
⅓	cup slivered almonds, toasted
½	cup fresh parsley leaves
5	garlic cloves, minced
1	onion, chopped fine
1	red bell pepper, stemmed, seeded, and chopped fine
	Kosher salt and pepper
2	tablespoons tomato paste
1	teaspoon smoked paprika
¼	teaspoon saffron threads, crumbled
⅛	teaspoon red pepper flakes
1½	pounds tomatoes, cored and chopped
1½	pounds littleneck clams, scrubbed
8	ounces mussels, scrubbed and debearded
12	ounces large sea scallops, tendons removed

1. Heat 1 tablespoon oil in medium saucepan over medium heat until shimmering. Add reserved shrimp shells and cook until lightly toasted, about 5 minutes. Stir in water and bay leaves, bring to simmer, and cook for 10 minutes. Off heat, cover and let steep until ready to use.

2. Pulse almonds in food processor to fine crumbs, about 10 pulses. Add parsley, 2 teaspoons garlic, and 2 tablespoons oil and pulse to coarse paste, about 15 pulses, scraping down sides of bowl as needed; transfer to bowl and set aside.

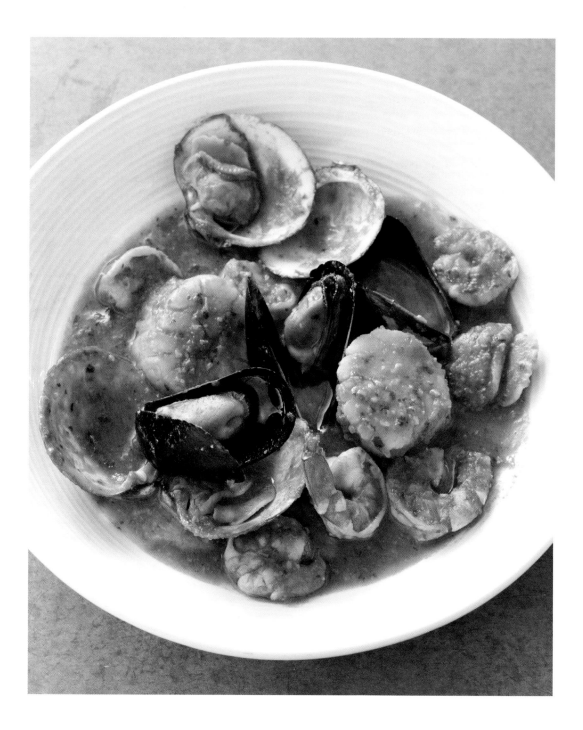

3. Heat remaining 2 tablespoons oil in Dutch oven over medium heat until shimmering. Add onion, bell pepper, and 1 teaspoon salt and cook until softened and lightly browned, 8 to 10 minutes. Stir in tomato paste, paprika, saffron, pepper flakes, and remaining garlic and cook until fragrant, about 1 minute.

4. Working in batches, process vegetable mixture and tomatoes in food processor until coarsely ground, about 1 minute; return to now-empty pot and bring to simmer over medium-low heat. Cook, stirring occasionally, until thickened, about 30 minutes.

5. Strain shrimp broth into pot, pressing on shells to extract as much liquid as possible, and return to simmer over medium-high heat. Add clams, cover, and cook until just beginning to open, about 4 minutes. Add mussels and scallops, cover, and continue to cook until most of clams have opened, about 3 minutes. Add shrimp, flip scallops, cover, and continue to cook until shrimp and scallops are opaque throughout and clams and mussels have opened, about 2 minutes.

6. Off heat, discard any unopened clams and mussels. Stir in almond mixture and season with salt and pepper to taste. Serve.

TEST KITCHEN TIP **BUILDING FLAVOR IN SHELLFISH STEW**

Since this seafood stew relies on simple ingredients, it's important to maximize every ingredient's flavor.

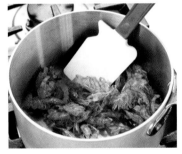

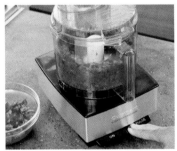

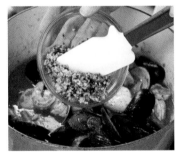

1. To create ultraflavorful shrimp stock, brown shrimp shells and then steep them in water. This extracts flavor from shells, which would otherwise be discarded.

2. We avoid canned tomatoes by pulsing fresh tomatoes with lightly caramelized onions, peppers, and aromatics to create a stew base. Cooking down this mixture thickens stew.

3. Once seafood has cooked, stir in picada to give stew brightness and bite.

New England Fish Chowder

Serves 4

👨‍🍳 **WHY THIS RECIPE WORKS** New England–style fish chowders are often loaded with heavy cream and potatoes. We wanted a paleo version that wouldn't weigh us down while still having the characteristic thick and creamy texture of the original. After testing a couple of different ways to thicken our soup, we found that pureeing cooked cauliflower into our base re-created the velvety consistency of dairy-based versions. We started by rendering a few strips of bacon in our pot and saving the crispy bacon bits for serving. To create a flavorful and creamy cooking medium for our fish, we sautéed a bit of onion and thyme before stirring in our cauliflower. Cooking the florets in clam juice reinforced the seafood flavor of the soup and allowed us to scrape up the flavorful browned bits on the bottom of the pot. We simmered the mixture until the cauliflower began to break down, transferred it to a blender, and pureed the base until it had the smooth consistency of a creamy soup. On returning the base to the pot, we added pieces of celery root, which were the perfect paleo stand-in for classic potatoes. When the celery root was tender, we added large chunks of cod fillets, reduced the heat to medium-low, covered the pot, and allowed the fish to gently cook through. Before serving, we stirred fresh parsley and lemon juice into the soup for brightness. Sprinkling crisp bacon over each serving provided a savory finishing touch. Halibut or haddock are good substitutes for the cod.

4   slices bacon, chopped
1   large onion, chopped
1   teaspoon minced fresh thyme
     or ¼ teaspoon dried
2   (8-ounce) bottles clam juice
2   cups water
8   ounces cauliflower florets,
     cut into ½-inch pieces
1   celery root (14 ounces), peeled and
     cut into ½-inch pieces
     Kosher salt and pepper
1   bay leaf
1½   pounds skinless cod fillets, 1 inch thick,
     cut into 2-inch pieces
1   tablespoon minced fresh parsley
1   teaspoon lemon juice

1. Cook bacon in Dutch oven over medium heat until crisp, 5 to 7 minutes. Using slotted spoon, transfer bacon to paper towel–lined plate; set aside for serving.

2. Add onion to fat left in pot and cook over medium heat until softened, about 8 minutes. Stir in thyme and cook until fragrant, about 30 seconds. Stir in clam juice and water, scraping up any browned bits, and bring to simmer. Stir in cauliflower and cook until cauliflower falls apart easily when poked with fork, about 20 minutes.

3. Process cauliflower mixture in blender until smooth, about 1 minute; return to now-empty pot and bring to simmer over medium heat. Stir in celery root, 1 teaspoon salt, ¼ teaspoon pepper, and bay leaf and cook until celery root is tender, 15 to 20 minutes.

4. Season cod with salt and pepper and nestle into soup. Reduce heat to medium-low, cover, and simmer gently until cod flakes apart when gently prodded with paring knife and registers 140 degrees, 5 to 7 minutes.

5. Off heat, discard bay leaf. Stir in parsley and lemon juice and season with salt and pepper to taste. Break up any remaining large pieces of cod. Sprinkle individual portions with crisp bacon before serving.

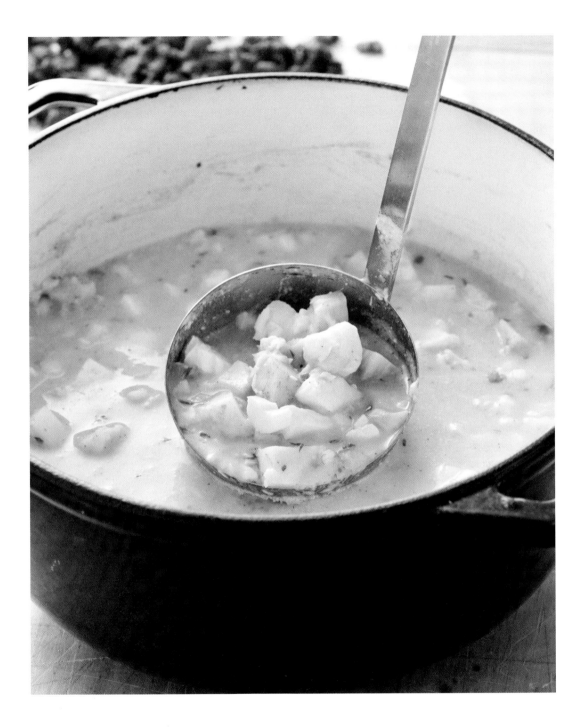

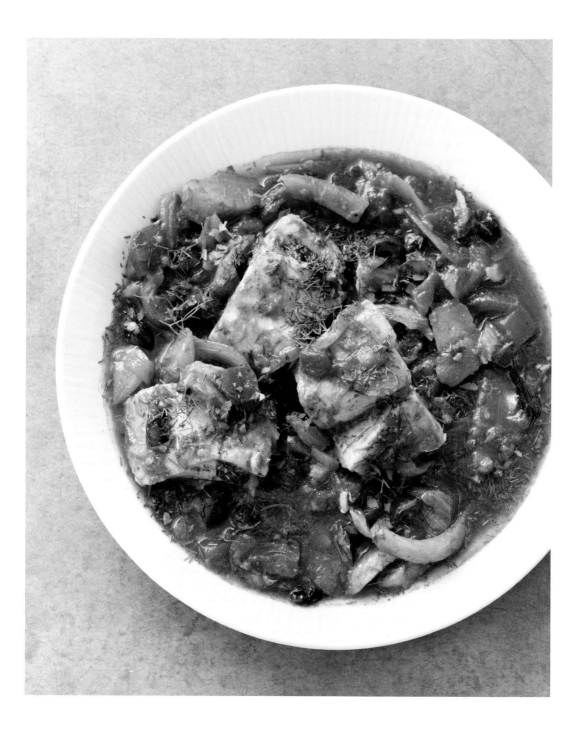

Slow-Cooker Moroccan Fish Tagine

Serves 4 to 6

WHY THIS RECIPE WORKS Traditional Moroccan tagines are slow-cooked stews that get their name from the earthenware pots in which they are cooked. The domed lids of tagine pots trap condensed moisture and return it to the pot as the dish simmers, gently steaming the contents in their own flavorful juices as they slowly intensify over time. Tagine recipes are a great fit for modern slow cookers, which similarly collect and reincorporate savory moisture while gently simmering their contents. For our fish tagine, we built the base of our complex, aromatic broth using fennel, onion, garlic, tomatoes, and warm spices, and we added subtle richness and depth with our Paleo Chicken Broth. We simmered this mixture until the broth was deeply flavorful and the fennel tender. We added the cod in the last 30 minutes to allow it to steam gently in the broth without overcooking. Chopped kalamata olives and sweet raisins added texture and lent a bright and tangy finish to our tagine. Halibut or haddock are good substitutes for the cod. You will need a 4- to 7-quart slow cooker for this recipe. Cayenne pepper gives this dish a spicy kick; for a milder dish, cut back to ⅛ teaspoon.

⅓ cup extra-virgin olive oil

2 fennel bulbs, ¼ cup fronds minced, stalks discarded, bulbs halved, cored, and sliced ¼ inch thick

1 onion, halved and sliced thin
Kosher salt and pepper

3 tablespoons tomato paste

4 garlic cloves, minced

2 teaspoons garam masala

1½ teaspoons paprika

¼ teaspoon cayenne pepper

2 cups Paleo Chicken Broth (page 16)

2 tomatoes, cored and chopped

2 (2-inch) strips lemon zest

½ cup pitted kalamata olives, chopped coarse

¼ cup raisins

1½ pounds skinless cod fillets, 1 inch thick, cut into 2-inch pieces

2 tablespoons minced fresh parsley

1. Heat 3 tablespoons oil in 12-inch skillet over medium heat until shimmering. Add sliced fennel, onion, and 1 teaspoon salt and cook until softened and lightly browned, 8 to 10 minutes. Stir in tomato paste, garlic, garam masala, paprika, and cayenne and cook until fragrant, about 1 minute. Stir in broth, scraping up any browned bits; transfer to slow cooker.

2. Stir in tomatoes and lemon zest. Cover and cook until flavors meld, 4 to 6 hours on low or 3 to 5 hours on high.

3. Discard lemon zest. Stir in olives and raisins, then season cod with salt and pepper and nestle into slow cooker. Cover and cook on high until cod flakes apart when gently prodded with paring knife and registers 140 degrees, 20 to 30 minutes.

4. Season with salt and pepper to taste. Sprinkle individual portions with parsley and fennel fronds and drizzle with remaining oil before serving.

TEST KITCHEN TIP **PITTING OLIVES**

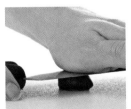

To loosen olive meat from pit, press olive firmly with flat side of knife. Remove pit with your fingers.

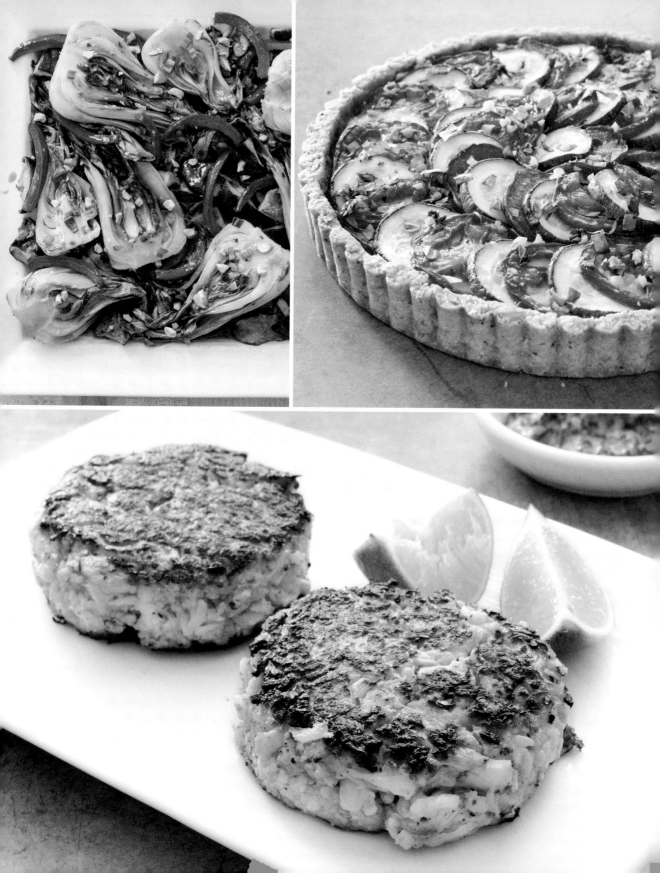

VEGETABLE MAINS
CHAPTER 6

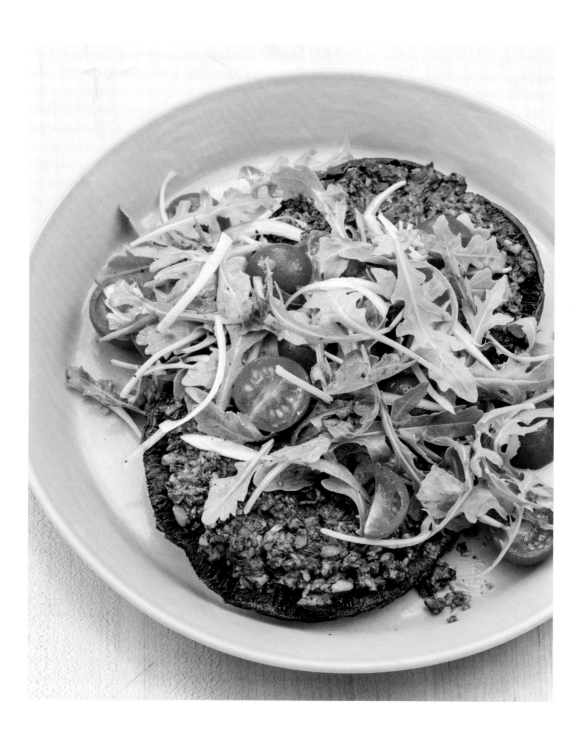

Stuffed Portobello Mushrooms

Serves 4

✓ **WHY THIS RECIPE WORKS** Stuffed portobello mushrooms are a substantial, satisfying vegetarian entrée, but the stuffings are often heavily dependent on cheese, bread crumbs, and other nonpaleo ingredients. We wanted to create a paleo stuffing with bold flavors and contrasting textures that would be simple to make. We opted for a Mediterranean flavor profile, but to keep the mushrooms' flavor in the spotlight, we used two whole mushroom caps as the base of our stuffing. Toasted pine nuts provided textural contrast without being distractingly crunchy; briny kalamata olives complemented the earthy mushrooms beautifully. Fresh parsley and lemon juice and zest offered layers of bright flavor. The food processor made quick work of turning our stuffing into a coarse, easily spreadable paste. Next, we turned our attention to the mushrooms themselves. We found that parcooking the mushrooms before stuffing them was necessary to get rid of excess moisture. Cutting slits in the caps and roasting them on a preheated baking sheet worked like a charm. Once the caps were stuffed and baked, we topped each one with a cool, bright salad of arugula, cherry tomatoes, and shallot tossed in a lemony dressing.

10 portobello mushroom caps (4 to 5 inches in diameter)
½ cup extra-virgin olive oil
    Kosher salt and pepper
½ cup pitted kalamata olives, chopped coarse
½ cup chopped fresh parsley
¼ cup pine nuts, toasted
2 garlic cloves, minced
2 teaspoons grated lemon zest plus 2 tablespoons juice
¼ teaspoon red pepper flakes
6 ounces cherry tomatoes, quartered
4 ounces (4 cups) baby arugula
1 shallot, sliced thin

1. Adjust oven rack to upper-middle position, place rimmed baking sheet on rack, and heat oven to 400 degrees. Using sharp knife, cut ¼-inch slits, spaced ½ inch apart, in crosshatch pattern on surface (non-gill side) of 8 mushrooms. Cut remaining 2 mushrooms into ½-inch pieces.

2. Brush both sides of mushroom caps with 2 tablespoons oil and sprinkle evenly with 2 teaspoons salt. Carefully place mushrooms, gill side up, on preheated sheet. Roast until mushrooms have released some of their juices and begin to brown around edges, 8 to 12 minutes. Flip mushrooms over and continue to roast until liquid has completely evaporated and caps are golden brown, 8 to 12 minutes. Remove mushrooms from oven.

3. Process mushroom pieces, olives, parsley, pine nuts, half of garlic, lemon zest and 1 tablespoon juice, pepper flakes, ¼ cup oil, ½ teaspoon salt, and ¼ teaspoon pepper in food processor to coarse paste, about 5 pulses.

4. Flip mushrooms gill side up and spoon filling into caps, pressing filling flat with back of spoon. Roast stuffed mushrooms until heated through, 10 to 15 minutes. Transfer mushrooms to serving platter.

5. Whisk remaining 2 tablespoons oil, remaining garlic, remaining 1 tablespoon lemon juice, ½ teaspoon salt, and ¼ teaspoon pepper together in large bowl. Add tomatoes, arugula, and shallot and toss to combine. Season with salt and pepper to taste. Top each mushroom with salad. Serve.

TEST KITCHEN TIP SCORING MUSHROOM CAPS

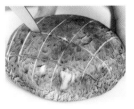

To encourage mushrooms to release excess moisture, use sharp knife to cut ¼-inch slits, spaced ½ inch apart, in crosshatch pattern on caps.

Cauliflower Cakes with Cilantro-Mint Sauce

Serves 4

✅ **WHY THIS RECIPE WORKS** Although cauliflower is often relegated to the realm of side dishes, we knew that this hearty vegetable would make an ideal base for a paleo-friendly vegetarian meal. Since many cauliflower cakes use flour or bread crumbs to bind the cakes together, we needed to come up with a viable alternative. Arrowroot flour and eggs made the cakes more cohesive, but they were still difficult to flip. A 30-minute rest in the refrigerator firmed up the cakes and made them easier to work with. Because many recipes include cheese, we needed to add bold flavor in other ways. Tasters liked warm spices like turmeric, coriander, and ginger. A bright, fresh sauce made with almond yogurt and fresh herbs completed the dish perfectly. We prefer to use homemade almond yogurt, but you can substitute your favorite unsweetened store-bought brand. This recipe calls for a 12-inch nonstick skillet; however, a well-seasoned cast-iron skillet can be used instead.

CILANTRO-MINT SAUCE

¾	cup minced fresh cilantro
¾	cup minced fresh mint
½	cup Paleo Almond Yogurt (page 23)
¼	cup finely chopped onion
1	tablespoon lime juice
1½	teaspoons honey
½	teaspoon ground cumin
	Kosher salt and pepper

CAKES

2	heads cauliflower (4 pounds), cored and cut into 1-inch florets (12 cups)
½	cup extra-virgin olive oil
	Kosher salt and pepper
1	teaspoon ground turmeric
1	teaspoon ground coriander
½	teaspoon ground ginger
2	large eggs, lightly beaten
2	scallions, sliced thin
2	garlic cloves, minced
1	teaspoon grated lime zest, plus lime wedges for serving
3	tablespoons arrowroot flour

1. FOR THE CILANTRO-MINT SAUCE Combine all ingredients in serving bowl and season with salt and pepper to taste; set aside.

2. FOR THE CAKES Adjust oven rack to middle position and heat oven to 450 degrees. Toss cauliflower, 2 tablespoons oil, 2 teaspoons salt, ¼ teaspoon pepper, turmeric, coriander, and ginger together in bowl. Spread cauliflower out over aluminum foil–lined rimmed baking sheet and roast, stirring occasionally, until well browned and tender, about 25 minutes. Transfer cauliflower to large bowl and let cool slightly. Reduce oven temperature to 200 degrees.

3. Line sheet with clean foil. Mash cauliflower coarsely with potato masher, then stir in beaten egg, scallions, garlic, and lime zest. Sprinkle flour over mixture and stir until well combined. Using wet hands, divide mixture into 8 equal portions, pack gently into ¾-inch-thick cakes, and place on prepared sheet. Refrigerate cakes until chilled and firm, about 30 minutes.

4. Line large plate with paper towels. Set wire rack in second rimmed baking sheet. Heat 3 tablespoons oil in 12-inch nonstick skillet over medium-low heat until shimmering. Gently lay 4 cakes in skillet and cook until golden brown and slightly crisp, about 5 minutes per side. Drain cakes briefly on prepared plate, then transfer to prepared rack and keep warm in oven. Repeat with remaining 3 tablespoons oil and remaining 4 cakes. Season cakes with salt and serve with sauce and lime wedges.

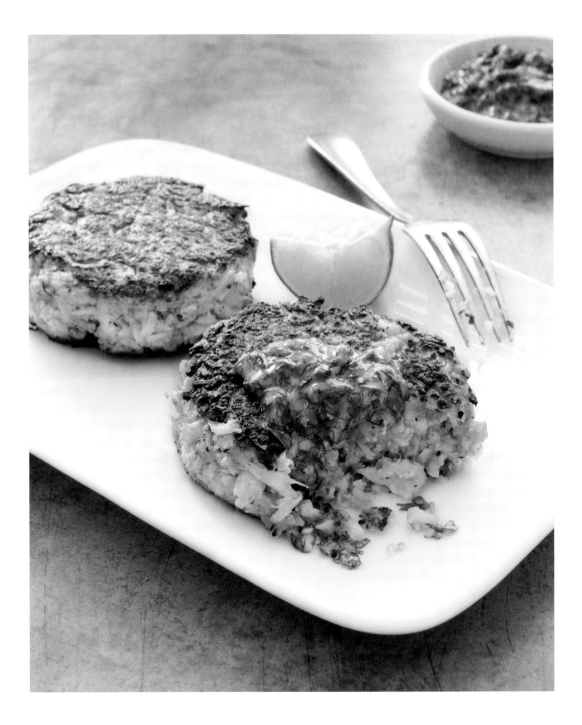

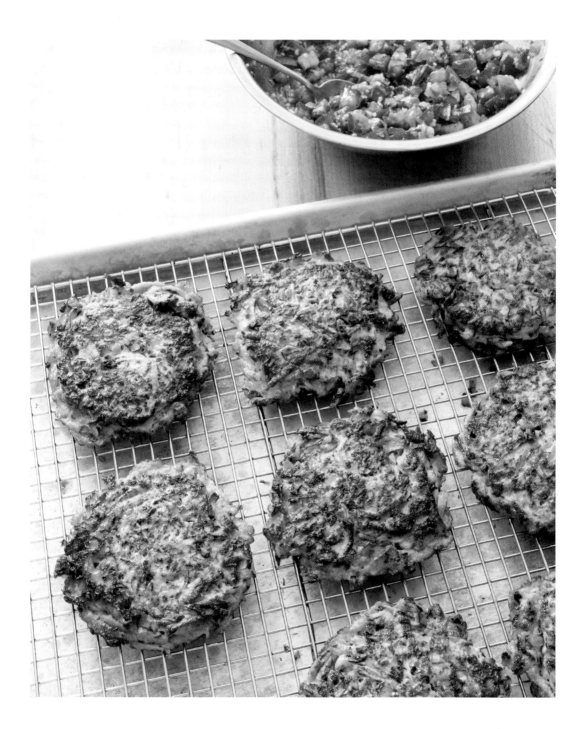

Zucchini Fritters with Fresh Tomato Salsa

Serves 4

✓ **WHY THIS RECIPE WORKS** Crispy zucchini fritters with a bright, flavorful tomato salsa make a delicious and simple vegetarian entrée. But since one of the key ingredients in many fritter recipes is cheese, which provides flavor and binding power, making a paleo version would require some creativity. First, to prevent the fritters from becoming soggy and falling apart, we rid the zucchini of excess moisture by salting it, letting it drain, and then squeezing it out in a clean dish towel. We wanted to avoid a heavy batter so the delicate flavor of the zucchini would shine through, so we turned to arrowroot flour and a few eggs. But without the cheese, our fritters were too small and a bit bland. The solution was adding shredded sweet potato to the zucchini mixture: It provided a hint of sweetness and helped make the fritters more substantial. We rounded out the flavor of the fritters with scallions, cilantro, jalapeño, and garlic. Finally, we put together a simple fresh salsa to serve alongside our fritters. This recipe calls for a 12-inch nonstick skillet; however, a well-seasoned cast-iron skillet can be used instead. Use a coarse grater or the shredding disk of a food processor to shred the zucchini and sweet potato. Make sure to squeeze the zucchini until it is completely dry, or the fritters will fall apart in the skillet. Do not let the zucchini sit for too long after it has been squeezed dry, or it will turn brown.

SALSA

- 2 tomatoes, cored and chopped
- 1 shallot, minced
- 2 tablespoons minced fresh cilantro
- 1 tablespoon extra-virgin olive oil
- 1 tablespoon lime juice
  Kosher salt and pepper

FRITTERS

- 1½ pounds zucchini, shredded
  Kosher salt and pepper
- 1 small sweet potato (8 ounces), peeled and shredded
- 3 large eggs, lightly beaten
- 7 tablespoons extra-virgin olive oil
- 2 scallions, minced
- 2 tablespoons minced fresh cilantro
- 1 jalapeño chile, stemmed, seeded, and minced
- 1 garlic clove, minced
- 1 teaspoon ground coriander
- 1 teaspoon ground cumin
- 3 tablespoons arrowroot flour

1. FOR THE SALSA Combine all ingredients in serving bowl and season with salt and pepper to taste; set aside.

2. FOR THE FRITTERS Adjust oven rack to middle position and heat oven to 200 degrees. Set wire rack in rimmed baking sheet. Toss zucchini with 2 teaspoons salt and let drain in fine-mesh strainer for 10 minutes. Wrap zucchini in clean dish towel and squeeze out excess liquid.

3. Combine dried zucchini, sweet potato, beaten eggs, 1 tablespoon oil, scallions, cilantro, jalapeño, garlic, coriander, cumin, 1 teaspoon salt, and ¼ teaspoon pepper in large bowl. Sprinkle flour over mixture and stir until well combined.

4. Heat 3 tablespoons oil in 12-inch nonstick skillet over medium-low heat until shimmering. Drop ⅓-cup portions of batter into skillet and use back of spoon to press batter into 3-inch-wide fritters (you should fit about 4 fritters in skillet at a time). Cook until golden brown and slightly crisp, about 4 minutes per side. Drain fritters briefly on paper towel–lined plate, then transfer to prepared rack and keep warm in oven. Repeat with remaining 3 tablespoons oil and remaining batter. Season fritters with salt and serve.

Spicy Stir-Fried Bok Choy and Shiitakes

Serves 4

✓ **WHY THIS RECIPE WORKS** We wanted a vegetarian paleo dinner that was so hearty and flavorful that we wouldn't even miss the meat. We decided to develop a vegetarian stir-fry that put crisp-tender bok choy in the spotlight. We aimed to bring out both the pleasantly bitter, earthy flavor of the leaves and the subtle sweetness of the stalks using complementary vegetables and a paleo-friendly sauce. First, we halved heads of baby bok choy and cooked them cut side down for several minutes to achieve a flavor-building sear. To avoid overcooking the bok choy, we set it aside while we cooked the rest of the vegetables and the aromatics. Shiitake mushrooms and red bell pepper, cooked until just beginning to brown, complemented the bok choy nicely. For aromatic interest and well-rounded flavor, we added ginger, garlic, red pepper flakes, and scallion whites to the veggies. Next, we turned our attention to creating a flavorful sauce that would tie all the ingredients together. As we had discovered in previous paleo stir-fry recipes, savory coconut aminos made a good replacement for soy sauce, and a bit of tapioca flour thickened the sauce nicely. We finished off our stir-fry with toasted cashews and fresh sliced scallion greens. For more information on coconut aminos, see page 11. This recipe calls for a 12-inch nonstick skillet; however, a well-seasoned cast-iron skillet can be used instead. Serve with Cauliflower Rice (page 288).

SAUCE

- ½ cup coconut aminos
- 3 tablespoons water
- 2 tablespoons rice vinegar
- 1½ tablespoons toasted sesame oil
- 2 teaspoons tapioca flour
- 1½ teaspoons honey
- 1 teaspoon kosher salt

STIR-FRY

- 3 tablespoons coconut oil
- 2 scallions, white parts minced, green parts sliced thin on bias
- 3 garlic cloves, minced
- 1 tablespoon grated fresh ginger
- ½ teaspoon red pepper flakes
- 6 heads baby bok choy (4 ounces each), halved
- 12 ounces shiitake mushrooms, stemmed and halved if small or quartered if large
- 1 red bell pepper, stemmed, seeded, and cut into ¼-inch-wide strips
- 2 tablespoons chopped toasted cashews

1. FOR THE SAUCE Whisk all ingredients together in bowl.

2. FOR THE STIR-FRY Combine 1 teaspoon coconut oil, scallion whites, garlic, ginger, and pepper flakes in bowl.

3. Heat 1 tablespoon coconut oil in 12-inch nonstick skillet over high heat until just smoking. Place half of bok choy cut side down in skillet in single layer. Cook, without moving, until lightly browned on first side, about 3 minutes. Flip bok choy and continue to cook until lightly browned on second side, about 2 minutes; transfer to large plate. Repeat with 1 tablespoon coconut oil and remaining bok choy; transfer to plate.

4. Heat remaining 2 teaspoons coconut oil in now-empty skillet over medium-high heat until just smoking. Add mushrooms and bell pepper and cook, stirring occasionally, until spotty brown, about 5 minutes. Push vegetables to sides of skillet. Add scallion mixture to center and cook, mashing mixture into skillet, until fragrant, about 30 seconds. Stir mixture into vegetables.

5. Whisk sauce to recombine, then add to skillet and cook, stirring constantly, until sauce is thickened, about 1 minute. Return bok choy and any accumulated juices to skillet and cook, turning bok choy as needed, until coated with sauce. Transfer to serving platter and sprinkle with cashews and scallion greens. Serve.

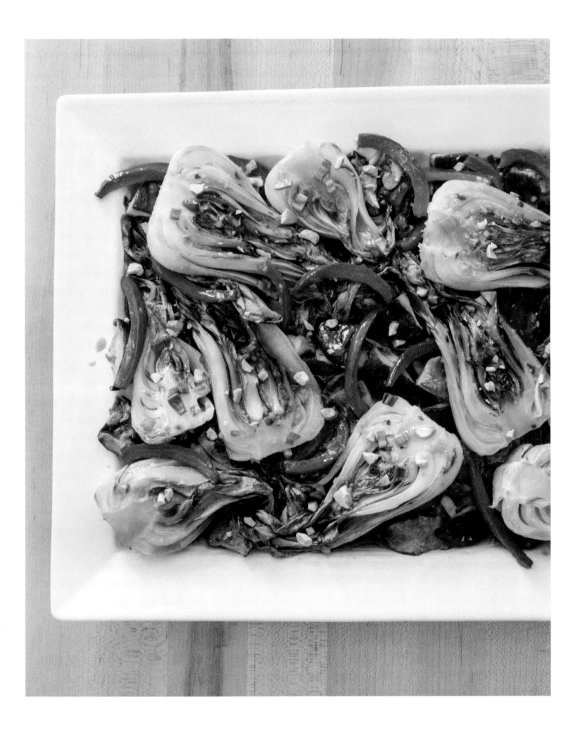

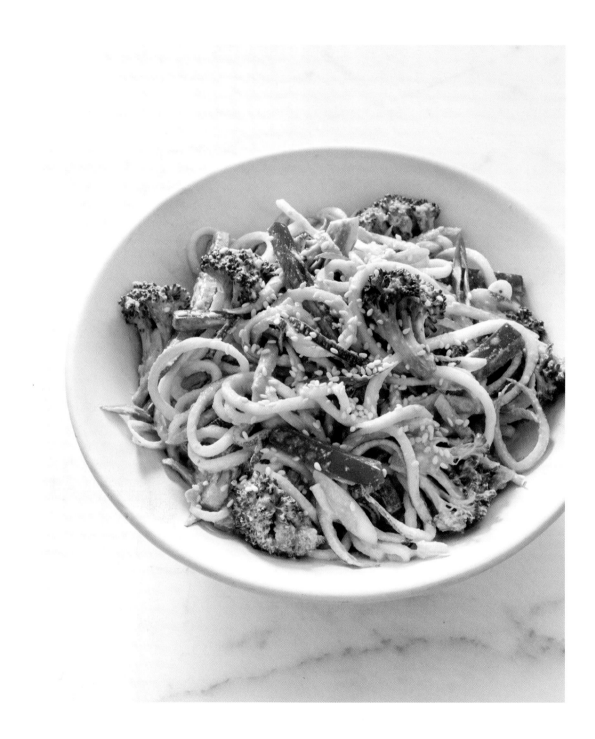

Zucchini "Noodle" Salad
with Tahini-Ginger Dressing

Serves 4 to 6

✅ **WHY THIS RECIPE WORKS** With their bold, Asian-inspired flavors and bountiful crisp-tender vegetables, cool noodle salads make perfect vegetarian lunches or dinners. But coming up with a paleo-friendly version presents an obvious challenge: Traditional Asian noodles are made from rice, wheat, or other nonpaleo ingredients. Although we considered making paleo noodles from almond, coconut, or tapioca flour, we decided instead to keep the recipe simple by using spiralized vegetables. We tested a wide range of vegetables to find which one provided the best texture and worked with the other ingredients in the recipe. Cucumber noodles contained too much liquid and made the sauce watery. Noodles made from sweet potatoes were dry and brittle. Zucchini noodles were the clear winner: The squash was easy to work with and produced long, satisfying noodles with a pleasant, neutral flavor. Next, we shifted our focus to how the noodles would be treated. We first tried boiling them, but they absorbed extra water that leached out into our finished entrée. Stir-frying the noodles proved no better. In the end, we found that leaving the zucchini noodles raw gave us a texture closer to that of real noodles; plus, tasters enjoyed their delicate flavor. To bulk up the salad, we added red bell pepper, shredded carrot, and sautéed broccoli. Since many noodle salad dressings rely on peanut butter as their base, we decided to replace it with paleo-friendly tahini, a nutty, buttery paste made from ground sesame seeds. Coconut aminos and other Asian-inspired ingredients like ginger, rice vinegar, and garlic rounded out the flavor of the dressing. For more information on coconut aminos, see page 11. If possible, use smaller, in-season zucchini, which have thinner skins and fewer seeds. For more information on spiralizing, see page 14. This recipe calls for a 12-inch nonstick skillet; however, a well-seasoned cast-iron skillet can be used instead.

½ cup tahini

5 tablespoons coconut aminos

2 tablespoons rice vinegar

4 teaspoons grated fresh ginger

1 tablespoon honey

2 teaspoons hot sauce
   Kosher salt and pepper

1 garlic clove, minced

2 tablespoons toasted sesame oil

12 ounces broccoli florets, cut into
   ½-inch pieces

3 pounds zucchini, trimmed

1 red bell pepper, stemmed, seeded,
   and cut into ¼-inch-wide strips

1 carrot, peeled and shredded

4 scallions, sliced thin on bias

1 tablespoon sesame seeds, toasted

1. Process tahini, coconut aminos, vinegar, ginger, honey, hot sauce, 1 teaspoon salt, and garlic in blender until smooth, about 30 seconds; transfer to large serving bowl.

2. Heat oil in 12-inch nonstick skillet over medium-high heat until shimmering. Add broccoli and cook until softened and spotty brown, about 5 minutes; transfer to plate and let cool slightly.

3. Using spiralizer, cut zucchini into ⅛-inch-thick noodles, then cut noodles into 12-inch lengths. Add zucchini, bell pepper, carrot, scallions, and broccoli to bowl with dressing and toss to combine. Sprinkle with sesame seeds. Serve.

Summer Squash "Spaghetti" with Roasted Cherry Tomato Sauce

Serves 4

✔ **WHY THIS RECIPE WORKS** Since pasta and canned tomatoes are not part of the paleo diet, we set out to develop an alternative to satisfy our craving for spaghetti with tomato sauce. Our first goal was to develop an aromatic, deeply flavorful sauce. We decided to use cherry tomatoes as our base, since they are available year round and are of more reliable quality than their larger cousins. We halved and roasted them, which drove off extra moisture and intensified their natural sweetness. Tossing the fresh tomatoes with a bit of tomato paste before roasting encouraged caramelization and gave the sauce a deeper, more rounded tomato flavor. Thinly sliced shallot, minced garlic, fresh oregano, and red pepper flakes, roasted with the tomatoes, provided an aromatic backbone for our sauce. Next, we focused on determining the right "pasta" to pair with this dish. Spaghetti squash seemed like a natural choice, but tasters weren't impressed: No matter how long we cooked the squash, the strands had a raw, almost crunchy quality that didn't resemble real spaghetti. Although zucchini worked fairly well, tasters ultimately preferred spiralized yellow summer squash; it had a soft texture and a pleasant chew similar to pasta, and its neutral flavor allowed our sauce to be the star. Roasting the spiralized squash and then transferring it to a colander allowed us to get rid of any excess moisture so our tomato sauce didn't become watered down. Shredded basil sprinkled on top before serving added some brightness and peppery notes. If possible, use smaller, in-season summer squash, which have thinner skins and fewer seeds. You can substitute zucchini for the summer squash, if desired. For more information on spiralizing, see page 14.

2 pounds cherry tomatoes, halved

1 shallot, sliced thin

3 tablespoons extra-virgin olive oil

5 garlic cloves, minced

1 tablespoon minced fresh oregano or 1 teaspoon dried

1 tablespoon tomato paste

Kosher salt and pepper

¼ teaspoon red pepper flakes

3 pounds yellow summer squash, trimmed

¼ cup chopped fresh basil

1. Adjust oven racks to upper-middle and lower-middle positions and heat oven to 375 degrees. Toss tomatoes, shallot, 2 tablespoons oil, garlic, oregano, tomato paste, 1 teaspoon salt, ¼ teaspoon pepper, and pepper flakes together in bowl. Spread tomato mixture out over aluminum foil–lined rimmed baking sheet and roast, without stirring, on lower rack until tomatoes are softened and skins begin to shrivel, about 30 minutes.

2. Meanwhile, using spiralizer, cut squash into ⅛-inch-thick noodles, then cut noodles into 12-inch lengths. Toss squash with 1 teaspoon salt and remaining 1 tablespoon oil on second rimmed baking sheet and roast on upper rack until tender, 20 to 25 minutes. Transfer squash to colander and shake to remove any excess liquid; transfer to large serving bowl. Add roasted tomato mixture and any accumulated juices to bowl with squash and gently toss to combine. Season with salt and pepper to taste. Sprinkle with basil and serve.

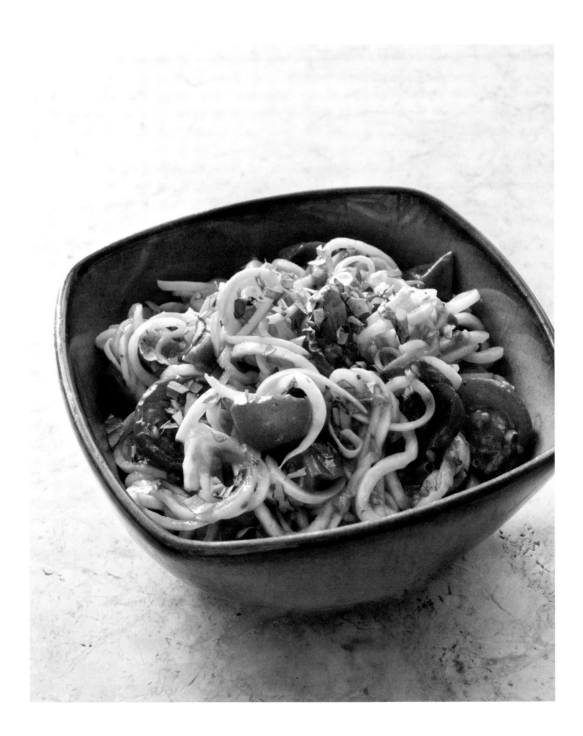

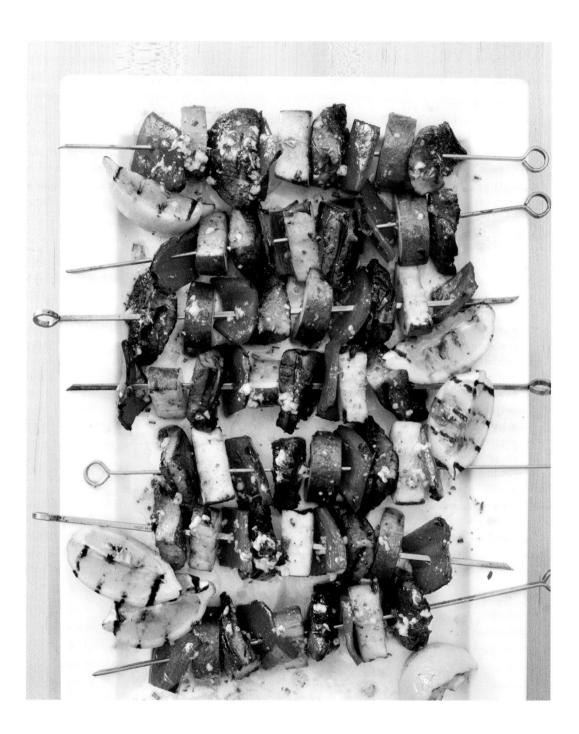

Grilled Vegetable Kebabs

Serves 4

✓ **WHY THIS RECIPE WORKS** When it comes to grilled kebabs, vegetables are often an afterthought—used as a filler on meat-heavy skewers. But this treatment often leads to mushy, burnt vegetables with no flavor of their own. We wanted to create a recipe that would put the vegetables front and center. We started by choosing the right vegetables. We wanted a good mix of flavors and textures, but we knew that not all veggies would hold up on the high heat of the grill. We started with bell peppers, which sweetened beautifully over the flames, and zucchini, which held its shape nicely and had a crunchy, satisfying texture. Portobello mushroom caps were the perfect addition to the kebabs; as they released their moisture over the flame, they picked up great char and developed a deep, meaty taste. Tossing grilled vegetables with a bold dressing can amp up their flavor considerably, but for our vegetable kebabs, we took the idea one step further. We tossed the vegetables with half of the dressing before skewering and grilling them, giving them great flavor from the start. We pumped up the complexity and nuance of the remaining dressing with juice from grilled lemons, and tossed it with the cooked vegetables for a punchy, bright finish. You will need eight 12-inch metal skewers for this recipe.

¼ cup extra-virgin olive oil

1 teaspoon Dijon mustard

1 teaspoon minced fresh rosemary

1 garlic clove, minced
 Kosher salt and pepper

6 portobello mushroom caps (4 to 5 inches in diameter), quartered

2 zucchini, halved lengthwise and sliced ¾ inch thick

2 red bell peppers, stemmed, seeded, and cut into 1½-inch pieces

2 lemons, quartered

1. Whisk oil, mustard, rosemary, garlic, 1 teaspoon salt, and ¼ teaspoon pepper together in large bowl. Transfer half of dressing to separate bowl and set aside for serving. Toss mushrooms, zucchini, and bell peppers with remaining dressing, then thread in alternating order onto eight 12-inch metal skewers.

2A. FOR A CHARCOAL GRILL Open bottom vent completely. Light large chimney starter half filled with charcoal briquettes (3 quarts). When top coals are partially covered with ash, pour evenly over grill. Set cooking grate in place, cover, and open lid vent completely. Heat grill until hot, about 5 minutes.

2B. FOR A GAS GRILL Turn all burners to high, cover, and heat grill until hot, about 15 minutes. Turn all burners to medium.

3. Clean and oil cooking grate. Place kebabs and lemon quarters on grill. Cook (covered if using gas), turning as needed, until vegetables are tender and well browned, 16 to 18 minutes. Transfer kebabs and lemon quarters to serving platter. Juice 2 lemon quarters into reserved dressing and whisk to combine. Pour dressing over kebabs and serve with remaining lemon quarters.

Tunisian-Style Grilled Vegetables

Serves 4 to 6

✓ **WHY THIS RECIPE WORKS** When following a meat-heavy paleo diet, a lighter, vegetable-based meal can be a welcome change. And while classic vegetable kebabs fit the bill, we wanted to develop a more unique, exotic take on grilled vegetables. We took inspiration from a Tunisian preparation of grilled and chopped vegetables like eggplant, zucchini, tomatoes, and bell peppers served in a boldly spiced dressing. Since getting good char was important to the flavor of the finished dish, we wanted to expose as much surface area as possible to the flames. Although some recipes called for grilling the vegetables whole, we found we could get more even, intense char flavor if we cut the eggplant, zucchini, and tomatoes in half and flattened the bell peppers. Scoring the eggplant and zucchini encouraged them to release moisture as they cooked, ensuring that our dressing wouldn't be watered down. As for the dressing, we needed to find a replacement for the traditional but hard-to-find spice blend known as *tabil*. A potent combination of coriander seeds, caraway seeds, cumin seeds, paprika, and cayenne worked well; using whole seeds instead of preground spices made the flavors even more intense. We brushed the vegetables with some of the spiced oil before grilling and bloomed the remaining spiced oil on the stovetop, adding garlic, lemon zest and juice, and a generous handful of fresh herbs to create a bright, lively dressing. Equal amounts of ground coriander and cumin can be substituted for the whole spices. Serve with hard-cooked eggs and olives.

DRESSING

- 2 teaspoons coriander seeds
- 1½ teaspoons caraway seeds
- 1 teaspoon cumin seeds
- 5 tablespoons extra-virgin olive oil
- ½ teaspoon paprika
- ⅛ teaspoon cayenne pepper
- 3 garlic cloves, minced
- ¼ cup chopped fresh parsley
- ¼ cup chopped fresh cilantro
- 2 tablespoons chopped fresh mint
- 1 teaspoon grated lemon zest plus 2 tablespoons juice
  Kosher salt

VEGETABLES

- 2 bell peppers (1 red and 1 green)
- 1 small eggplant, halved lengthwise
- 1 zucchini, halved lengthwise
- 4 plum tomatoes, cored and halved lengthwise
  Kosher salt and pepper
- 2 shallots, unpeeled

1. FOR THE DRESSING Grind coriander seeds, caraway seeds, and cumin seeds in spice grinder until finely ground. Whisk ground spices, oil, paprika, and cayenne together in bowl. Measure out 3 tablespoons of oil mixture and set aside. Heat remaining oil mixture and garlic in small skillet over low heat, stirring occasionally, until fragrant and small bubbles appear, 8 to 10 minutes. Transfer to large serving bowl and let cool, about 10 minutes, then whisk in parsley, cilantro, mint, and lemon zest and juice. Season dressing with salt to taste; set aside for serving.

2. FOR THE VEGETABLES Using sharp knife, slice ¼ inch off tops and bottoms of bell peppers and remove cores. Make slit down 1 side of each bell pepper and then press flat into 1 long strip, removing ribs and remaining seeds with knife as needed. Cut slits in flesh of eggplant and zucchini, spaced ½ inch apart, in crosshatch pattern, being careful to cut down to but not through skin. Brush interior of bell peppers and cut sides of eggplant, zucchini, and tomatoes with reserved spiced oil and season with salt.

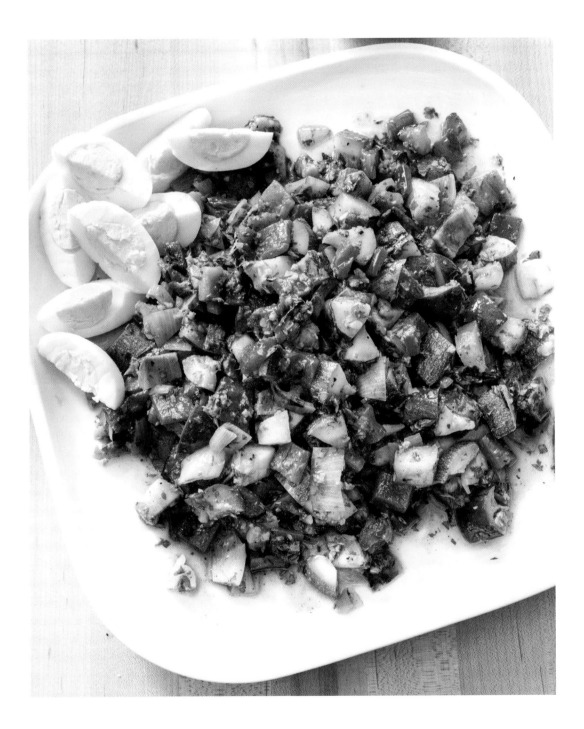

3A. FOR A CHARCOAL GRILL Open bottom vent completely. Light large chimney starter three-quarters filled with charcoal briquettes (4½ quarts). When top coals are partially covered with ash, pour evenly over grill. Set cooking grate in place, cover, and open lid vent completely. Heat grill until hot, about 5 minutes.

3B. FOR A GAS GRILL Turn all burners to high, cover, and heat grill until hot, about 15 minutes. Turn all burners to medium-high.

4. Clean and oil cooking grate. Place bell peppers, eggplant, zucchini, and tomatoes cut side down on grill. Place shallots on grill. Cook (covered if using gas), turning as needed, until vegetables are tender and slightly charred, 8 to 16 minutes. Transfer eggplant, zucchini, tomatoes, and shallots to baking sheet as they finish cooking; place bell peppers in bowl, cover with plastic wrap, and let steam to loosen skins.

5. Let vegetables cool slightly. Peel bell peppers, tomatoes, and shallots. Chop all vegetables into ½-inch pieces, add to bowl with dressing, and gently toss to coat. Season with salt and pepper to taste. Serve warm or at room temperature.

TEST KITCHEN TIP **PREPARING TUNISIAN-STYLE GRILLED VEGETABLES**

To achieve plenty of flavorful char on our vegetables, we maximize the veggies' surface area with a few key cuts.

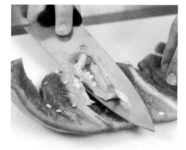

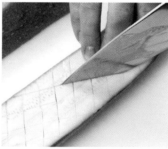

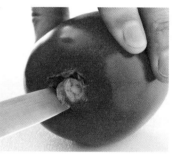

1. To ensure bell peppers char evenly and thoroughly, trim off top and bottom, then remove stem and seeds. Cut through 1 side of pepper, then press flat and trim away any remaining ribs.

2. Using tip of chef's knife (or paring knife), score cut side of halved zucchini and eggplant in ½-inch crosshatch pattern, cutting down to but not through skin. This encourages moisture to escape, preventing soggy vegetables.

3. Remove core of tomato using paring knife, then halve lengthwise. Plum tomatoes are best since they hold their shape when grilled.

Tomato and Zucchini Tart

Serves 8

☑ **WHY THIS RECIPE WORKS** We set the bar pretty high for ourselves with this vegetable tart: We had to create a paleo-friendly crust that was rich and crisp, not to mention a creamy, satisfying filling without using cheese. First we set out to tackle the tart shell, and, drawing on previous paleo baking recipes, assumed that a combination of different flours would be necessary for the right texture. Almond flour, with its pleasant flavor and high protein content, provided an ideal base, but when used alone it cooked up dense and greasy. Adding some highly absorbent coconut flour made the shell crisper and less oily, but it gave the tart a pliable texture that tasters didn't like. A half-cup of arrowroot flour solved this problem, lightening the texture of the tart and helping it to crisp beautifully in the oven. A small amount of baking soda further lightened the shell and encouraged good browning. Our next challenge was to determine the fat and liquid components of the shell. Using an egg white instead of a whole egg provided structural support without making the tart taste eggy. A tablespoon of water comprised the remainder of the liquid, while a generous amount of olive oil gave the tart great savory flavor and richness. Some lemon zest and juice rounded out the tart shell's flavor with subtle, fresh notes. The dough was too fragile to roll out; luckily, we found we could simply press it into the tart pan before parbaking. Next, we turned our attention to the filling. We decided to use our Paleo Cashew Nut Cheese as a creamy base. Tasters thought the puree on its own was a bit bland, so we boosted its flavor by stirring in extra olive oil and lemon juice as well as some chopped fresh herbs. We cut tomatoes and zucchini into thin slices, then salted them and let them drain so they wouldn't leach moisture into the tart. Shingling them on the tart made for a beautiful presentation, and drizzling them with some garlic-infused oil boosted their flavor and ensured that they wouldn't dry out in the oven.

CRUST

- 2 cups (6 ounces) almond flour
- ½ cup (2 ounces) arrowroot flour
- 2 tablespoons coconut flour
- ½ teaspoon baking soda
- ½ teaspoon kosher salt
- ½ teaspoon pepper
- 6 tablespoons extra-virgin olive oil
- 1 large egg white
- 1 tablespoon water
- 2 teaspoons grated lemon zest plus 1 tablespoon juice

FILLING

- 3 plum tomatoes, cored and sliced ¼ inch thick
- 1 small zucchini (6 ounces), sliced ¼ inch thick
  Kosher salt and pepper
- 3 tablespoons extra-virgin olive oil
- 1 garlic clove, minced
- 1 recipe Paleo Cashew Nut Cheese (page 24)
- 1 tablespoon lemon juice
- 3 tablespoons chopped fresh basil
- 2 tablespoons minced fresh oregano

1. FOR THE CRUST Adjust oven rack to middle position and heat oven to 350 degrees. Whisk almond flour, arrowroot flour, coconut flour, baking soda, salt, and pepper together in large bowl. In separate bowl, whisk oil, egg white, water, and lemon zest and juice together until thoroughly combined. Stir oil mixture into flour mixture with rubber spatula until dough comes together.

2. Sprinkle walnut-size clumps of dough evenly into 9-inch tart pan with removable bottom. Working outward from center, press dough into even layer, sealing any cracks. Working around edge, press dough firmly into corners of pan with your fingers. Go around edge once more, pressing dough up sides and into fluted ridges. Use your thumb to level off top edge. Use excess dough to patch any holes. Lay plastic wrap over dough and smooth out any bumps using palm of your hand. Remove plastic and, using fork, poke dough bottom at 2-inch intervals. Place pan on rimmed baking sheet and bake until crust is golden brown, 25 to 30 minutes, rotating sheet halfway through baking. (A few small cracks may appear in crust.) Let tart shell cool on sheet for at least 10 minutes before filling. Increase oven temperature to 425 degrees.

3. FOR THE FILLING While crust bakes, spread tomatoes and zucchini out over several layers of paper towels, sprinkle with 1 teaspoon salt, and let drain for 30 minutes. Combine 2 tablespoons oil and garlic in small bowl. In separate bowl, combine nut cheese, lemon juice, 2 tablespoons basil, oregano, ½ teaspoon salt, and remaining 1 tablespoon oil. Season with salt and pepper to taste.

4. Spread nut cheese mixture evenly over bottom of tart shell. Blot vegetables dry with paper towels and shingle attractively on top of nut cheese mixture in concentric circles, alternating tomatoes and zucchini. Drizzle with garlic-oil mixture. Bake tart on sheet until vegetables are slightly wilted, 25 to 30 minutes, rotating sheet halfway through baking.

5. Let tart cool on sheet for at least 10 minutes or up to 2 hours. To serve, remove outer metal ring of pan, slide thin metal spatula between tart and pan bottom, and carefully slide tart onto serving platter or cutting board. Sprinkle with remaining 1 tablespoon basil before serving.

TEST KITCHEN TIP **MAKING A TOMATO AND ZUCCHINI TART**

Rolling out and fitting a paleo dough into a tart pan can be challenging, so we opt for a simpler press-in style crust, which bakes up tender and flavorful. Soaked and pureed cashews make a perfect creamy filling.

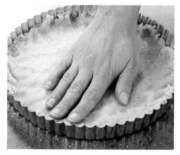

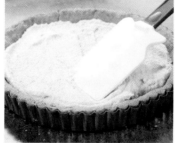

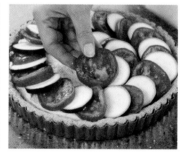

1. To ensure crust of even thickness, work outward from center, pressing clumps of dough evenly into tart pan. Working around edge, press dough firmly into corners and up fluted sides. Level off top edge and use excess dough to patch any holes.

2. To boost flavor, combine nut cheese with lemon juice, basil, and oregano. Spread nut cheese mixture evenly over bottom of prebaked and cooled tart shell.

3. Salt tomatoes and zucchini so they don't leach moisture into tart and water down filling. Shingle tomatoes and zucchini attractively in concentric circles, starting at outside edge and working inward.

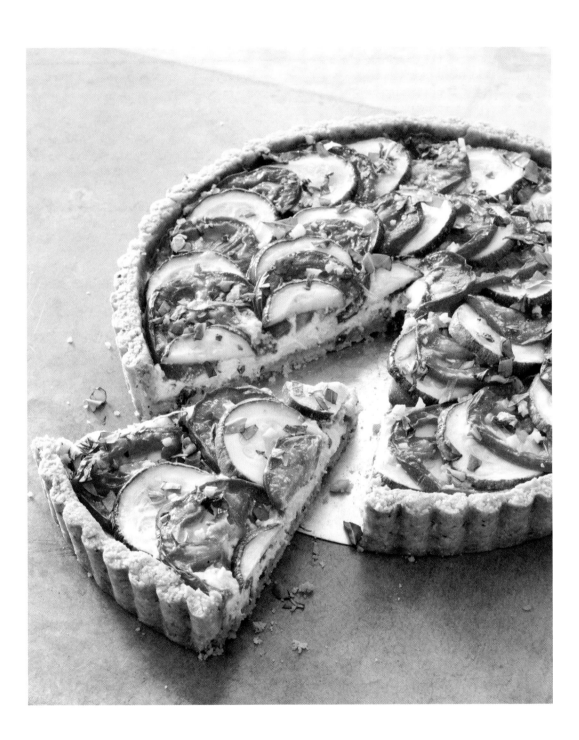

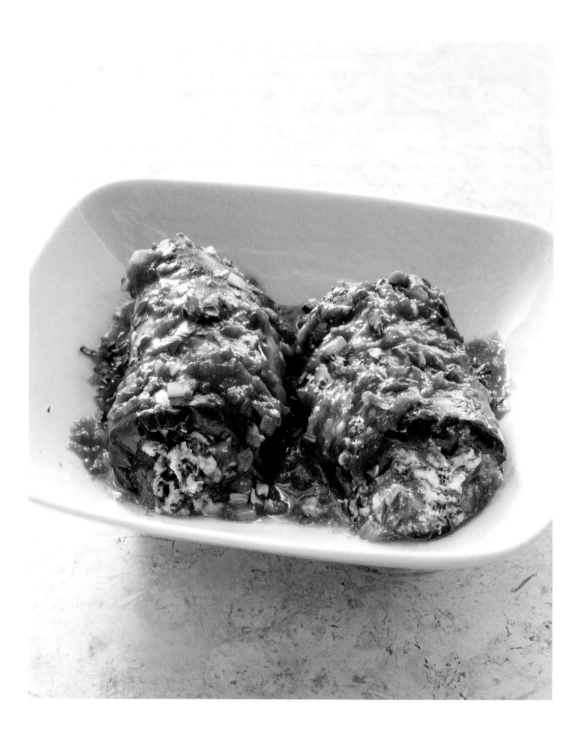

Slow-Cooker Italian-Style Eggplant Bundles

Serves 4 to 6

✓ **WHY THIS RECIPE WORKS** Looking for a unique way to prepare eggplant, we were inspired by a classic Italian dish known as eggplant *involtini,* in which slices of eggplant are rolled around a creamy ricotta filling and covered in a savory tomato sauce. To make it work, we would need to replace the cheese and canned tomatoes that are usually integral to this comforting dish. Since we were already making drastic changes, we decided to make one more and move the process to a slow cooker. We focused first on the filling. We were happy to find that our Paleo Cashew Nut Cheese, a puree made from soaked cashews, made a perfect stand-in for fresh ricotta. Spinach, fresh basil, and lemon kept the richness of the filling in check. For our sauce, we found we could replace canned tomatoes with a combination of tomato paste and processed fresh tomatoes. To rid the eggplant of excess moisture, we sliced it into long planks and then microwaved it until the planks were pliable enough to roll around our filling. The eggplant cooked to supple, velvety perfection in the slow cooker. Select shorter, wider eggplants for this recipe. You will need a 5½- to 7-quart oval slow cooker for this recipe.

3	pounds eggplant, trimmed
2	pounds tomatoes, cored and quartered
1	onion, chopped fine
1	(6-ounce) can tomato paste
¼	cup extra-virgin olive oil
8	garlic cloves, minced
2	teaspoons minced fresh oregano or ½ teaspoon dried
	Kosher salt and pepper
⅛	teaspoon red pepper flakes
1	recipe Paleo Cashew Nut Cheese (page 24)
10	ounces frozen chopped spinach, thawed and squeezed dry
¼	cup plus 1 tablespoon chopped fresh basil
1	tablespoon lemon juice

1. Line large plate with double layer of coffee filters. Slice each eggplant lengthwise into ½-inch-thick planks (you should have 12 planks). Trim rounded surface from each end piece so it lies flat. Arrange half of eggplant in single layer on prepared plate and microwave until eggplant is dry to touch and slightly shriveled, about 10 minutes, flipping eggplant halfway through microwaving. Transfer eggplant to cutting board. Line plate with clean coffee filters and repeat with remaining eggplant; transfer to cutting board.

2. Working in batches, process tomatoes in food processor until smooth. Microwave onion, tomato paste, 2 tablespoons oil, 2 tablespoons garlic, oregano, 1½ teaspoons salt, and pepper flakes in large bowl, stirring occasionally, until onion is softened and mixture is fragrant, about 5 minutes. Stir processed tomatoes into onion mixture until well combined. Transfer two-thirds of sauce to slow cooker.

3. Combine nut cheese, spinach, ¼ cup basil, lemon juice, 1 teaspoon salt, remaining 2 tablespoons oil, and remaining garlic in bowl. Season eggplant with salt and pepper. With widest ends of eggplant slices facing you, evenly distribute nut cheese mixture on bottom third of each slice. Gently roll up each eggplant slice and place seam side down in tomato sauce. Spread remaining sauce evenly over eggplant. Cover and cook until eggplant is tender, 3 to 4 hours on low or 2 to 3 hours on high. Sprinkle with remaining 1 tablespoon basil and serve.

TEST KITCHEN TIP

SLICING EGGPLANT FOR INVOLTINI

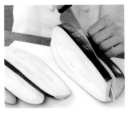

To make planks that can be rolled around filling, lay each eggplant on its side and slice it lengthwise into ½-inch-thick planks (you should have about 12 planks).

Braised Squash and Winter Greens with Coconut Curry

Serves 4

🗹 **WHY THIS RECIPE WORKS** Aromatic, savory coconut curry should have rich, unmistakable coconut flavor, but this is often achieved using canned coconut milk—a nonstarter on the paleo diet. We set our sights on developing a one-pot recipe for a flavorful, vegetable-laden coconut curry made with paleo ingredients. We decided first on the vegetables and settled on robust kale, sweet butternut squash, and crisp red bell peppers. To cook the vegetables to perfect tenderness, we opted to braise them. We built a flavorful base for our braise with aromatics like onion, garlic, and ginger. A hefty dollop of paleo-friendly curry paste gave our braise multidimensional flavor. Next, we turned our attention to the coconut. Shredded unsweetened coconut gave the braise a solid, coconutty backbone but also left chewy, gritty bits in the finished dish. We decided instead to make a coconut "broth" by processing our braising liquid in a blender and then straining out the solids. We used this broth in two ways: We braised the vegetables in it and we also used it to create a quick sauce, which we thickened with arrowroot flour. We stirred the sauce in at the end of cooking for a bold punch of flavor. A bit of lime juice provided welcome brightness. For more information on Thai red curry paste, see page 12. Serve with Cauliflower Rice (page 288).

¼ cup coconut oil
1½ pounds butternut squash, peeled, seeded, and cut into 1-inch pieces (6 cups)
1 onion, chopped fine
   Kosher salt and pepper
¼ cup Thai red curry paste
3 garlic cloves, minced
2 teaspoons grated fresh ginger
5 cups water
2 cups unsweetened shredded coconut
2 pounds kale, stemmed and cut into 1-inch strips
2 red bell peppers, stemmed, seeded, and cut into 1-inch pieces
2 tablespoons arrowroot flour
2 teaspoons lime juice, plus extra for seasoning
2 scallions, sliced thin

1. Heat 2 tablespoons oil in Dutch oven over medium heat until shimmering. Add squash and cook, stirring occasionally, until lightly browned, 5 to 7 minutes; transfer to bowl.

2. Add remaining 2 tablespoons oil to now-empty pot and return to medium heat until shimmering. Add onion and 2 teaspoons salt and cook until softened, about 5 minutes. Stir in curry paste, garlic, and ginger and cook until fragrant, about 30 seconds. Stir in water and coconut, scraping up any browned bits, and bring to simmer. Cook until coconut is softened, about 5 minutes.

3. Working in batches, process coconut mixture in blender until coconut is finely ground, about 2 minutes. Strain mixture through fine-mesh strainer set over bowl, pressing on solids to extract as much liquid as possible; discard spent pulp. Measure out ½ cup coconut broth and set aside.

4. Bring remaining coconut broth to simmer in now-empty pot over medium heat. Stir in kale, 1 handful at a time, and cook until just beginning to wilt, about 5 minutes. Stir in browned squash and any accumulated juices. Cover, reduce heat to medium-low, and cook, stirring occasionally, until kale is wilted, about 15 minutes.

5. Stir in bell pepper, cover, and cook until vegetables are tender, about 10 minutes.

6. Whisk reserved coconut broth and flour together in bowl, stir into vegetables, and cook until sauce thickens slightly, about 2 minutes. Stir in lime juice and scallions and season with salt, pepper, and extra lime juice to taste. Serve.

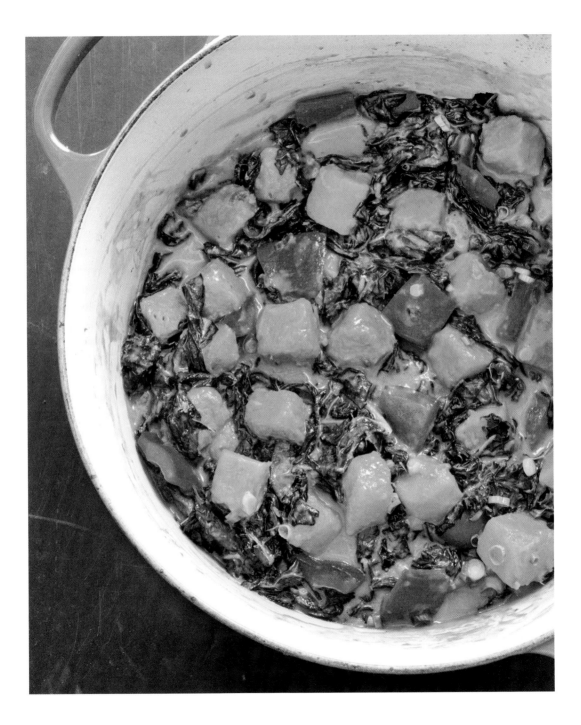

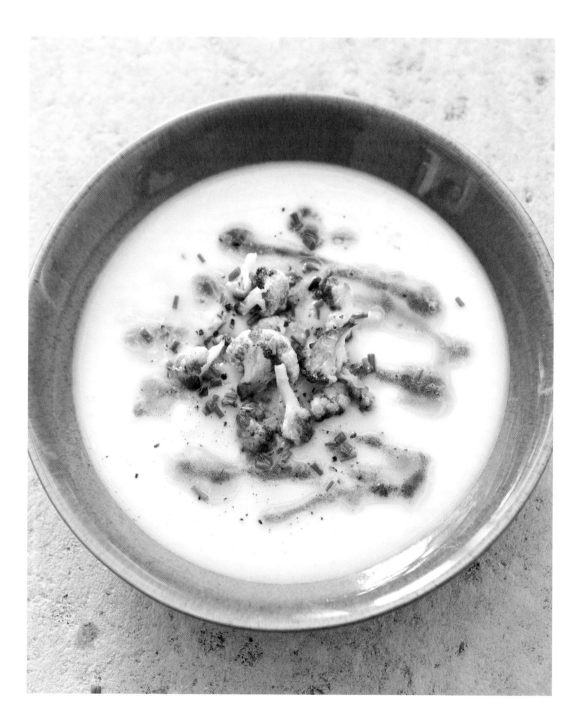

Creamy Cauliflower Soup

Serves 4 to 6

✓ **WHY THIS RECIPE WORKS** We wanted a recipe for a creamy, rich cauliflower soup, but since cream is not part of the paleo diet, we needed to get creative. During testing, we discovered that cauliflower is low in fiber, so it easily breaks down when cooked. This in turn meant that we could create a velvety-smooth puree without any cream at all. To keep the flavor of the cauliflower at the fore, we cooked it in water instead of broth. We found that the amount of time the cauliflower spent in the water greatly affected its flavor. In the end, we decided to add the cauliflower to the simmering water in two stages so that we got both the grassy flavor of just-cooked cauliflower and the sweeter, nuttier flavor of longer-cooked cauliflower. Our next task was to choose some complementary flavorings for the soup. We opted to skip the spice rack entirely, and instead bolstered the soup with sautéed onion and leek. Finally, we browned some cauliflower florets in ghee and used both as flavorful garnishes. White wine vinegar may be substituted for the sherry vinegar. Be sure to thoroughly trim the cauliflower's core of green leaves and leaf stems, which can be fibrous and can contribute to a grainy texture in the soup.

1	head cauliflower (2 pounds)
½	cup ghee
1	leek, white and light green parts only, halved lengthwise, sliced thin, and washed thoroughly
1	small onion, halved and sliced thin
	Kosher salt and pepper
5	cups water, plus extra as needed
½	teaspoon sherry vinegar
3	tablespoons minced fresh chives

1. Pull off outer leaves of cauliflower and trim stem. Using paring knife, cut around core to remove; slice core thin and set aside. Cut heaping 1 cup of ½-inch florets from head of cauliflower; set aside. Cut remaining cauliflower crosswise into ½-inch-thick slices.

2. Heat 3 tablespoons ghee in large saucepan over medium-low heat until shimmering. Add leek, onion, and 2 teaspoons salt and cook, stirring frequently, until softened, 5 to 7 minutes. Stir in water, sliced cauliflower core, and half of sliced cauliflower and bring to simmer. Reduce heat to medium-low and simmer gently for 15 minutes. Stir in remaining sliced cauliflower, return to simmer, and cook until cauliflower is tender and crumbles easily, 15 to 20 minutes.

3. Meanwhile, heat remaining 5 tablespoons ghee in 8-inch skillet over medium heat until shimmering. Add reserved florets and cook, stirring frequently, until golden brown and tender, 6 to 8 minutes. Off heat, use slotted spoon to transfer florets to small bowl. Toss florets with vinegar and season with salt to taste. Reserve ghee in skillet for garnishing.

4. Working in batches, process soup in blender until smooth, about 45 seconds. Return pureed soup to clean saucepan and bring to simmer over medium heat. Adjust soup consistency with extra hot water as needed (soup should have thick, velvety texture but should be thin enough to settle with flat surface after being stirred) and season with salt to taste. Garnish individual bowls with browned florets, drizzle of ghee, chives, and pepper before serving.

TEST KITCHEN TIP **PUREEING SOUPS SAFELY**

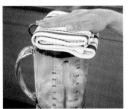

When pureeing hot soups, do not fill blender jar more than two-thirds full. Hold lid with folded dish towel and pulse several times before blending continuously.

Italian Vegetable Stew

Serves 6 to 8

✅ **WHY THIS RECIPE WORKS** Known as *ciambotta* in Italy, this stew makes for a hearty one-bowl meal. To make a paleo version, we'd have to find a substitute for the canned tomatoes that are usually the backbone of the stew, as well as a replacement for the commonly added russet potatoes. We found that a combination of fresh tomatoes and tomato paste created the flavorful base we were after. Browning the tomato paste intensified its flavor. Chopped plum tomatoes, simmered in plenty of water, broke down into a tomatoey broth. We cooked the tomatoes for at least 40 minutes to ensure they didn't have a raw flavor. Although this stew was flavorful, it was too thin. Since eggplant has a natural tendency to fall apart with long cooking, we let it simmer with the tomatoes to create a heartier, more substantial broth. Microwaving the eggplant before adding it to the pot ensured that it didn't leach excess moisture into the stew. Mellow-flavored celery root made a perfect stand-in for russet potatoes. To keep the zucchini and bell peppers crisp-tender and not mushy, we browned them and set them aside, adding them back only at the end of the cooking time. A quick basil-oregano pesto provided freshness and balance to our savory stew.

PESTO

- ½ cup chopped fresh basil
- ½ cup fresh oregano leaves
- 2 tablespoons extra-virgin olive oil
- 4 garlic cloves, minced
- ¼ teaspoon red pepper flakes

STEW

- 12 ounces eggplant, peeled and cut into ½-inch pieces
  Kosher salt
- 5 tablespoons extra-virgin olive oil
- 2 zucchini, halved lengthwise, seeded, and cut into ½-inch pieces
- 2 red or yellow bell peppers, stemmed, seeded, and cut into ½-inch pieces
- 1 large onion, chopped
- 5 tablespoons tomato paste
- 4 cups water
- 1½ pounds plum tomatoes, cored and cut into ½-inch pieces
- 1 celery root (14 ounces), peeled and cut into ½-inch pieces
- 1 cup chopped fresh basil

1. FOR THE PESTO Process all ingredients in food processor to smooth paste, about 1 minute, scraping down sides of bowl as needed; set aside.

2. FOR THE STEW Line large plate with double layer of coffee filters. Toss eggplant with 2 teaspoons salt and spread evenly over prepared plate. Microwave until eggplant is dry to touch and slightly shriveled, 8 to 12 minutes, tossing halfway through microwaving.

3. Heat 2 tablespoons oil in Dutch oven over medium-high heat until shimmering. Add zucchini, bell peppers, and 1 teaspoon salt and cook, stirring occasionally, until vegetables are softened and lightly browned, 8 to 10 minutes; transfer to bowl.

4. Add 2 tablespoons oil to now-empty pot and return to medium-high heat until shimmering. Add eggplant and onion and cook, stirring occasionally, until eggplant is lightly browned, about 2 minutes. Push vegetables to sides of pot. Add tomato paste and remaining 1 tablespoon oil to center and cook, stirring often, until tomato paste begins to brown, about 2 minutes. Stir in water, scraping up any browned bits. Stir in tomatoes and celery root, bring to gentle simmer, and cook until eggplant and tomatoes are completely broken down and celery root is tender, 40 to 50 minutes.

5. Off heat, stir in pesto and zucchini–bell pepper mixture, cover, and let sit until flavors meld, about 20 minutes. Stir in basil and season with salt to taste. Serve.

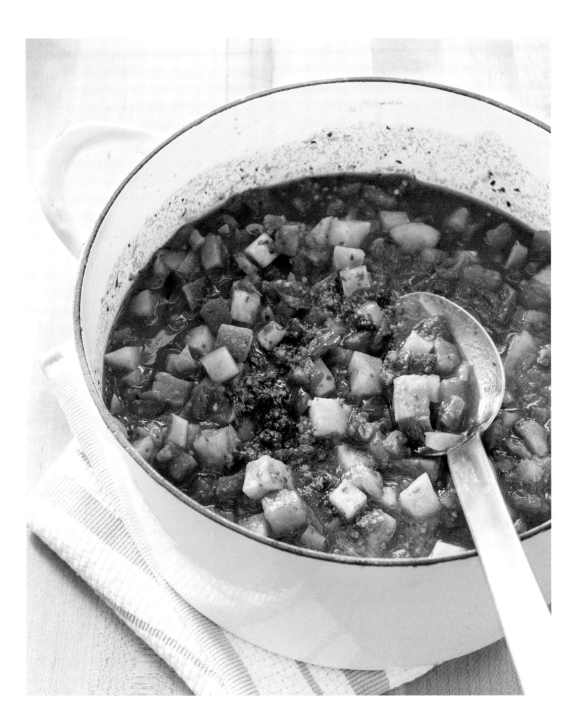

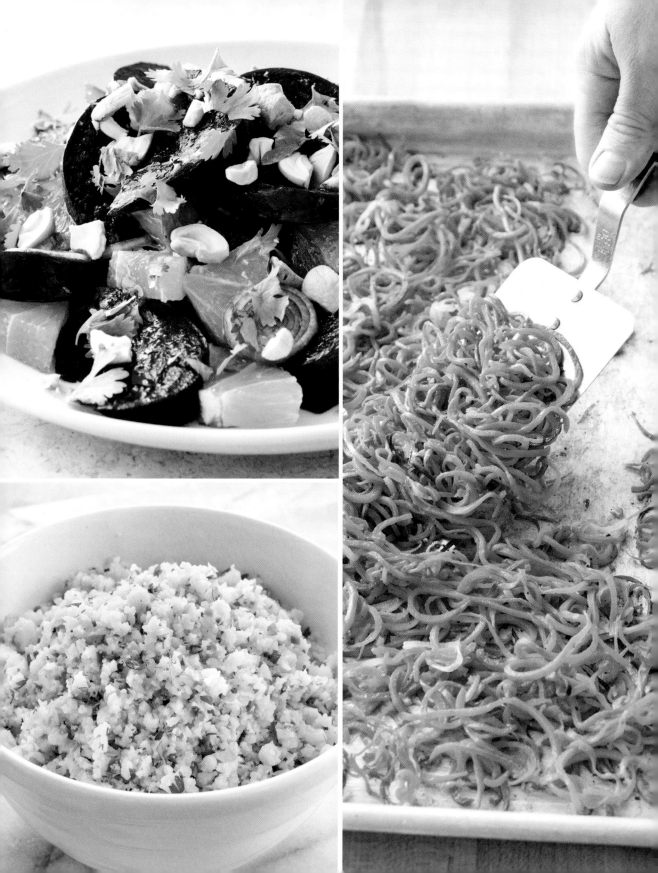

VEGETABLE SIDES

CHAPTER 7

Roasted Artichokes with Lemon Vinaigrette

Serves 4

✓ **WHY THIS RECIPE WORKS** We wanted a dish that would highlight the delicate flavor and buttery texture of whole artichokes. While they're often steamed, roasting better accentuated their naturally nutty flavor. To keep the artichokes from oxidizing and turning brown as we worked, we dropped them in lemon water. We roasted them covered so that the heat wouldn't dry them out; placing them in the baking dish cut side down encouraged flavorful browning. Roasting lemons along with the artichokes deepened the lemons' flavor; the juice made a perfect base for a tangy vinaigrette. A rasp-style grater makes quick work of turning the garlic to a paste. If your artichokes are larger than 8 to 10 ounces, strip away another layer or two of the toughest outer leaves. The tender inner leaves, heart, and stem are entirely edible. To eat the tough outer leaves, use your teeth to scrape the flesh out from the underside of each leaf. These artichokes taste great warm or at room temperature.

3   lemons
4   artichokes (8 to 10 ounces each)
9   tablespoons extra-virgin olive oil
     Kosher salt and pepper
½   teaspoon garlic, minced to paste
½   teaspoon Dijon mustard
2   tablespoons minced fresh parsley

1. Adjust oven rack to lower-middle position and heat oven to 475 degrees. Cut 1 lemon in half, squeeze halves into container filled with 2 quarts water, then add spent halves.

2. Working with 1 artichoke at a time, trim stem about ¾ inch long and cut off top quarter of artichoke. Break off bottom 3 or 4 rows of tough outer leaves by pulling them downward. Using paring knife, trim outer layer of stem and base, removing any dark green parts. Cut artichoke in half lengthwise, then remove fuzzy choke and any tiny inner purple-tinged leaves using small spoon. Submerge prepped artichokes in lemon water. Trim ends off remaining 2 lemons and halve crosswise.

3. Brush 13 by 9-inch baking dish with 1 tablespoon oil. Drain artichokes, leaving some water clinging to leaves, and toss with 2 tablespoons oil, 1½ teaspoons salt, and pinch pepper in bowl. Gently rub oil and seasonings between leaves.

4. Arrange artichoke halves cut side down and lemon halves cut side up in prepared dish. Cover tightly with aluminum foil and roast until cut sides of artichokes begin to brown and bases and leaves are tender when poked with tip of paring knife, 25 to 30 minutes.

5. Transfer artichokes to serving dish. Let roasted lemons cool slightly, then squeeze into fine-mesh strainer set over bowl, extracting as much juice and pulp as possible; press firmly on solids to yield 1½ tablespoons juice. Whisk garlic, mustard, and ½ teaspoon salt into juice and season with pepper to taste. Whisking constantly, gradually drizzle in remaining 6 tablespoons oil until emulsified. Whisk in parsley. Drizzle dressing over artichokes and serve.

TEST KITCHEN TIP **PREPARING ARTICHOKES**

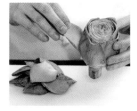

1. Cut off top quarter of artichoke. Break off bottom 3 or 4 rows of outer leaves by pulling them downward. Trim outer layers of stem and base.

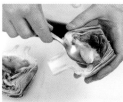

2. Halve artichoke lengthwise, then remove fuzzy choke and any tiny inner purple-tinged leaves using small spoon.

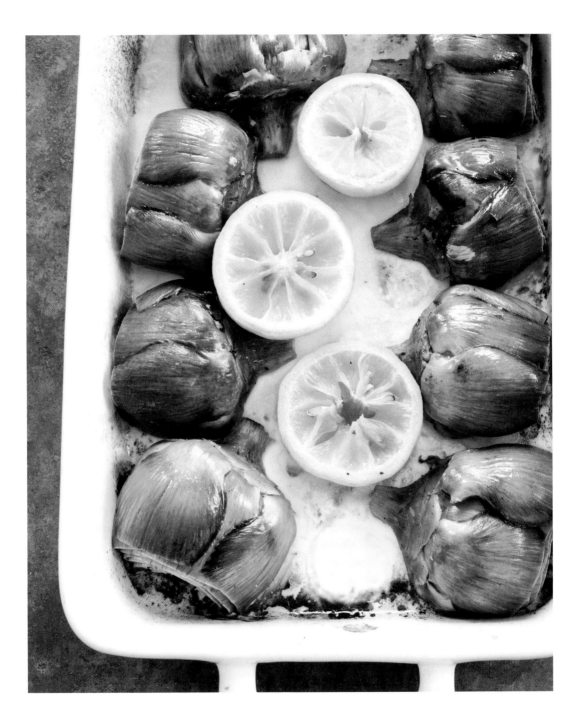

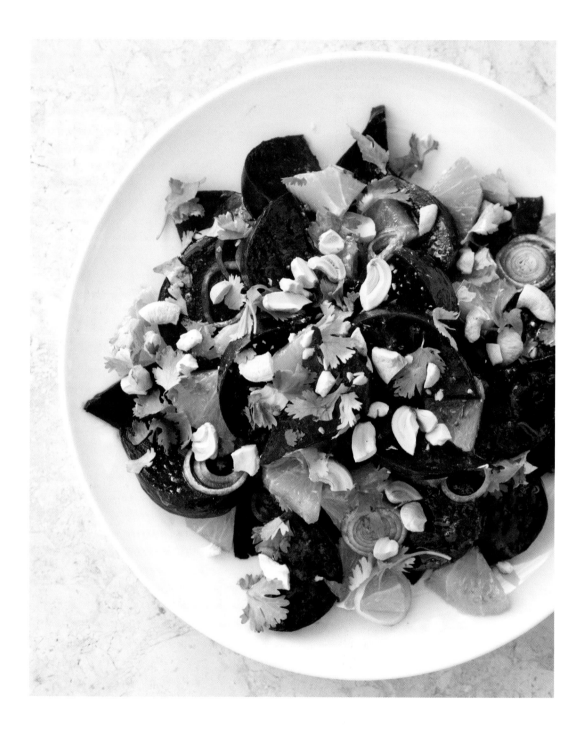

Slow-Cooker Braised Beets with Oranges

Serves 4

✓ **WHY THIS RECIPE WORKS** Roasting beets can take up to an hour, which is a long time for the oven to be occupied by a simple side, and steaming them can lead to a loss in flavor. Moving ours to the slow cooker both freed up the oven and guaranteed beets with an undiluted, earthy flavor. Wrapping the beets in aluminum foil and including ½ cup of water in the slow cooker ensured that they cooked through evenly. Rather than skin the beets when they were raw—which can be a messy endeavor—we waited until they were cooked and simply rubbed the skins off with paper towels. Cutting our beets into fork-friendly wedges ensured that they were easy to eat. To complement the tender, deeply flavored beets, we added toasted cashews for nutty crunch and cilantro and orange slices for freshness and balance. A simple vinaigrette of extra-virgin olive oil, sweet orange zest and juice, spicy ginger, and tangy vinegar brought the dish to life. To ensure even cooking, we recommend using beets that are similar in size—roughly 3 inches in diameter. You will need a 4- to 7-quart slow cooker for this recipe.

1½ pounds beets, trimmed

3 oranges (2 whole, plus 2 teaspoons orange zest and 3 tablespoons juice)

2 tablespoons extra-virgin olive oil

1 tablespoon honey

1 tablespoon grated fresh ginger

2 teaspoons white wine vinegar
 Kosher salt and pepper

1 shallot, sliced thin

¼ cup fresh cilantro leaves

2 tablespoons coarsely chopped toasted cashews

1. Wrap beets individually in aluminum foil and place in slow cooker. Add ½ cup water, cover, and cook until beets are tender, 6 to 7 hours on low or 4 to 5 hours on high.

2. Transfer beets to cutting board, open foil, and let cool; discard cooking liquid. Rub off beet skins with paper towels and cut beets into ½-inch-thick wedges.

3. Cut away peel and pith from 2 whole oranges. Quarter oranges, then slice crosswise into ½-inch-thick pieces. Whisk orange zest and juice, oil, honey,

ginger, vinegar, and ½ teaspoon salt together in large serving bowl. Add beets, oranges, and shallot and toss to combine. Season with salt and pepper to taste. Sprinkle with cilantro and cashews. Serve.

VARIATION

Slow-Cooker Braised Beets with Oranges and Tarragon

Omit ginger. Substitute 3 tablespoons chopped fresh tarragon for cilantro and 2 tablespoons coarsely chopped toasted pistachios for cashews.

TEST KITCHEN TIP **REMOVING BEET SKINS**

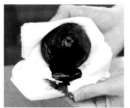

Once beets are completely cooled, cradle each beet in your hand with several layers of paper towels, then gently rub off skin.

Broccoli Salad

Serves 4 to 6

✓ **WHY THIS RECIPE WORKS** Most recipes for broccoli salad rely on a mayonnaise-based dressing that overwhelms the flavor of the broccoli. For our paleo version, we decided to skip the mayo entirely and instead find a simple substitute that would allow the broccoli to shine. We landed on creamy, mild-flavored avocado as the base for our dressing, and punched up its flavor with fresh orange zest and juice, tangy vinegar, and aromatic garlic. A little extra-virgin olive oil ensured that the dressing came out smooth. While most recipes leave the broccoli raw, we found that blanching it briefly in boiling water improved both flavor and appearance. We added the hardier stems to the cooking water before the florets so both were tender at the same time. Drying the broccoli in a salad spinner got rid of excess moisture so our dressing didn't get watered down. Toasted pecans brought pleasant crunchiness while rehydrated dried cherries added sweet-tart pops to the salad. If you don't own a salad spinner, lay the broccoli on a clean dish towel to dry in step 2. When prepping the broccoli, be sure to keep the stems and florets separate.

½   **cup dried cherries**

1½   **pounds broccoli, florets cut into 1-inch pieces, stalks peeled and sliced ¼ inch thick**

1   **avocado, halved, pitted, and cut into ½-inch pieces**

2   **tablespoons extra-virgin olive oil**

1   **tablespoon white wine vinegar**

1   **garlic clove, minced**

1   **teaspoon grated orange zest plus 3 tablespoons juice**

    Kosher salt and pepper

½   **cup pecans, toasted and chopped coarse**

1   **shallot, sliced thin**

2   **tablespoons minced fresh parsley**

1. Bring 3 quarts water to boil in Dutch oven. Fill large bowl halfway with ice and water. Remove ½ cup boiling water and combine with cherries in small bowl; cover, let sit for 5 minutes, and then drain.

2. Meanwhile, add broccoli stalks to boiling water and cook for 1 minute. Add florets and cook until slightly tender, about 1 minute. Drain broccoli, transfer to ice water, and let sit until chilled, about 5 minutes. Drain broccoli again, transfer to salad spinner, and spin to remove excess moisture.

3. Process avocado, oil, vinegar, garlic, orange zest and juice, 1 teaspoon salt, and ¼ teaspoon pepper in food processor until smooth, scraping down sides of bowl as needed; transfer to large serving bowl. Add broccoli, soaked cherries, pecans, shallot, and parsley and toss to combine. Season with salt and pepper to taste. Serve.

VARIATION

Broccoli Salad with Cherry Tomatoes and Pepitas

Omit cherries and vinegar. Substitute 1½ teaspoons lime zest and 3 tablespoons lime juice (2 limes) for orange zest and juice and add ½ teaspoon chipotle chile powder to food processor with avocado. Substitute ½ cup toasted pepitas for pecans and 2 tablespoons minced fresh cilantro for parsley and add 1 cup cherry tomatoes, halved, to dressing with broccoli.

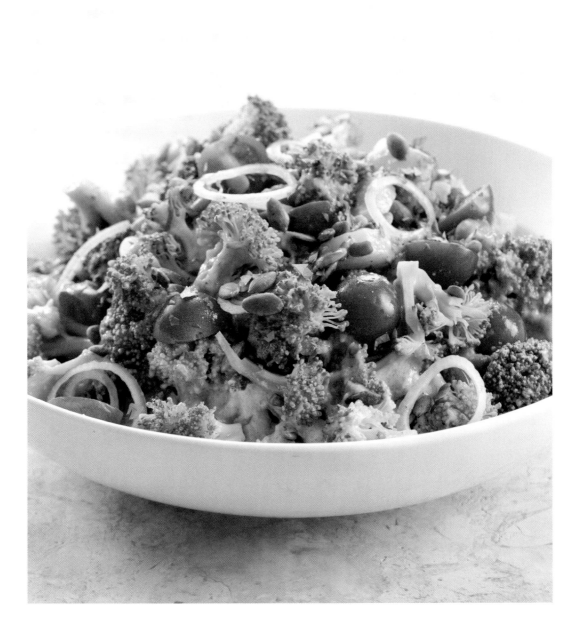

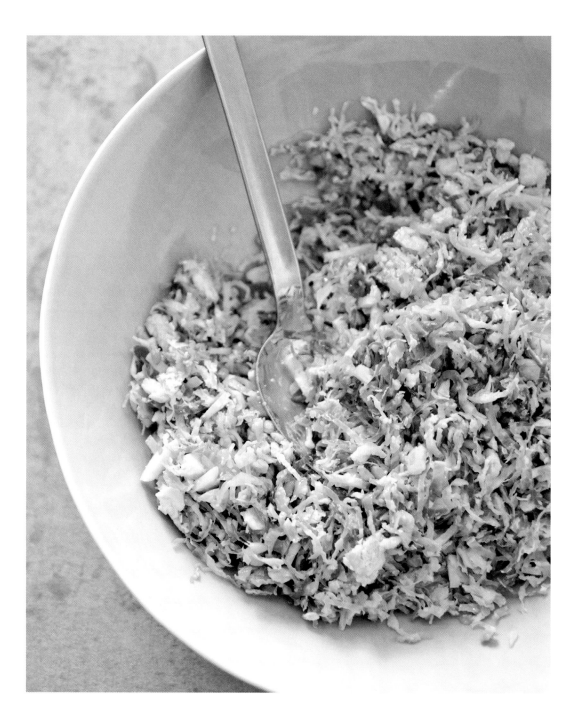

Brussels Sprout Salad

Serves 4

✓ **WHY THIS RECIPE WORKS** While roasting can bring out the intense flavor of Brussels sprouts, we don't always want to turn on the oven to enjoy this versatile vegetable. We wanted a light, bright, raw preparation that was just as delicious. To get the texture just right, we found that slicing the "little cabbages" superthin was key—leaving the sprouts whole or cutting them into larger chunks left us with underseasoned sprouts and a salad that didn't feel cohesive. Letting the shredded sprouts sit in the dressing for at least 30 minutes softened their raw crunch and seasoned them deeply. A simple, bright lemon vinaigrette, rounded out with aromatic shallot and mustard, complemented the earthy sprouts nicely. Adding toasted pine nuts just before serving provided a layer of crunch and nutty richness. Slicing the sprouts as thin as possible is important to the success of this dish.

3	tablespoons extra-virgin olive oil
2	tablespoons lemon juice
1	small shallot, minced
1	tablespoon Dijon mustard
1	garlic clove, minced
	Kosher salt and pepper
1	pound Brussels sprouts, trimmed, halved, and sliced very thin
½	cup pine nuts, toasted

1. Whisk oil, lemon juice, shallot, mustard, garlic, and 1 teaspoon salt together in large serving bowl. Add Brussels sprouts and toss to coat. Let salad sit for at least 30 minutes or up to 2 hours.

2. Stir pine nuts into salad and season with salt and pepper to taste. Serve.

VARIATIONS

Brussels Sprout Salad with Apple and Hazelnuts

Substitute ⅓ cup hazelnuts, toasted, skinned, and chopped, for pine nuts and add 1 small Granny Smith apple, cored and cut into 2-inch-long matchsticks, to Brussels sprouts with hazelnuts.

Brussels Sprout Salad with Currants and Almonds

Substitute ⅓ cup toasted slivered almonds for pine nuts and add ¼ cup currants to Brussels sprouts with almonds.

TEST KITCHEN TIP **SLICING BRUSSELS SPROUTS**

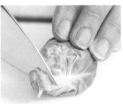

1. Trim stem ends of Brussels sprouts using sharp knife.

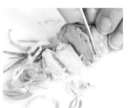

2. To ensure thorough seasoning, cut sprouts in half and slice very thin.

Roasted Carrot "Noodles"

Serves 4

✓ **WHY THIS RECIPE WORKS** We set out to create a simple and versatile carrot side that would work with a wide range of dishes. Roasting carrots draws out their natural sugars and intensifies their flavor—but the high heat can cause them to become dry, shriveled, and jerky-like. Using a spiralizer to cut the carrots into uniform ⅛-inch noodles ensured that the carrots cooked evenly, and cooking them covered for half the roasting time steamed them slightly and prevented them from drying out. We then uncovered the baking sheet and returned it to the oven to allow the noodles' surface moisture to evaporate, encouraging light caramelization and creating perfectly tender noodles. We kept the flavorings simple to allow the carrots' flavor to shine—just a handful of fresh thyme for earthy notes and a spoonful of honey to accent the carrots' natural sweetness. For the best noodles, use carrots that measure at least ¾ inch across at the thinnest end and 1½ inches across at the thickest end. For more information on spiralizing, see page 14.

2 **pounds carrots, trimmed and peeled**
2 **tablespoons extra-virgin olive oil**
2 **teaspoons minced fresh thyme**
1 **teaspoon honey**
  Kosher salt and pepper

1. Adjust oven rack to middle position and heat oven to 375 degrees. Using spiralizer, cut carrots into ⅛-inch-thick noodles, then cut noodles into 12-inch lengths. Toss carrots with 1 tablespoon oil, thyme, honey, 1 teaspoon salt, and ½ teaspoon pepper on rimmed baking sheet. Cover carrots tightly with aluminum foil and roast for 15 minutes. Remove foil and continue to roast until carrots are tender, 10 to 15 minutes.

2. Transfer carrots to serving platter, drizzle with remaining 1 tablespoon oil, and season with salt and pepper to taste. Serve.

VARIATIONS

Roasted Carrot "Noodles" with Garlic, Pepper Flakes, and Basil
Substitute 2 thinly sliced garlic cloves and ½ teaspoon red pepper flakes for thyme. Toss roasted carrots with oil and 1 tablespoon chopped fresh basil before serving.

Roasted Carrot "Noodles" with Shallot, Dill, and Orange
Substitute 1 thinly sliced shallot for thyme. Toss roasted carrots with oil, 1 tablespoon minced fresh dill, 1 teaspoon orange zest, and 1 tablespoon orange juice before serving.

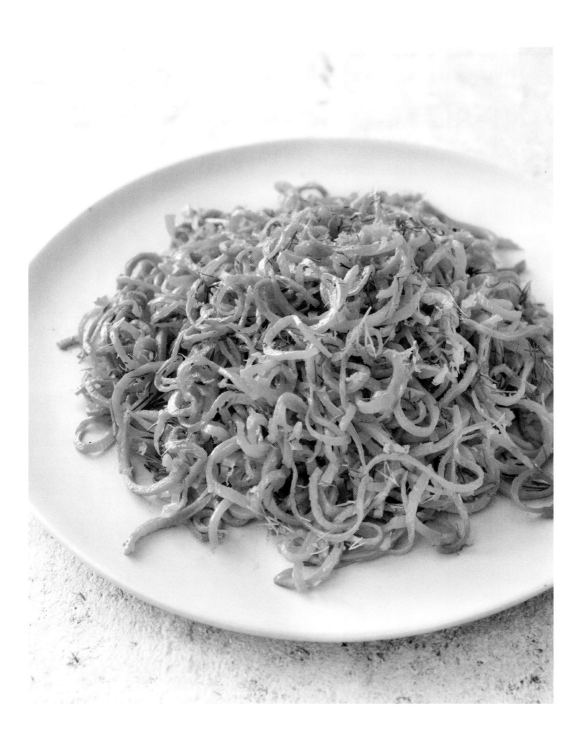

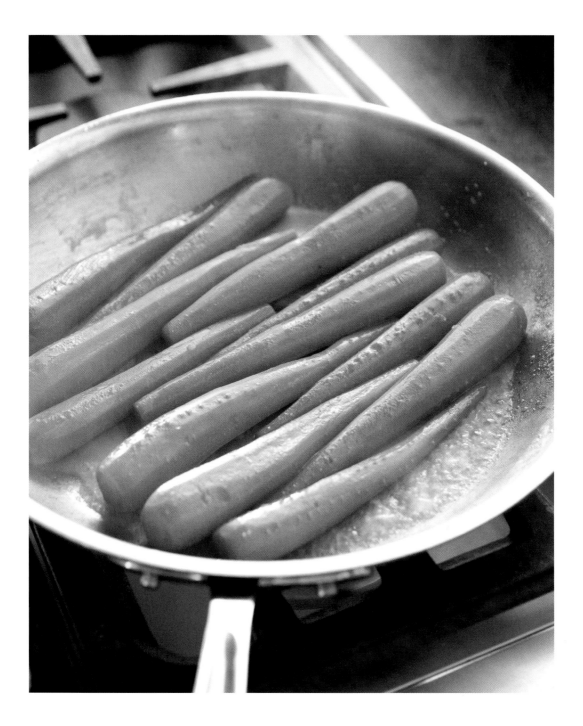

Slow-Cooked Whole Carrots

Serves 4 to 6

✓ **WHY THIS RECIPE WORKS** For sweet, tender carrots that would be impressive enough for company, we wanted to cook them whole—without the carrots becoming mushy or waterlogged. We first tried simmering them in water, but the tapered shape of the carrots made them cook unevenly and so the thinner ends overcooked by the time the thick ends were tender. Our science editor told us that cooking the carrots at a low temperature first would help them stay consistently firm through the rest of cooking by causing an enzymatic reaction that makes the carrots resistant to breaking down. With this in mind, we let the carrots "steep" off the heat for the first 20 minutes of cooking. We also topped the carrots with a circle of parchment paper during cooking to ensure that the moisture in the pan was evenly distributed. We finished cooking the carrots at a gentle simmer to evaporate the liquid and concentrate the carrots' flavor so that they tasted great when served on their own or with a flavorful relish. Use carrots that measure ¾ to 1¼ inches across at the thickest end.

3   **cups water**
1   **tablespoon extra-virgin olive oil**
1   **teaspoon kosher salt**
12 **carrots (1½ to 1¾ pounds), peeled**

1. Cut parchment paper into 11-inch circle, then cut 1-inch hole in center, folding paper as needed.

2. Bring water, oil, and salt to simmer in 12-inch skillet over high heat. Off heat, add carrots, top with parchment, cover skillet, and let sit for 20 minutes.

3. Uncover, leaving parchment in place, and bring to simmer over high heat. Reduce heat to medium-low and cook until most of water has evaporated and carrots are very tender, about 45 minutes.

4. Discard parchment, increase heat to medium-high, and cook carrots, shaking skillet often, until lightly glazed and no water remains, 2 to 4 minutes. Transfer carrots to serving platter and serve.

VARIATIONS

Slow-Cooked Whole Carrots with Green Olive and Raisin Relish

Microwave ⅓ cup raisins and 1 tablespoon water in bowl until hot, about 1 minute; let sit for 5 minutes. Stir in ½ cup chopped green olives, 1 minced shallot, 2 tablespoons extra-virgin olive oil, 1 tablespoon red wine vinegar, 1 tablespoon minced fresh parsley, ½ teaspoon ground fennel, and ½ teaspoon kosher salt. Spoon relish over carrots before serving.

Slow-Cooked Whole Carrots with Onion-Balsamic Relish

Heat 3 tablespoons extra-virgin olive oil in medium saucepan over medium heat until shimmering. Add 1 finely chopped red onion and ½ teaspoon kosher salt and cook until soft and brown, about 15 minutes. Stir in 2 minced garlic cloves and cook for 30 seconds. Stir in 2 tablespoons balsamic vinegar and cook for 1 minute. Let cool for 15 minutes. Stir in 2 tablespoons minced fresh mint. Spoon relish over carrots before serving.

TEST KITCHEN TIP **FOLDING PARCHMENT**

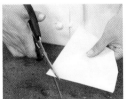

1. Cut parchment into 11-inch circle, then cut 1-inch hole in center, folding paper as needed to cut out hole.

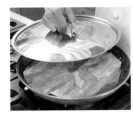

2. Lay parchment circle on top of carrots, underneath lid, to help retain and evenly distribute moisture during cooking.

Cauliflower Rice

Serves 4

✓ **WHY THIS RECIPE WORKS** In paleo cooking, cauliflower is often used in place of rice, since it's easy to process the florets into rice-size granules and it cooks up pleasantly fluffy. To make our cauliflower rice foolproof, we first needed to figure out the best way to chop the florets to the right size. We found that using the food processor made quick work of breaking down the florets and created a fairly consistent texture. Working in batches helped to ensure that all of the florets broke down evenly. Next, we needed to give our neutral-tasting cauliflower a boost in flavor; a shallot and a small amount of chicken broth did the trick. To ensure that the cauliflower was tender but still maintained a pleasant, rice-like chew, we first steamed the "rice" in a covered pot, then finished cooking it uncovered to evaporate any remaining moisture. We also decided to develop a couple of flavorful variations so that our cauliflower rice could accompany any number of meals. For the first one, we opted for a generously spiced curry profile and added sliced almonds for crunch and nuttiness. We also created a Tex-Mex inspired version with spicy fresh jalapeños, cumin, and cilantro. This recipe can be doubled; use a Dutch oven and increase the cooking time to about 25 minutes in step 2.

1   **head cauliflower (2 pounds), cored and cut into 1-inch florets (6 cups)**
1   **tablespoon extra-virgin olive oil**
1   **shallot, minced**
½   **cup Paleo Chicken Broth (page 16)**
     Kosher salt and pepper
2   **tablespoons minced fresh parsley (optional)**

1. Working in 2 batches, pulse cauliflower in food processor until finely ground into ¼- to ⅛-inch pieces, 6 to 8 pulses, scraping down sides of bowl as needed; transfer to bowl.

2. Heat oil in large saucepan over medium-low heat until shimmering. Add shallot and cook until softened, about 3 minutes. Stir in processed cauliflower, broth, and 1½ teaspoons salt. Cover and cook, stirring occasionally, until cauliflower is tender, 12 to 15 minutes.

3. Uncover and continue to cook until cauliflower rice is almost completely dry, about 3 minutes. Off heat, stir in parsley, if using, and season with salt and pepper to taste.

VARIATIONS

Curried Cauliflower Rice

Add ¼ teaspoon ground cardamom, ¼ teaspoon ground cinnamon, and ¼ teaspoon ground turmeric to saucepan with shallot. Substitute 1 tablespoon minced fresh mint for parsley and stir ¼ cup toasted sliced almonds into cauliflower rice with mint.

Tex-Mex Cauliflower Rice

Add 2 minced jalapeños, 1 minced garlic clove, 1 teaspoon ground cumin, and 1 teaspoon ground coriander to saucepan with shallot. Substitute 2 tablespoons minced fresh cilantro for parsley and stir 1 teaspoon lime juice into cauliflower rice with cilantro.

TEST KITCHEN TIP **MAKING CAULIFLOWER RICE**

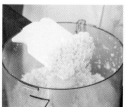

Working in batches, pulse cauliflower in food processor until finely ground into ¼- to ⅛-inch pieces.

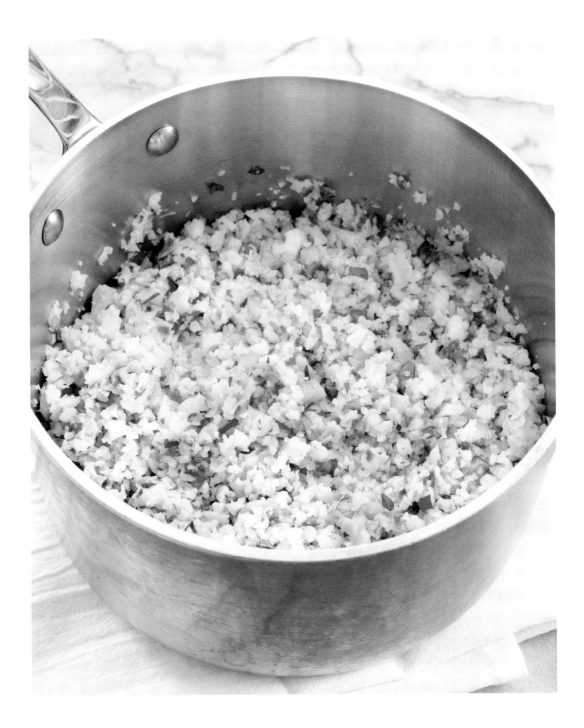

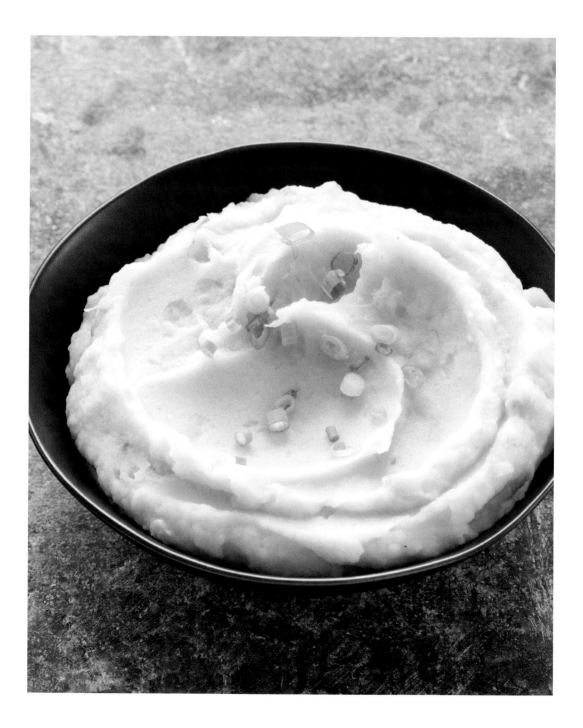

Celery Root Puree

Serves 4

✓ **WHY THIS RECIPE WORKS** In search of a paleo-friendly alternative to classic mashed potatoes, we mashed, milled, riced, and pureed a variety of different root vegetables—everything from parsnips to turnips to celery root. We tasted each vegetable on its own and in combination. In the end, tasters preferred the pleasantly mild flavor and velvety texture of celery root pureed in the food processor. To develop creaminess and character in our puree without the butter and cream typically used in mashed potatoes, we started by lightly sautéing our celery root in ghee, which concentrated its earthy flavor and added richness. To bring out even more depth of flavor, we simmered it in our homemade Paleo Chicken Broth, which we perfumed with some garlic, thyme, and bay leaf. To finish, we processed our celery root along with all of the rich, aromatic broth. Although starchy potatoes can turn gluey when whipped in a food processor, the celery root broke down beautifully into a perfectly smooth, luscious puree.

¼   **cup ghee**
4   **pounds celery root, peeled and cut into 1-inch pieces**
6   **garlic cloves, lightly crushed and peeled**
½   **cup Paleo Chicken Broth (page 16)**
2   **sprigs fresh thyme**
1   **bay leaf**
    Kosher salt and pepper

1. Melt ghee in large saucepan over medium heat. Add celery root and garlic and cook, stirring occasionally, until celery root is softened and lightly browned, 10 to 12 minutes. (If after 4 minutes celery root has not started to brown, increase heat to medium-high.)

2. Stir in broth, thyme sprigs, bay leaf, and 2 teaspoons salt. Reduce heat to low, cover, and cook, stirring occasionally, until celery root falls apart when poked with fork, about 40 minutes. Off heat, remove lid and allow steam to escape for 2 minutes.

3. Discard thyme sprigs and bay leaf. Working in batches, transfer contents of pot to food processor and process until smooth, about 2 minutes, scraping down sides of bowl as needed; transfer to serving bowl. Season with salt and pepper to taste. Serve.

VARIATION

Celery Root Puree with Horseradish and Scallions

Stir 2 tablespoons prepared horseradish and 4 thinly sliced scallions into celery root puree before serving.

TEST KITCHEN TIP **PEELING CELERY ROOT**

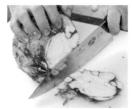

1. Using chef's knife, cut ½ inch from both root end and opposite end of celery root.

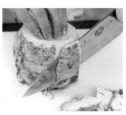

2. Turn celery root so 1 cut side rests on board. To peel, cut from top to bottom, rotating celery root while removing wide strips of skin.

Fennel Salad with Onion and Capers

Serves 4 to 6

✅ **WHY THIS RECIPE WORKS** We wanted a quick, flavorful salad that put often-overlooked fennel in the spotlight. Raw fennel has an appealingly crunchy texture and a mild licorice flavor that we wanted to bring out using contrasting flavors and textures. We quickly learned that to prevent tough, fibrous strands, it was important to slice the fennel thin. We wanted to keep the salad simple and bright; sliced red onion and a handful of briny capers complemented the fennel nicely. We created a lively dressing with honey, lemon, and Dijon. Letting the vegetables sit in the dressing softened their raw crunch and seasoned them deeply. Right before serving, we tossed in fresh whole parsley leaves, whose subtle flavor added balance and an herby freshness.

¼ cup extra-virgin olive oil

3 tablespoons lemon juice

2 teaspoons Dijon mustard

2 teaspoons honey

Kosher salt and pepper

2 fennel bulbs, stalks discarded, bulbs halved, cored, and sliced thin lengthwise

½ red onion, halved through root end and sliced thin crosswise

3 tablespoons capers, rinsed and minced

½ cup fresh parsley leaves

Whisk oil, lemon juice, mustard, honey, 2 teaspoons salt, and 1 teaspoon pepper together in large bowl. Add fennel, onion, and capers and toss to combine. Cover and refrigerate for 30 minutes. Stir in parsley and season with salt and pepper to taste. Serve.

VARIATIONS

Fennel Salad with Radishes and Tarragon

Omit capers. Add 6 thinly sliced radishes to dressing with fennel and substitute ¼ cup minced fresh tarragon for parsley.

Fennel Salad with Orange and Olives

Cut away peel and pith from 1 orange. Quarter orange, then slice crosswise into ½-inch-thick pieces. Substitute ¼ cup chopped pitted brine-cured black olives for capers and add orange to salad with parsley.

TEST KITCHEN TIP **PREPARING FENNEL**

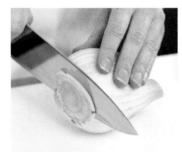

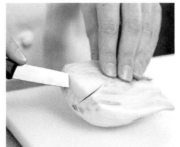

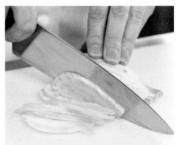

1. After cutting off stalks and feathery fronds, cut thin slice from base of fennel bulb and remove any tough blemished layers.

2. Cut bulb in half vertically through base, then use small knife to remove pyramid-shaped core.

3. Slice each half into thin slices to ensure best texture.

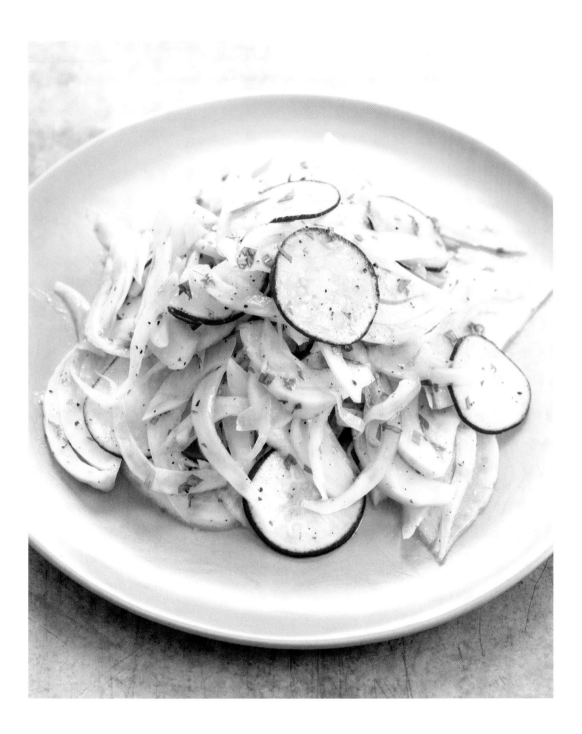

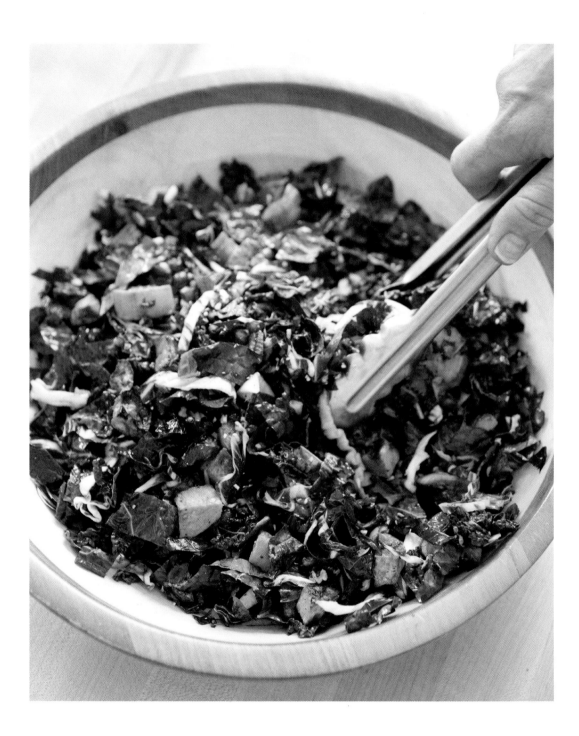

Kale Salad with Roasted Sweet Potatoes and Pomegranate

Serves 4 to 6

✔ WHY THIS RECIPE WORKS We love the earthy flavor of raw kale, but its texture can be a little tough. Many recipes call for tossing it with dressing and letting it tenderize in the fridge overnight. This method didn't deliver the tender leaves we were after, and the long sitting time wasn't very convenient. We discovered another technique that worked better and faster: massaging. Squeezing and massaging the kale broke down the cell walls in much the same way that heat would, darkening the leaves and turning them silky. Caramelized roasted sweet potatoes, shredded radicchio, crunchy pecans, a sprinkling of pomegranate seeds, and a flavorful balsamic vinaigrette turned our salad into a hearty side dish. Tuscan kale (also known as dinosaur or Lacinato kale) is more tender than curly-leaf and red kale; if using curly-leaf or red kale, increase the massaging time to 5 minutes. Do not use baby kale.

- 1½ **pounds sweet potatoes, peeled, quartered lengthwise, and sliced crosswise ½ inch thick**
- ⅓ **cup extra-virgin olive oil**
  Kosher salt and pepper
- 1 **small shallot, minced**
- 1 **tablespoon honey**
- 1 **tablespoon balsamic vinegar**
- 12 **ounces Tuscan kale, stemmed and sliced crosswise into ½-inch-wide strips (7 cups)**
- ½ **head radicchio (5 ounces), cored and sliced thin**
- ½ **cup pecans, toasted and chopped**
- ½ **cup pomegranate seeds**

1. Adjust oven rack to middle position and heat oven to 400 degrees. Toss sweet potatoes with 1 tablespoon oil and season with salt and pepper. Lay potatoes in single layer on rimmed baking sheet and roast until bottom edges are browned on both sides, 25 to 30 minutes, flipping potatoes halfway through roasting. Transfer potatoes to plate and let cool for 20 minutes.

2. Whisk shallot, honey, vinegar, ½ teaspoon salt, and ¼ teaspoon pepper together in large bowl. Whisking constantly, gradually drizzle in remaining oil until emulsified.

3. Place kale in large bowl or on counter. Vigorously squeeze and massage kale with your hands until leaves are uniformly darkened and slightly wilted, about 1 minute. Add kale, radicchio, and roasted sweet potatoes to vinaigrette and gently toss to combine. Transfer salad to serving platter and sprinkle with pecans and pomegranate seeds. Serve.

TEST KITCHEN TIP **MASSAGING KALE**

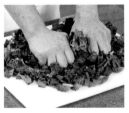

Vigorously squeeze and massage kale with your hands on counter or in large bowl until leaves are uniformly darkened and wilted, about 1 minute.

Roasted Mushrooms

Serves 4

✓ **WHY THIS RECIPE WORKS** From earthy and smoky to deep and woodsy, mushrooms have an amazing range of flavors and textures. We decided to develop a simple side that would showcase this versatile ingredient. We found that a combination of full-flavored cremini and meaty, smoky shiitakes gave us the deepest, most well-rounded flavor. As for our cooking method, we quickly ruled out work-intensive sautéing, which required us to cook the mushrooms in multiple batches to achieve good browning. Instead, we turned to the oven, roasting the mushrooms until they were deeply browned. But this presented a new problem: Since roasting concentrates flavor, the seasoning became more noticeable. Tasters immediately picked up on the fact that the mushrooms were unevenly seasoned—some were inedibly salty, while others were quite bland. To remedy this, we brined the mushrooms briefly in salted water before cooking. This not only ensured even seasoning in all of the mushrooms, but also seasoned them more deeply and thoroughly than salt alone. The excess water easily evaporated away during cooking. Finally, we coated the mushrooms in a simple vinaigrette of olive oil and lemon juice, and stirred in pine nuts for crunch and nuttiness and parsley for complementary freshness.

Kosher salt and pepper

1½ pounds cremini mushrooms, trimmed and left whole if small, halved if medium, or quartered if large

1 pound shiitake mushrooms, stemmed, caps larger than 3 inches halved

3 tablespoons extra-virgin olive oil

1 teaspoon lemon juice

2 tablespoons pine nuts, toasted

2 tablespoons chopped fresh parsley

1. Adjust oven rack to lowest position and heat oven to 450 degrees. Dissolve 3 tablespoons salt in 2 quarts room-temperature water in large container. Add cremini mushrooms and shiitake mushrooms to brine, cover with plate or bowl to submerge, and let stand for 10 minutes.

2. Drain mushrooms in colander and pat dry with paper towels. Toss mushrooms with 2 tablespoons oil on rimmed baking sheet, then spread into even layer. Roast until liquid from mushrooms has completely evaporated, 35 to 45 minutes.

3. Remove sheet from oven (be careful of escaping steam when opening oven) and, using thin metal spatula, carefully stir mushrooms. Return to oven and continue to roast until mushrooms are deeply browned, 5 to 10 minutes longer.

4. Whisk remaining 1 tablespoon oil and lemon juice together in large bowl. Add mushrooms and toss to coat. Stir in pine nuts and parsley and season with salt and pepper to taste. Serve immediately.

VARIATION

Roasted Mushrooms with Sesame and Scallions

Substitute 2 teaspoons toasted sesame oil for remaining 1 tablespoon extra-virgin olive oil in step 4. Substitute 1½ teaspoons rice vinegar for lemon juice, 2 teaspoons toasted sesame seeds for pine nuts, and 2 thinly sliced scallions for parsley.

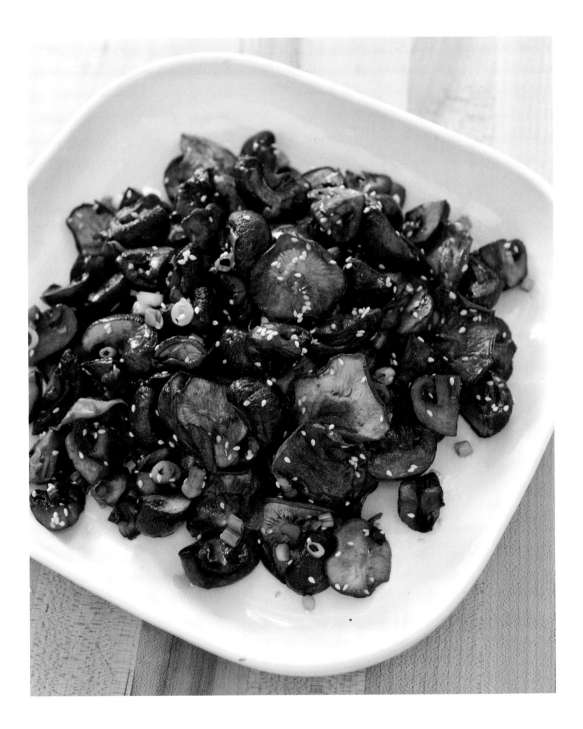

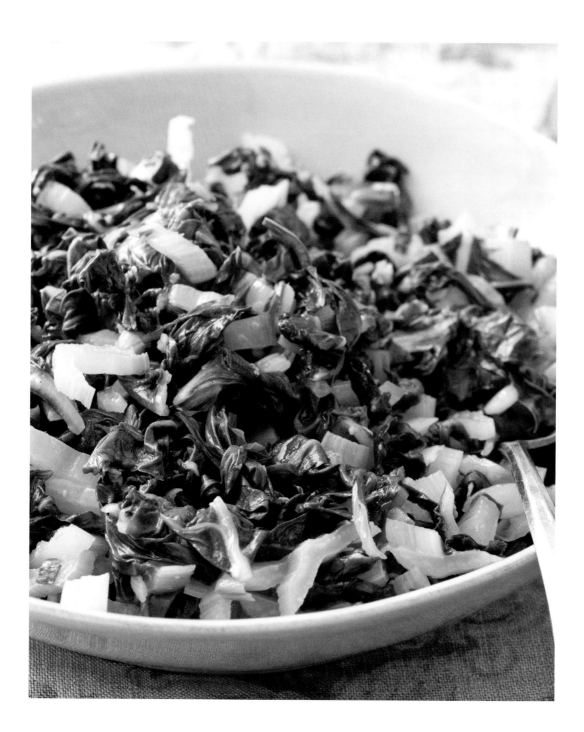

Garlicky Swiss Chard

Serves 4 to 6

✓ **WHY THIS RECIPE WORKS** We wanted a one-pot approach to cooking hearty, flavorful Swiss chard. To avoid watery, overcooked chard, we started cooking the greens in a covered pot just until they wilted down. Then we uncovered the pot and continued to cook the greens until all the liquid evaporated. Cutting the tough stems smaller than the tender leaves meant that we could throw both in the pot at the same time and still get evenly cooked results. Plenty of garlic, sautéed in olive oil before the chard was added, gave this simple side a big hit of flavor, while a splash of mild white wine vinegar and red pepper flakes added brightness and subtle heat. You can use any variety of chard for this recipe. The recipe is easily doubled and cooked in two batches.

2	tablespoons plus 1 teaspoon extra-virgin olive oil
6	garlic cloves, minced
2	pounds Swiss chard, stems sliced crosswise ¼ inch thick, leaves sliced into ½-inch-wide strips
	Kosher salt and pepper
⅛	teaspoon red pepper flakes
1	teaspoon white wine vinegar

1. Heat 2 tablespoons oil and garlic in Dutch oven over medium-low heat, stirring occasionally, until garlic is light golden, about 3 minutes. Stir in chard, ½ teaspoon salt, and pepper flakes. Increase heat to high, cover, and cook, stirring occasionally, until chard is wilted but still bright green, 2 to 4 minutes.

2. Uncover and continue to cook, stirring often, until liquid evaporates, 4 to 6 minutes. Stir in vinegar and remaining 1 teaspoon oil and season with salt and pepper to taste. Transfer to bowl and serve.

TEST KITCHEN TIP **PREPPING HEARTY GREENS**

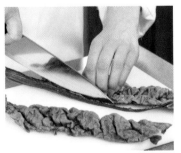

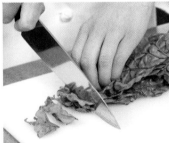

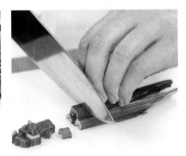

1. Cut leafy green portion away from either side of stalk using chef's knife.

2. Stack several leaves on top of one another and slice ½ inch wide. Wash and dry leaves after slicing, using salad spinner.

3. Wash stems thoroughly, then trim and cut into ¼-inch-thick pieces.

Slow-Cooker Mashed Sweet Potatoes

Serves 6

✔ **WHY THIS RECIPE WORKS** With their deep, natural sweetness and vibrant orange flesh, sweet potatoes can round out many a meal—from rich spicy stews to smoky grilled meats. We wanted a recipe for mashed sweet potatoes that would allow these humble tubers to shine. Using a slow cooker trapped moisture, allowing us to use just enough water to steam the potatoes without watering down the mash. We thinly sliced the potatoes and pressed a piece of parchment on top of them so that the moisture would be evenly distributed. To keep the recipe simple and streamlined, we mashed the sweet potatoes by hand right in the slow cooker. Finally, we added richness and a slight nutty flavor by folding in a bit of ghee. This dish can be held on the warm setting for up to 2 hours; loosen with hot water as needed before serving. You will need a 5½- to 7-quart slow cooker for this recipe.

3   pounds sweet potatoes, peeled and
    sliced ¼ inch thick
½   cup water, plus extra as needed
    Kosher salt and pepper
3   tablespoons ghee, melted

1. Combine potatoes, water, and 1 teaspoon salt in slow cooker. Grease 16 by 12-inch sheet of parchment paper and press firmly onto potatoes, folding down edges as needed. Cover and cook until potatoes are tender, 5 to 6 hours on low or 3 to 4 hours on high.

2. Discard parchment. Mash potatoes with potato masher until smooth. Fold in melted ghee and season with salt and pepper to taste. Serve.

VARIATIONS

Slow-Cooker Mashed Sweet Potatoes with Garam Masala and Ginger

Add 2 teaspoons garam masala to slow cooker with potatoes. Fold ⅓ cup raisins, ¼ cup toasted sliced almonds, and 2 teaspoons grated fresh ginger into mashed potatoes with ghee.

Slow-Cooker Mashed Sweet Potatoes with Cilantro and Lime

Substitute 3 tablespoons extra-virgin olive oil for ghee. Fold 3 tablespoons minced fresh cilantro, 1 teaspoon grated lime zest, and 2 teaspoons lime juice into mashed sweet potatoes with olive oil. Season with additional lime juice to taste.

TEST KITCHEN TIP

CREATING A PARCHMENT SHIELD

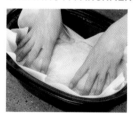

To create parchment shield, press 16 by 12-inch sheet of greased parchment firmly onto potatoes, folding down edges as needed.

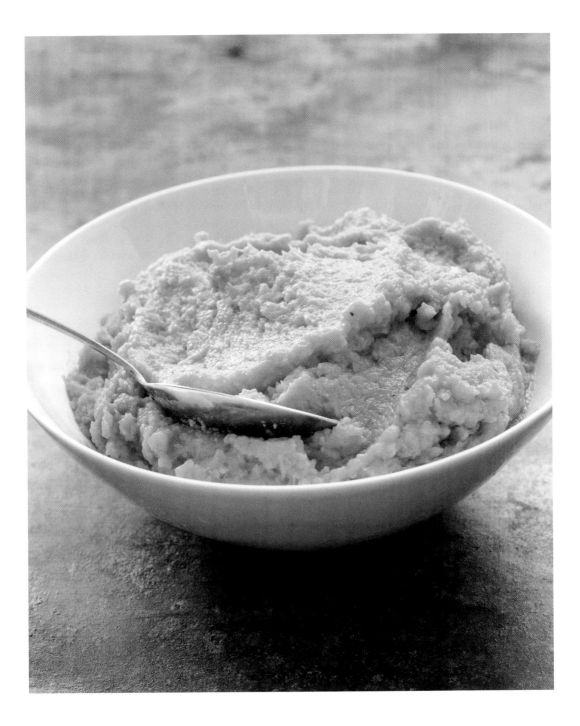

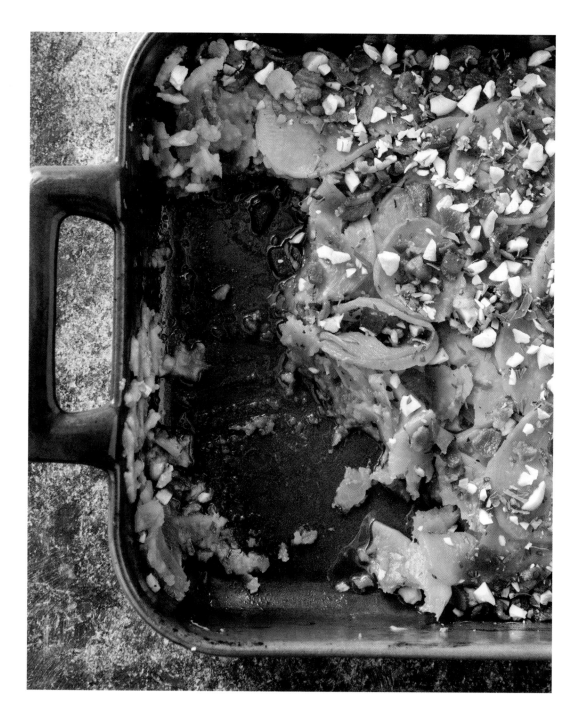

Sweet Potato Gratin

Serves 6 to 8

☑ **WHY THIS RECIPE WORKS** A classic potato gratin makes a hearty, comforting side dish, but the white potatoes, creamy sauce, and cheesy topping put it out of reach for anyone on the paleo diet. We wanted to make a paleo-friendly gratin with all the flavor and appeal of traditional ones. To replace typical russet potatoes, we decided to use earthy sweet potatoes. Next, we set out to find a way to build flavor and richness without relying on a cream sauce. We tested gratins made with a cashew-based cream, but the process was too laborious for the mediocre results. Instead, we decided to forgo the sauce entirely; we added savory depth and heartiness with bacon. We cooked the bacon and reserved the fat; we tossed some of the fat with the potatoes before they went into the casserole dish, and used the rest of the fat to sauté onions until they were deep golden. We layered the onions with the potatoes, and poured chicken broth over the top of the casserole to give the gratin a thick, luxurious consistency. Baking the gratin covered for most of the baking time ensured that the potatoes were tender and creamy, not dry. Finally, we replaced the typical cheesy topping with a mixture of crispy bacon, toasted cashews, and fresh parsley, which gave the dish both extra flavor and a nice textural element.

6   slices bacon, chopped
3   pounds sweet potatoes, peeled and sliced ⅛ inch thick
2   teaspoons minced fresh thyme
    Kosher salt and pepper
2   onions, halved and sliced thin
2   garlic cloves, minced
1   cup Paleo Chicken Broth (page 16)
⅓   cup raw cashews, toasted and chopped fine
2   tablespoons minced fresh parsley

1. Adjust oven rack to upper-middle position and heat oven to 400 degrees. Grease 13 by 9-inch baking dish. Cook bacon in 12-inch skillet over medium heat until crisp, 8 to 10 minutes. Using slotted spoon, transfer bacon to paper towel–lined plate; set aside. (You should have 5 tablespoons fat; if not, add extra-virgin olive oil as needed to equal 5 tablespoons.)

2. Toss potatoes with 3 tablespoons fat from skillet, 1 teaspoon thyme, 1 teaspoon salt, and ½ teaspoon pepper; set aside.

3. Heat fat left in skillet over medium heat until shimmering. Add onions, ½ teaspoon salt, and ¼ teaspoon pepper and cook until softened and well browned, 10 to 15 minutes. Stir in garlic and remaining 1 teaspoon thyme and cook until fragrant, about 30 seconds. Stir in ¼ cup broth, scraping up any browned bits, and cook until almost completely evaporated, about 1 minute.

4. Arrange half of potatoes in prepared dish, spread onion mixture in even layer over potatoes, and distribute remaining potatoes over onions. Pour remaining ¾ cup broth over potatoes. Cover dish tightly with aluminum foil and bake for 45 minutes.

5. Remove foil and continue to bake until potatoes are completely tender, about 15 minutes. Let cool for 15 minutes. Sprinkle gratin with crisp bacon, cashews, and parsley. Serve.

Roasted Butternut Squash with Cilantro and Sesame

Serves 4 to 6

✔ **WHY THIS RECIPE WORKS** While butter and brown sugar are common accompaniments to roasted squash, we sought to create a paleo-friendly, savory preparation that would be simple and delicious. We peeled the squash thoroughly to remove not only the tough outer skin but also the rugged fibrous layer of white flesh just beneath, ensuring supremely tender squash. To encourage the squash slices to caramelize, we used a hot 425-degree oven, placed the baking sheet on the lowest oven rack, and let the squash bake until almost all of the moisture had evaporated and the slices were beautifully caramelized. Finally, we selected a mix of toppings that added crunch, brightness, and visual appeal. A simple vinaigrette of olive oil and lemon juice added flavor and tang. Coriander and sesame seeds, toasted to bring out their flavor, added a textured crunch and nuttiness, while thyme added a subtle, herbal aroma. Finally, cilantro added bright freshness. For the best texture it's important to remove the fibrous flesh just below the squash's skin. This dish can be served warm or at room temperature.

2½-3   **pounds butternut squash**
3   **tablespoons ghee, melted**
    Kosher salt and pepper
4   **teaspoons extra-virgin olive oil**
1   **teaspoon lemon juice**
¼   **cup fresh cilantro leaves**
1   **teaspoon minced fresh thyme**
    or ¼ teaspoon dried
1   **teaspoon sesame seeds, toasted**
1   **teaspoon coriander seeds,**
    toasted and crushed

1. Adjust oven rack to lowest position and heat oven to 425 degrees. Using sharp vegetable peeler or chef's knife, remove skin and fibrous threads from squash just below skin (peel until squash is completely orange with no white flesh remaining, roughly ⅛ inch deep). Halve squash lengthwise and scrape out seeds. Place squash cut side down on cutting board and slice crosswise ½ inch thick.

2. Toss squash with melted ghee, 1 teaspoon salt, and ½ teaspoon pepper and arrange on rimmed baking sheet in single layer. Roast squash until side touching sheet toward back of oven is well browned, 25 to 30 minutes. Rotate sheet and continue to bake until side touching sheet toward back of oven is well browned, 6 to 10 minutes. Remove squash from oven and use metal spatula to flip each piece. Continue to roast until squash is very tender and side touching sheet is browned, 10 to 15 minutes. Transfer squash to serving platter.

3. Whisk oil, lemon juice, and ¼ teaspoon salt together in bowl, then drizzle over squash. Sprinkle with cilantro, thyme, sesame seeds, and coriander seeds. Serve.

TEST KITCHEN TIP
PEELING BUTTERNUT SQUASH

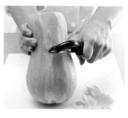

Trim ends of squash. Use vegetable peeler or knife to remove skin and fibrous layer from squash until squash has no white flesh remaining.

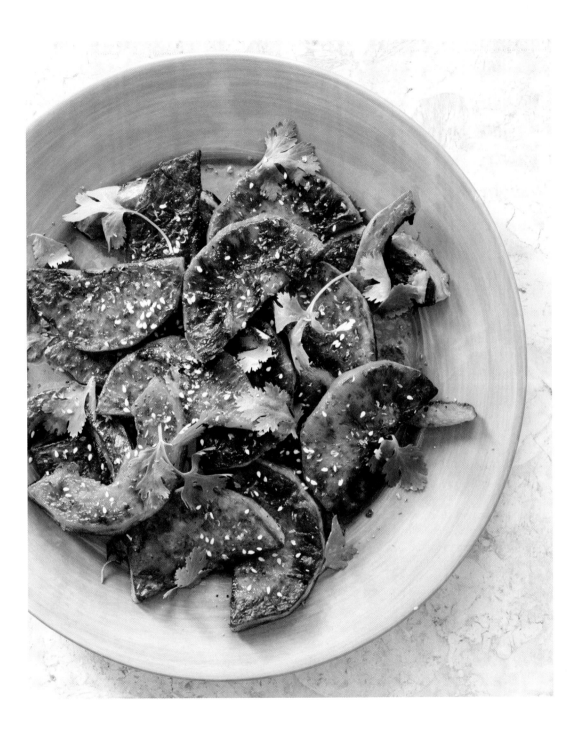

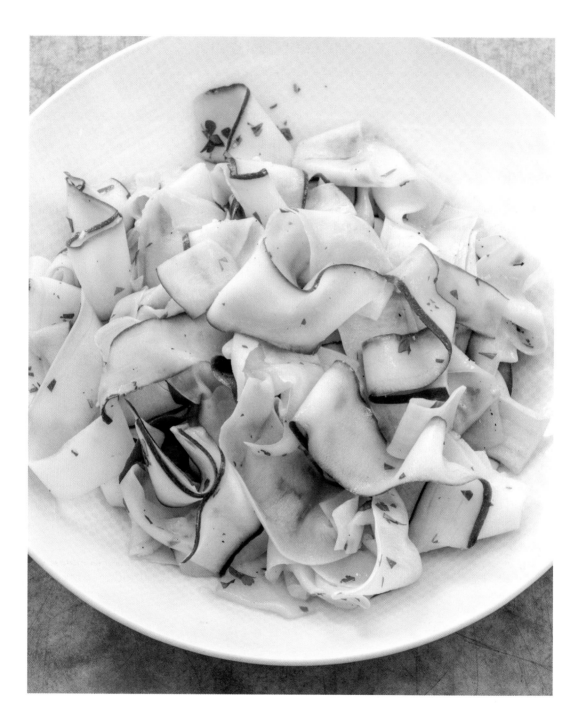

Sautéed Summer Squash Ribbons

Serves 4

✔ WHY THIS RECIPE WORKS Summer squash and zucchini make great side dishes; they cook quickly and have creamy, delicately flavored flesh that pairs perfectly with most proteins. But summer squash and zucchini contain a lot of excess moisture that can inhibit browning and result in a mushy, unpleasant texture. To avoid this, many recipes call for salting and draining or shredding and wringing the squash to remove moisture, but these steps can be time-consuming for what should be a simple side dish. We found that we could avoid the extra work by starting with very thinly sliced squash. We used a peeler to make evenly thin "ribbons," discarding the waterlogged seeds. The ultrathin ribbons browned and cooked so quickly that they didn't have time to break down and release their liquid. The delicate cooked squash needed little embellishment; a quick, tangy vinaigrette of extra-virgin olive oil, garlic, and lemon and a sprinkle of fresh parsley rounded out the flavors. We like a mix of summer squash and zucchini, but you can use just one or the other. The thickness of the squash ribbons may vary depending on the peeler used; we developed this recipe with our winning Kuhn Rikon Original Swiss peeler, which produces ribbons that are 1/32 inch thick. Steeping the minced garlic in lemon juice mellows the garlic's bite; do not skip this step. To avoid overcooking the squash, start checking for doneness at the lower end of the cooking time.

1 small garlic clove, minced

1 teaspoon grated lemon zest plus
    1 tablespoon juice

4 (6- to 8-ounce) yellow squash or zucchini,
    trimmed

2 tablespoons plus 1 teaspoon extra-virgin
    olive oil
    Kosher salt and pepper

1½ tablespoons chopped fresh parsley

1. Combine garlic and lemon juice in large bowl and set aside for at least 10 minutes. Using vegetable peeler, shave each squash lengthwise into ribbons: Shave off 3 ribbons from 1 side, then turn squash 90 degrees and shave off 3 more ribbons. Continue to turn and shave ribbons until you reach seeds; discard core.

2. Whisk 2 tablespoons oil, ½ teaspoon salt, ⅛ teaspoon pepper, and lemon zest into garlic/lemon juice mixture.

3. Heat remaining 1 teaspoon oil in 12-inch nonstick skillet over medium-high heat until just smoking. Add squash and cook, tossing occasionally with tongs, until squash has softened and is translucent, 3 to 4 minutes. Transfer squash to bowl with dressing, add parsley, and toss to coat. Season with salt and pepper to taste. Transfer to serving platter and serve immediately.

VARIATION

Sautéed Summer Squash Ribbons with Mint and Pistachios

Omit lemon zest and substitute 1½ teaspoons cider vinegar for lemon juice. Substitute ⅓ cup chopped fresh mint for parsley and sprinkle squash with 2 tablespoons toasted and chopped pistachios before serving.

TEST KITCHEN TIP **MAKING SQUASH RIBBONS**

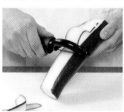

Using vegetable peeler, shave 3 ribbons from squash. Turn squash 90 degrees. Continue shaving ribbons and turning squash until you reach seeds.

Nutritional Information for Our Recipes

Analyzing recipes for their nutritional values is a tricky business, and we did our best to be as realistic and accurate as possible throughout this book. We were absolutely strict about measuring when cooking and never resorted to guessing or estimating. And we never made the portion sizes unreasonably small to make the nutritional numbers appear lower. We also didn't play games when analyzing the recipes in the nutritional program to make the numbers look better. To calculate the nutritional values of our recipes per serving, we used The Food Processor SQL by ESHA Research. When using this program, we entered all the ingredients, including optional ones, using weights for important ingredients such as meat, cheese, and most vegetables. We also used all of our preferred brands in these analyses. Yet there are two tricky ingredients to be mindful of when analyzing a recipe—salt and fat—that require some special rules of their own.

When the recipe called for seasoning with an unspecified amount of salt and pepper (often raw meat), we added 1 teaspoon salt and ¼ teaspoon pepper to the analysis. We did not, however, include additional salt or pepper in our analysis when the food was "seasoned to taste" at the end of cooking. As for fat, it can be difficult to accurately predict the amount of oil retained during cooking. We compared our recipes, without any added cooking fat, to similar foods in The Food Processor SQL to estimate how much fat was absorbed during cooking. We then added the estimated amount of fat back into our nutritional analysis to calculate our final numbers.

Note: Unless otherwise indicated, information applies to a single serving. If there is a range in the serving size in the recipe, we used the highest number of servings to calculate the nutritional values.

	Cal	Fat (g)	Sat Fat (g)	Chol (mg)	Carb (g)	Protein (g)	Fiber (g)	Sodium (mg)
PALEO BASICS								
Ghee*	130	14	9	40	0	0	0	0
Paleo Chicken Broth**	20	0	0	0	0	4	0	276
Paleo Beef Broth**	53	0	0	0	0	13	0	248
Paleo Vegetable Broth**	9	0	0	0	0	1	0	288
Paleo Mayonnaise*	50	5	1	25	0	0	0	40
Paleo Ketchup*	35	0	0	0	10	0	0	160
Paleo Barbecue Sauce*	15	1	0	0	2	0	0	65
Paleo Dijon Mustard*	25	1.5	0	0	2	1	1	140
Paleo Whole-Grain Mustard*	25	1	0	0	2	1	0	105
Paleo Tomato Sauce**	130	6	1	0	17	4	5	450
Paleo Coconut Milk**	60	5	5	0	1	0	0	150
Paleo Almond Milk**	40	3	0	0	2	1	1	180

*Serving size for these items is 1 tablespoon.
**Serving size for these items is 1 cup.
***Serving size for pie crust is ⅛ of crust.

	Cal	Fat (g)	Sat Fat (g)	Chol (mg)	Carb (g)	Protein (g)	Fiber (g)	Sodium (mg)
Paleo Almond Yogurt**	40	3	0	0	2	1	1	180
Paleo Cashew Nut Cheese*	60	6	1	0	3	2	0	35
Paleo Wraps	190	14	2	30	12	5	3	210
Paleo Sandwich Rolls	400	28	3	45	33	11	8	460
Paleo Single-Crust Pie Dough***	270	22	8	0	16	7	4	170

APPETIZERS AND SNACKS

	Cal	Fat (g)	Sat Fat (g)	Chol (mg)	Carb (g)	Protein (g)	Fiber (g)	Sodium (mg)
Whipped Cashew Nut Dip with Roasted Red Peppers and Olives	220	19	3	0	10	5	1	370
Whipped Cashew Nut Dip with Chipotle and Lime	200	17	3	0	9	5	1	210
Whipped Cashew Nut Dip with Sun-Dried Tomatoes and Rosemary	210	18	3	0	10	5	1	230
Baba Ghanoush	80	6	1	0	8	2	3	210
Sweet Potato Hummus	140	9	1.5	0	12	2	2	240
Parsnip Hummus	140	9	1.5	0	12	2	3	220
Chicken Liver Pâté	210	17	9	185	4	8	1	360
Seeded Crackers	260	22	3	0	11	7	4	180
Kale Chips	70	3.5	0	0	8	3	2	320
Ranch-Style Kale Chips	70	3.5	0	0	9	3	2	320
Spicy Sesame-Ginger Kale Chips	80	4.5	0.5	0	9	3	2	320
Spiced Nuts	270	20	3.5	0	18	9	2	240
Curry-Spiced Nuts	270	20	3.5	0	17	9	2	240
Chipotle-Spiced Nuts	270	20	3.5	0	17	9	2	240
Orange and Fennel–Spiced Nuts	270	20	3.5	0	17	9	2	240
Prosciutto-Wrapped Stuffed Dates	220	11	1.5	15	29	7	3	430
Prosciutto-Wrapped Stuffed Dates with Pistachios and Balsamic Vinegar	210	8	1.5	15	31	7	3	430
Beef Jerky	80	2.5	1	30	3	10	1	530
Spinach and Bacon–Stuffed Mushrooms	250	21	4	5	11	7	2	370
Beef Satay with Spicy Almond Sauce	230	13	2.5	55	6	22	2	490

	Cal	Fat (g)	Sat Fat (g)	Chol (mg)	Carb (g)	Protein (g)	Fiber (g)	Sodium (mg)
APPETIZERS AND SNACKS (CONT.)								
Oven-Baked Buffalo Wings	270	20	8	130	2	18	0	910
Oven-Baked Honey-Mustard Wings	290	20	8	130	9	18	0	630
Broiled Shrimp Cocktail with Tarragon Sauce	190	17	8	85	1	8	0	470
BREAKFAST FAVORITES								
Sweet Potato and Celery Root Hash with Fried Eggs	500	32	14	420	35	19	6	860
Poached Eggs in Spicy Tomato Sauce	310	20	4.5	370	18	15	3	1040
Scrambled Eggs with Easy Homemade Sausage and Bell Pepper	320	25	11	420	3	19	1	350
Scrambled Eggs with Easy Homemade Sausage and Asparagus	320	25	11	420	2	20	1	350
Family-Size Omelet with Bacon and Spinach	400	32	11	410	6	21	1	680
Family-Size Omelet with Bacon, Tomato, and Bell Pepper	410	32	11	410	8	21	2	660
Leek and Prosciutto Frittata	300	19	8	405	12	19	1	760
Wild Mushroom Frittata	240	17	4	370	6	15	1	240
Spiced Breakfast Casserole with Tomatoes and Swiss Chard	270	19	8	270	14	13	4	660
Homemade Breakfast Sausage	110	7	4	45	1	10	0	180
Homemade Apple-Fennel Breakfast Sausage	120	7	4	45	2	10	0	180
Blueberry Muffins	330	20	4.5	45	36	8	5	280
Applesauce-Spice Muffins	350	21	5	45	37	8	5	280
Pancakes	440	34	8	90	26	13	5	240
Blueberry Pancakes	460	34	8	90	29	13	6	240
Nut and Seed Granola	320	24	9	0	22	5	5	65
Tropical Nut and Seed Granola	340	27	10	0	22	6	5	65
All-Morning Energy Bars	170	11	1.5	0	15	6	3	95
Almond Yogurt Parfaits	410	26	2.5	0	37	13	12	140
Almond Yogurt Parfaits with Pineapple and Kiwi	460	29	3	0	46	15	10	140
Almond Yogurt Parfaits with Dates, Oranges, and Bananas	580	26	2.5	0	83	14	14	135

	Cal	Fat (g)	Sat Fat (g)	Chol (mg)	Carb (g)	Protein (g)	Fiber (g)	Sodium (mg)
POULTRY								
Chicken "Noodle" Soup	190	8	3	75	7	22	2	690
Slow-Cooker Southwestern Chicken Soup	250	12	2	60	11	25	5	760
Chicken Salad with Bacon and Tomatoes	280	17	4.5	75	4	26	1	470
Thai Chicken Lettuce Wraps	230	8	4.5	105	13	25	2	710
Nut-Crusted Chicken Breasts	740	46	20	265	32	49	6	700
Chicken with Mexican Pumpkin Seed Sauce	650	39	9	175	11	63	4	620
Pan-Roasted Chicken Breasts with Zucchini and Cherry Tomatoes	500	23	6	170	11	62	3	630
Grilled Greek-Style Chicken Kebabs	600	34	5	165	19	53	3	670
Grilled Chipotle-Lime Chicken Breasts with Shaved Zucchini and Avocado Salad	520	33	5	125	14	41	6	650
Grilled Lemon-Garlic Chicken Breasts with Fennel and Arugula Salad	640	36	7	165	16	64	6	690
Rustic Braised Chicken with Mushrooms	420	17	4.5	175	9	56	2	560
Slow-Cooker Curried Chicken Thighs with Acorn Squash	510	28	5	160	30	36	4	730
Slow-Cooker Caribbean Chicken Drumsticks	400	25	11	220	6	39	1	560
Braised Chicken Thighs with Swiss Chard and Carrots	570	32	9	245	25	45	8	1240
Latin-Style Chicken and Cauliflower Rice	400	18	2.5	125	18	44	6	990
Stir-Fried Chicken and Broccoli with Sesame-Orange Sauce	440	27	9	85	23	31	6	610
Gingery Stir-Fried Chicken with Asparagus and Bell Pepper	440	26	9	85	20	33	4	600
Batter-Fried Chicken Fingers	500	31	21	110	21	36	2	410
Honey-Mustard Dipping Sauce*	50	0	0	0	13	0	0	160
Ranch Dipping Sauce*	5	0	0	0	0	0	0	60
One-Pan Roast Chicken with Root Vegetables	710	38	15	210	37	56	9	990
Roast Chicken with Mushroom Pan Sauce	550	32	9	170	6	55	1	690
Peruvian Roast Chicken with Sweet Potatoes	690	29	7	165	50	56	9	840
Roast Cornish Game Hens	570	40	11	280	1	48	0	1840
Pan-Seared Duck Breasts with Melon Relish	460	22	6	230	20	43	3	450
Turkey Breast with Shallot-Porcini Gravy	530	22	6	185	6	72	1	450

*Serving size for these items is 1 tablespoon.

	Cal	Fat (g)	Sat Fat (g)	Chol (mg)	Carb (g)	Protein (g)	Fiber (g)	Sodium (mg)
BEEF, PORK, LAMB, AND MORE								
Ultimate Beef Stew	420	15	4.5	145	14	53	3	400
Slow-Cooker Oxtail Soup	270	8	3	100	13	35	3	710
Bison Chili	390	23	8	80	24	25	6	630
Ultimate Burgers	350	22	10	125	0	37	0	780
Ultimate Burgers with Caramelized Onions and Bacon	490	33	14	145	7	41	2	960
Steak Tips with Mushroom-Onion Gravy	380	19	4.5	110	10	39	2	810
Grilled Beef and Vegetable Kebabs	560	34	9	160	12	54	3	400
Spicy Thai Grilled Beef Salad	290	10	4	95	12	37	3	700
Seared Flank Steak with Chimichurri Sauce	540	42	9	95	3	35	1	920
Tuscan-Style Steaks with Garlicky Spinach	630	41	11	190	6	56	3	520
Pan-Seared Steaks with Tomato and Watercress Salad	410	21	5	120	8	46	2	390
Pepper-Crusted Venison with Béarnaise Sauce	810	64	27	340	2	54	0	1030
Shredded Beef Tacos with Cabbage Slaw	670	38	7	160	38	47	11	1340
Zucchini "Spaghetti" and Meatballs	560	35	9	125	32	31	7	600
Butternut Squash "Spaghetti" and Meatballs	730	43	12	125	61	29	11	590
Shepherd's Pie	530	20	9	115	16	72	5	1370
Spicy Korean-Style Stir-Fried Beef	350	18	12	80	18	28	5	610
French Pot Roast with Mustard-Parsley Sauce	370	14	4	130	13	46	4	620
Slow-Cooker Italian-Style Pot Roast	380	16	6	140	11	47	3	550
Pomegranate-Braised Beef Short Ribs	480	25	10	115	24	38	1	720
Osso Buco	330	21	2.5	70	11	26	3	670
Orange Chipotle–Glazed Pork Chops	360	11	3	150	10	51	0	390
Maple-Glazed Pork Chops	430	11	3	150	28	51	0	460
Spiced Pork Tenderloins	240	11	2.5	90	1	32	0	630
Grilled Stuffed Pork Tenderloins	280	10	2.5	100	6	37	1	420
One-Pot Pork Roast with Apples and Shallots	410	15	3.5	120	25	44	5	290
Slow-Roasted Pork with Red Pepper Chutney	340	18	6	100	12	29	1	670
Slow-Cooker "Barbecued" Spareribs	660	48	17	180	13	44	2	1110
Stir-Fried Sesame Pork and Eggplant	440	29	9	75	19	28	4	1010

	Cal	Fat (g)	Sat Fat (g)	Chol (mg)	Carb (g)	Protein (g)	Fiber (g)	Sodium (mg)
Greek Lamb Meatballs with Cauliflower Rice	610	45	19	125	20	38	6	1080
Grilled Lamb Chops with Asparagus	490	38	8	95	6	31	2	500
Slow-Cooker Indian-Style Lamb Curry	370	19	8	145	3	45	1	490
Roast Butterflied Leg of Lamb	340	21	7	135	0	36	0	530
SEAFOOD								
Salmon Cakes with Spicy Cucumber Salad	420	29	17	125	10	30	2	700
Crab Cakes	270	12	1.5	165	4	31	1	850
Chile-Marinated Calamari Salad with Oranges	300	15	2	350	14	25	3	540
Shrimp Ceviche	210	15	2	105	5	12	1	630
Garlicky Roasted Shrimp with Anise	190	11	4	195	3	20	0	1000
Garlicky Roasted Shrimp with Cumin, Ginger, and Sesame	210	12	2	180	2	20	0	1000
Shrimp Scampi	300	20	4.5	115	16	17	3	1030
Seared Scallops with Butternut Squash Puree	350	15	9	65	34	23	5	1240
Grilled Bacon-Wrapped Scallops with Celery and Apple Salad	390	26	5	45	18	19	2	1130
Oven-Steamed Mussels with Coconut Curry	620	25	15	125	41	56	3	1830
Oven-Steamed Mussels Marinara	580	23	4	125	34	58	5	1740
Smoky Braised Clams with Kale	560	13	3	145	35	76	6	2940
Oven-Roasted Salmon with Tomato Relish	350	18	2.5	105	4	39	1	370
Oven Roasted Salmon with Grapefruit-Basil Relish	380	17	2.5	105	17	40	6	370
Cod Baked in Foil with Leeks and Carrots	320	15	9	95	12	32	2	550
Seared Trout with Brussels Sprouts and Bacon	550	34	12	135	18	45	7	1300
Whole Roasted Snapper with Citrus Vinaigrette	500	37	5	65	5	35	1	950
Grilled Swordfish Skewers with Charred Eggplant and Tomato Salad	480	30	5	110	18	37	8	670
Grilled Fish Tacos with Pineapple Salsa	710	44	6	135	50	35	9	910
Spanish Shellfish Stew	370	18	2.5	95	17	35	3	1370
New England Fish Chowder	330	13	4	95	17	37	4	1210
Slow-Cooker Moroccan Fish Tagine	280	14	2	50	16	24	4	620

	Cal	Fat (g)	Sat Fat (g)	Chol (mg)	Carb (g)	Protein (g)	Fiber (g)	Sodium (mg)
VEGETABLE MAINS								
Stuffed Portobello Mushrooms	390	36	4.5	0	15	7	5	930
Cauliflower Cakes with Cilantro-Mint Sauce	390	25	4.5	95	34	13	11	760
Zucchini Fritters with Fresh Tomato Salsa	360	25	4.5	140	26	9	5	690
Spicy Stir-Fried Bok Choy and Shiitakes	270	19	10	0	22	5	3	1080
Zucchini "Noodle" Salad with Tahini-Ginger Dressing	260	17	2.5	0	24	9	6	580
Summer Squash "Spaghetti" with Roasted Cherry Tomato Sauce	200	12	1.5	0	23	7	7	580
Grilled Vegetable Kebabs	190	15	2	0	13	5	4	330
Tunisian-Style Grilled Vegetables	170	12	1.5	0	14	3	5	200
Tomato and Zucchini Tart	480	41	5	0	23	11	5	450
Slow-Cooker Italian-Style Eggplant Bundles	400	25	4	0	37	11	12	890
Braised Squash and Winter Greens with Coconut Curry	470	24	19	0	61	11	13	1270
Creamy Cauliflower Soup	220	19	11	30	11	3	4	430
Italian Vegetable Stew	190	13	2	0	17	3	5	350
VEGETABLE SIDES								
Roasted Artichokes with Lemon Vinaigrette	350	28	4	0	23	8	11	720
Slow-Cooker Braised Beets with Oranges	220	9	1.5	0	33	4	7	280
Slow-Cooker Braised Beets with Oranges and Tarragon	220	9	1.5	0	32	5	7	270
Broccoli Salad	220	16	2	0	19	5	7	230
Broccoli Salad with Cherry Tomatoes and Pepitas	200	15	2.5	0	13	8	7	220
Brussels Sprout Salad	270	22	2.5	0	15	6	5	400
Brussels Sprout Salad with Apple and Hazelnuts	240	18	2	0	19	6	6	400
Brussels Sprout Salad with Currants and Almonds	230	15	2	0	21	6	6	400
Roasted Carrot "Noodles"	160	8	1	0	23	2	6	440
Roasted Carrot "Noodles" with Garlic, Pepper Flakes, and Basil	170	8	1	0	24	2	7	440

	Cal	Fat (g)	Sat Fat (g)	Chol (mg)	Carb (g)	Protein (g)	Fiber (g)	Sodium (mg)
Roasted Carrot "Noodles" with Shallot, Dill, and Orange	170	8	1	0	25	2	7	440
Slow-Cooked Whole Carrots	80	2.5	0	0	14	1	4	290
Slow-Cooked Whole Carrots with Green Olive and Raisin Relish	170	9	1	0	22	2	5	540
Slow-Cooked Whole Carrots with Onion-Balsamic Relish	160	10	1.5	0	17	2	4	380
Cauliflower Rice	100	4	1	0	13	5	5	520
Curried Cauliflower Rice	130	7	1	0	14	6	6	520
Tex-Mex Cauliflower Rice	100	4.5	1	0	14	5	5	570
Celery Root Puree	300	15	9	20	37	7	7	430
Celery Root Puree with Horseradish and Scallions	310	15	9	20	39	7	8	460
Fennel Salad with Onion and Capers	130	10	1.5	0	10	1	3	560
Fennel Salad with Radishes and Tarragon	130	10	1.5	0	10	1	3	460
Fennel Salad with Orange and Olives	140	10	1.5	0	13	2	4	500
Kale Salad with Roasted Sweet Potatoes and Pomegranate	320	19	2.5	0	34	5	7	180
Roasted Mushrooms	180	14	1.5	0	10	6	0	160
Roasted Mushrooms with Sesame and Scallions	150	11	1.5	0	10	5	1	160
Garlicky Swiss Chard	80	6	1	0	7	3	2	320
Slow-Cooker Mashed Sweet Potatoes	200	7	4	10	33	3	5	280
Slow-Cooker Mashed Sweet Potatoes with Garam Masala and Ginger	250	9	4.5	10	41	4	6	280
Slow-Cooker Mashed Sweet Potatoes with Cilantro and Lime	200	7	1	0	33	3	5	280
Sweet Potato Gratin	240	11	3.5	15	30	6	5	460
Roasted Butternut Squash with Cilantro and Sesame	140	8	3.5	5	18	2	3	240
Sautéed Summer Squash Ribbons	110	9	1	0	8	3	3	150
Sautéed Summer Squash Ribbons with Mint and Pistachios	130	10	1.5	0	9	4	3	150

Conversions and Equivalents

Some say cooking is a science and an art. We would say that geography has a hand in it, too. Flours and sugars manufactured in the United Kingdom and elsewhere will feel and taste different from those manufactured in the United States. So we cannot promise that the pie crust you bake in Canada or England will taste the same as a pie crust baked in the States, but we can offer guidelines for converting weights and measures. We also recommend that you rely on your instincts when making our recipes. Refer to the visual cues provided. If the pie dough hasn't "come together," as described, you may need to add more water—even if the recipe doesn't tell you to. You be the judge.

The recipes in this book were developed using standard U.S. measures following U.S. government guidelines. The charts below offer equivalents for U.S. and metric measures. All conversions are approximate and have been rounded up or down to the nearest whole number.

EXAMPLE

1 teaspoon	=	4.9292 milliliters, rounded up to 5 milliliters
1 ounce	=	28.3495 grams, rounded down to 28 grams

VOLUME CONVERSIONS

U.S.	METRIC
1 teaspoon	5 milliliters
2 teaspoons	10 milliliters
1 tablespoon	15 milliliters
2 tablespoons	30 milliliters
¼ cup	59 milliliters
⅓ cup	79 milliliters
½ cup	118 milliliters
¾ cup	177 milliliters
1 cup	237 milliliters
1¼ cups	296 milliliters
1½ cups	355 milliliters
2 cups (1 pint)	473 milliliters
2½ cups	591 milliliters
3 cups	710 milliliters
4 cups (1 quart)	0.946 liter
1.06 quarts	1 liter
4 quarts (1 gallon)	3.8 liters

WEIGHT CONVERSIONS

OUNCES	GRAMS
½	14
¾	21
1	28
1½	43
2	57
2½	71
3	85
3½	99
4	113
4½	128
5	142
6	170
7	198
8	227
9	255
10	283
12	340
16 (1 pound)	454

CONVERSIONS FOR INGREDIENTS COMMONLY USED IN PALEO BAKING

Baking is an exacting science. Because measuring by weight is far more accurate than measuring by volume, and thus more likely to produce reliable results, in our recipes we provide ounce measures in addition to cup measures for many ingredients. Refer to the chart below to convert these measures into grams.

INGREDIENT	OUNCES	GRAMS
1 cup almond flour	3	85
1 cup coconut flour	4	113
1 cup arrowroot flour	4	113
1 cup tapioca flour	4	113
1 cup coconut sugar	5	142
1 cup maple sugar	5	142
1 cup cocoa powder	3	85
1 tablespoon ghee	½	14
1 cup ghee	8	227
1 tablespoon coconut oil	½	14
1 cup coconut oil	8	227

OVEN TEMPERATURES

FAHRENHEIT	CELSIUS	GAS MARK
225	105	¼
250	120	½
275	135	1
300	150	2
325	165	3
350	180	4
375	190	5
400	200	6
425	220	7
450	230	8
475	245	9

CONVERTING TEMPERATURES FROM AN INSTANT-READ THERMOMETER

We include doneness temperatures in many of the recipes in this book. We recommend an instant-read thermometer for the job. Refer to the above table to convert Fahrenheit degrees to Celsius. Or, for temperatures not represented in the chart, use this simple formula:

Subtract 32 degrees from the Fahrenheit reading, then divide the result by 1.8 to find the Celsius reading.

EXAMPLE

"Roast chicken until thighs register 175 degrees."
To convert:

175°F − 32 = 143°
143° ÷ 1.8 = 79.44°C, rounded down to 79°C

Index

Note: Page references in *italics* indicate recipe photographs.